CONTRIBUTORS TO THE UK EDITION

Barbara Dunn, SRN, SCM, RCNT, RNT, DipN

Nurse Tutor, Nurse Education Centre, St Luke's Hospital, Guildford

Leonard Evans, BA, SRN, ONC, RCNT, RNT

Senior Tutor, Royal Orthopaedic Hospital, Birmingham

Cynthia Gilling, SRN, SCM, RNT

Assistant Director of Nurse Education, The Princess Alexandra School of Nursing, The London Hospital, London

Susan A Gowers, SRN, RCNT

Senior Nursing Officer (Capital Planning), Trent Regional Health Authority, formerly Senior Nursing Officer, Royal Marsden Hospital, London

Rosemarie Hawkins, SRN

Department of Occupational Medicine, Cardiothoracic Institute, Brompton Hospital, London

Morgan Hicks, SRN, OND, RCNT, Cert Ed, RNT

Tutor, Charing Cross Hospital School of Nursing, Charing Cross Hospital, London

Elizabeth Keighley, SRN, RSCN, RCNT, DipN

Clinical Teacher, JBCNS Course in Neuromedical/Neurosurgical Nursing, Cambridge School of Nursing, Addenbrooke's Hospital, Cambridge

Geraldine Matthison, SRN

Formerly Sister, Endocrine Unit, St Thomas's Hospital, London

Margaret Reed, SRN, DipN, Cert Ed, RNT

Tutor (Continuing and Inservice Education), Cambridge School of Nursing, Addenbrooke's Hospital, Cambridge

Lynette Stone, BA, SRN, SCM (NSW)

Nursing Officer (Outpatients), St John's Hospital for Diseases of the Skin, London

LIPPINCOTT MANUAL OF MEDICAL-SURGICAL NURSING

Volume 3

LILLIAN SHOLTIS BRUNNER,
RN, MSN, ScD, FAAN
Consultant in Nursing, Schools of
Nursing: Bryn Mawr Hospital and
Presbyterian-University of
Pennsylvania Medical Center; formerly
Assistant Professor of Surgical Nursing,
Yale University School of Nursing

DORIS SMITH SUDDARTH,
RN, BSNE, MSN
Consultant in Health Occupations, Job
Corps Health Office, U.S. Department
of Labor; formerly Coordinator of the
Curriculum, Alexandria Hospital
School of Nursing

THE LIPPINCOTT MANUAL
OF MEDICAL-SURGICAL NURSING

VOLUME 3

Lillian S. Brunner and Doris S. Suddarth

Harper & Row, Publishers
London

Cambridge San Francisco
Hagerstown Mexico City
Philadelphia Sao Paulo
New York Sydney

Harper & Row Ltd
28 Tavistock Street
London WC2E 7PN

Reprinted 1984, 1985

British Library Cataloguing in Publication Data

Brunner, Lillian
  Lippincott manual of medical-surgical nursing.
  Vol. 3
  1. Nursing
  I. Title   II. Suddarth, Doris
  610.73   RT41

ISBN 0-06-318209-2

Typeset by Inforum Ltd, Portsmouth
Printed and Bound by The Bath Press, Avon

NOTE:
The publishers wish to state that, whilst every effort has been made
to ensure the accuracy and correctness of the information
contained herein, the authors of the original work from which this
adaptation is taken cannot be held responsible for any changes
made to the original text in the course of the adaptation.

CONTENTS

Volume 3

Foreword ix

1 Conditions of the Nervous System
   Elizabeth Keighley 1

2 Ear Disorders
   Cynthia Gilling 81

3 Eye Disorders
   Morgan Hicks 99

4 Musculoskeletal Conditions
   Leonard Evans 139

5 Conditions of the Kidney, Urinary Tract and Reproductive System
   Cynthia Gilling 215

Index 391

Volume 1

Foreword   ix

1   Total Patient Care   1
    Barbara Dunn

2   Rehabilitation Concepts   9
    Barbara Dunn

3   The Ageing Person   51
    Barbara Dunn

4   Care of the Surgical Patient   69
    Cynthia Gilling

5   Emergency Nursing   153
    Cynthia Gilling

6   Communicable Diseases   207
    Barbara Dunn

7   Care of the Patient with Cancer   277
    Susan Gowers

8   Skin Disorders   307
    Lynette Stone

9   Allergy Problems   379
    Rosemarie Hawkins

Index   395

Volume 2

Foreword   ix

1   Conditions of the Cardiovascular System   1
    Margaret Reed

2   Blood Disorders   181
    Margaret Reed

3   Conditions of the Respiratory Tract   233
    Barbara Dunn

4   Disorders of the Digestive System   367
    Cynthia Gilling

5   Metabolic and Endocrine Disorders   521
    Geraldine Matthison

Index   589

FOREWORD

In recent years, there have been many American nursing books introduced on to the British market. Although most of these are very well presented, the differences in terminology and in some nursing practices have been great disadvantages.

The *Lippincott Manual*, which is very widely used in America, has been completely adapted for the UK by trained nurses in this country, each having a specialized knowledge in a particular field.

The information is tabulated for easy reference and we believe that these three volumes of medical-surgical nursing will form a useful source of information for both learners and trained nurses. We would like to thank our professional colleagues for their willing help and advice while we were gathering this information.

The first volume of *The Lippincott Manual of Medical-Surgical Nursing* introduces the basic nursing concepts within the framework of the nursing process. Other sections in this volume refer to conditions which are encountered in every sphere of nursing, such as the elderly patient, the cancer patient and those undergoing surgery.

The second volume introduces interrelated subjects, such as the cardiovascular system, disorders of the blood and respiratory system and, in the latter part, disorders of the digestive system, metabolism and the endocrine system. Although in the past, the emphasis may have been on the medical treatment of many of these disorders, modern investigations, a greater knowledge of physiology and improved techniques mean that surgery can now cure or alleviate many conditions. A full awareness of the physiological reasons for specialized nursing care is essential to all those concerned with caring for the patient in hospital and planning rehabilitation.

The third volume is concerned with two closely related groups of subjects. The first group consists of disorders of the nervous system itself, and the special senses of hearing and sight. Some of the disorders of the musculoskeletal system are also due to problems of nervous control. The second part of this volume has sections on the kidney, urinary tract and reproductive disorders. New techniques for treating patients with these disorders have been included and, importantly, the physiological changes which occur as a result of these problems are detailed.

Together these volumes will provide a valuable source of information, so that nurses will be able to understand fully the reasons for the decisions they make when planning the total care of their patients.

Barbara Dunn, 1982

Chapter 1

CONDITIONS OF THE NERVOUS SYSTEM

Diagnosis of Neurological Conditions	2
Guidelines: Assisting the Patient Undergoing a Lumbar Puncture	8
Special Neurological Nursing Considerations	11
Nursing Management of the Patient with a Head Injury	11
Nursing Management of the Patient with Increasing Intracranial Pressure	14
Guidelines: Administering a Tepid Sponge for Fever	16
Nursing Management of the Unconscious Patient	18
Nursing Management of the Patient Having a Convulsion	22
Nursing Management of the Patient Undergoing Intracranial Surgery	23
Cranial Nerve Involvement	26
Bell's Palsy	26
Trigeminal Neuralgia (Tic Douloureux)	28
Cerebrovascular Disease	30
Stroke or Cerebral Vascular Accident (CVA)	31
Aphasia	38
Subarachnoid Haemorrhage	40
Cerebral Aneurysm (Intracranial Aneurysm)	41
Brain Abscess	43
Brain Tumour	44
The Epilepsies	47
Status Epilepticus	51
Parkinson's Disease	52
Multiple Sclerosis	55
Myasthenia Gravis	58
Acute Infectious Polyneuritis (Landry–Guillain-Barré Syndrome)	62
Fractures and Dislocations of the Spine	63
Prolapsed Intravertebral Disc (Slipped Disc)	67
Management of the Patient Following a Laminectomy	71
Paraplegia	72
Intractable Pain	74
Further Reading	78

DIAGNOSIS OF NEUROLOGICAL CONDITIONS

Radiological Procedures

Skull x-ray

Skull x-ray reveals shape, density, vascular markings, intracranial calcification, fractures and some tumours.

Computerized Axial Tomography

Computerized axial tomography is an imaging method in which the head is scanned in successive layers by a narrow beam of x-ray. It provides a cross-sectional view of the brain and distinguishes differences in the densities of various brain tissues. A computer printout is obtained of the absorption values of the tissues in the plane that is being scanned. This same information is also shown on a cathode ray tube for additional radiological evaluation.

1   Lesions are seen as variations in tissue density differing from the surrounding normal brain tissue.
2   Abnormalities of tissue density indicate possible tumour masses, brain infarction, ventricular displacement; useful in patients with head injury, suspected brain tumour, hydrocephalus.
3   May be done with intravenous contrast medium enhancement to more accurately define boundaries of certain lesions and indicate presence of otherwise undetectable lesions.
4   *Patient preparation.*
   a. Inquire about allergies and any previous adverse reaction to contrast agent.
   b. No special preparation is required; this is a noninvasive technique that can be done on an outpatient basis.
   c. Instruct the patient that he must lie perfectly still while the testing is being carried out; he cannot talk or move his face as this distorts the picture.

Cerebral Angiography

X-ray study of the vascular system of the brain (cerebral circulation) by the injection of contrast material into a selected artery.

1   Contrast material may be injected into common carotid, vertebral or subclavian artery, or arch of the aorta. Selective catherization may be done via a femoral or brachial artery.
2   After injection of selected artery, x-rays are made of arterial and venous phases of circulation through brain and head.
3   Useful in demonstrating position of arteries, intracranial aneurysms, presence or absence of abnormal vasculature, haematomas, tumours.
4   Nursing responsibilities.
   a. Before angiogram.
      (1) Fast the patient prior to the procedure—follow guidelines of anaesthetist responsible for the patient.
      (2) Reinforce the doctor's explanation of the procedure.
      (3) Prepare patient as for anaesthetic (remove or cover rings, remove false teeth, etc). This procedure may be done using local anaesthetic.

Nursing support.

a. *Before angiogram* (performed under local anaesthetic).

(1) Withhold meal preceding test.

(2) Patient may be given sedative before going to x-ray department—may help minimize intensity of burning sensation felt along course of injected vessel.

(3) Instruct the patient:

(a) Try to lie quietly during injection.

(b) A burning sensation, lasting for a few seconds, may possibly be felt behind the eyes, or in jaw, teeth, tongue and lips.

b. *Following angiogram* (performed under either method).

(1) Make repeated observations for neurological deficits—motor or sensory deterioration, alterations in level of responsiveness, weakness on one side, speech disturbances, arrhythmias, blood pressure fluctuation.

(2) Observe injection site for haematoma formation; apply an ice cap intermittently—to relieve swelling and discomfort.

(3) Evaluate peripheral pulses—changes may develop if there is haematoma formation at puncture site or embolization to a distant artery.

(4) Note colour and temperature of involved extremity.

Brain Scan

Following intake (oral or intravenous) of radiopharmaceutical, the radioactivity subsequently transmitted through the skull is scanned by a rectilinear scanner which prints out a picture based on the number of counts received from the brain as it scans (or a gamma camera, which prints out image without actually scanning, may be used; this is a more recent imaging device).

1   Patient is treated with potassium perchlorate to block the radiopharmaceutical uptake in the thyroid, salivary glands, choroid plexus and gastrointestinal mucosa.

2   Brain scanning is useful in early detection and evaluation of intracranial neoplasms, stroke, abscess, follow-up of surgical or radiation therapy of brain.

3   This test is based on the principle that a radiopharmaceutical may diffuse through a disrupted blood-brain barrier into the abnormal cerebral tissue. (Normal brain tissue is relatively impermeable.) There is an increased uptake of radioactive material at the site of pathology.

4   *Nursing responsibility.*

a. Explain to patient that he will be expected to lie quietly during the procedure.

b. This is a noninvasive procedure.

Air Studies

A gaseous replacement of the fluid within the ventricles and subarachnoid systems as a contrast medium because air is less dense than fluid to roentgen rays.

NOTE: These investigations are now rarely used since the introduction of computerized axial tomography.

1   *Pneumoencephalogram*—withdrawal of cerebrospinal fluid and injection of air or other gas by means of a lumbar puncture.

a. Demonstrates ventricular system and subarachnoid space overlying the hemispheres and basal cisterns.

b. Useful in diagnosing degenerative cerebral atrophy and in detecting mass lesions at the base of the brain.

2 *Fractional pneumoencephalogram*—withdrawal of small amounts of fluid and injection of small amounts of air to visualize the ventricular system.

3 *Ventriculogram*—withdrawal of cerebrospinal fluid and injection of air or gas directly into the lateral ventricles through openings in the skull.

    a. Trephines (burr holes) are made through a scalp incision; ventricles are punctured by a special needle.

    b. The cerebrospinal fluid is replaced with air, the cannulae are withdrawn and the scalp wounds are closed.

    c. If a lesion is present, there is a change in the size, shape or position of the ventricular, subarachnoid or cisternal spaces.

4 *Nursing management following pneumoencephalogram or ventriculogram:*

    a. Watch the patient for increasing intracranial pressure.

      (1) Disturbances of intracranial pressure may cause serious complications.

      (2) Prepare for ventricular tap and prompt decompression.

    b. Take vital signs as frequently as clinical condition indicates and until stabilized.

    c. Assess for complaints of headache, fever and for signs of shock.

      (1) Place ice cap on head intermittently.

      (2) Give analgesics as directed—duration of headache depends on the speed with which the intracranial air is absorbed. Headache is reduced if patient lies flat in bed.

      (3) Nausea and vomiting may follow air studies.

      (4) Parenteral fluids may be necessary for first 24 hours.

5 Procedure done under general anaesthetic.

    Patient preparation before pneumoencephalogram.

      (1) Fast following guidelines of anaesthetist responsible.

      (2) Reinforce doctor's explanation.

      (3) Prepare patient for anaesthetic.

Echoencephalography

The recording of echoes from the deep structures within the skull (generated by the transmission of ultrasound (high frequency) waves) to determine the position of midline structures of the brain and the distance from the midline to the lateral ventricular wall or the third ventricular wall.

1 Useful for detecting a shift of the cerebral midline structures caused by subdural haematoma, intracerebral haemorrhage, massive cerebral infarction and neoplasms; can display dilation of ventricles; useful in evaluation of hydrocephalus.

2 Ultrasonic transducers are positioned over specified areas of the head; the echoes are imaged and stored on the oscilloscope.

3 *Nursing responsibilities.*

    a. There is no special patient preparation.

    b. Explain that this is a noninvasive test and that some type of gel (electrode jelly) may be used to eliminate the air gap between the transducer and the head.

NOTE: This test is still used in some hospitals, but needs a skilled operator to obtain an accurate echo image. It has been somewhat superseded by computerized axial tomography.

Myelography

The injection of contrast medium into the spinal subarachnoid space usually by lumbar puncture for radiological examination, outlines the spinal subarachnoid space and shows distortion of the spinal cord or dural sac by tumours, cysts, prolapsed intravertebral discs or other lesions.

1 After injection of the contrast medium, the head of the table is tilted down and the course of the contrast medium is observed radioscopically.
2 Contrast material may be removed after test completion by syringe and needle aspiration; patient may complain of sharp pain down leg during aspiration if a nerve root has been aspirated against a needle point—needle point is rotated or an adjustment in needle depth is made.

   With newer water soluble contrast agents a smaller needle can be used (less likely to produce headache).
3 *Nursing responsibilities.*
   a. *Before test.*
      (1) Reinforce doctor's explanation of procedure; explain that it is usually not painful and that the x-ray table will be tilted in varying positions during the study.
      (2) Omit the meal preceding myelography.
      (3) Patient's legs may be wrapped with elastic compression bandages to eliminate hypotension during procedure.
      (4) Patient may be given light sedative prior to test to help him cope with a rather lengthy (2 hour) procedure.
   b. *Post-test.*
      (1) Instruct the patient to lie in prone position for several hours; he may be kept in bed in supine position (turning from side to side) for 12–24 hours.
      (2) Advise patient to drink liberal quantities of fluid—for rehydration and replacement of cerebrospinal fluid and to decrease incidence of postlumbar puncture headache (thought to be due to escape of spinal fluid).
      (3) Assess neurological and vital signs; note motor and sensory deviations from normal.
      (4) Check on patient's ability to micturate.
      (5) Watch for fever, stiff neck, photophobia or other signs of chemical or bacterial meningitis.

Radiculography

The above information applies also to radiculography. This term is generally used when the lower nerve roots (cauda equina) have been examined, whereas myelography refers to examination of the spinal cord itself.

NOTE: If a water-soluble dye has been used for either of these tests, e.g. Amipaque, then the patients will return from the x-ray department sitting up and should remain so for at least the next 6 hours.

Discography

Injection of radiopaque substance directly into the intervertebral disc. This study can be used in patients suspected of having herniated disc disease but is infrequently done.

Electroencephalography (EEG)

Records, by means of electrodes applied on the scalp surface (or by microelectrodes placed within brain tissue), the electrical activity which is generated in the brain.

1   Provides physiological assessment of cerebral activity; useful in diagnosis of the epilepsies.
2   Electrodes are arranged on the scalp to permit the recording of activity in various head regions; the amplified activity of the neurones is recorded on a continuously moving paper sheet.
   a. For baseline recording the patient lies quietly with his eyes closed.
   b. For activation procedures (done to elicit abnormal electrical activities) patient may be asked to hyperventilate for 3–4 min, look at a bright flashing light or receive an injection of medication (Metrazol).
   c. EEG may also be made during sleep and upon awakening.
3   Pharyngeal (electrode inserted through nose; rests on mucosa of pharyngeal roof) and sphenoidal (inserted transcutaneously with tips resting on sphenoid bone near foramen ovale) electrodes are used when epileptogenic area is inaccessible to conventional scalp preparation.
4   Patient preparation for routine recording.
   a. Antiepileptic medication and tranquillizers may be withheld before EEG—many departments prefer patients to continue with medication and allow for this when interpreting EEG patterns.
   b. Reassure patient that he will not receive an electrical shock, that the EEG takes approximately 45–60 min (more for a sleep EEG), and that the EEG is *not* a form of treatment or a test of intelligence or insanity.

Electromyography (EMG)

The introduction of needle electrodes into the skeletal muscles to study changes in electric potential of muscles and nerves leading to them. These are shown on an oscilloscope and amplified by a loudspeaker for simultaneous visual and auditory analysis and comparison.

1   Useful in determining the presence of a neuromuscular disorder; helps distinguish weakness due to neuropathy from that due to other causes.
2   *Nursing responsibilities.*
   a. No special patient preparation is required.
   b. Explain to the patient that he will experience a sensation similar to that of an intramuscular injection as the needle is inserted into the muscle.

Cranial Nerve Tests

For neurological examinations for testing cranial nerves see Table 1.1.

Lumbar Puncture

Insertion of a needle into lumbar subarachnoid space and withdrawal of cerebrospinal fluid for diagnostic and therapeutic purposes.

Table 1.1. Neurological Examination for Testing Cranial Nerves

Nerve	Equipment	Clinical Examination
1 Olfactory	Four small bottles of volatile oils, such as (1) peppermint, (2) oil of cloves, (3) coffee, (4) aniseed	Instruct the patient to sniff and to identify the odours. Each nostril is tested separately. The patient is asked if he perceives the smell and if he can identify it
2 Optic	Ophthalmoscope	In a darkened room the patient is asked to look straight ahead at a distant object while the examiner looks for papill-oedema, optic atrophy and retinal and vascular lesions Special equipment is used for examination of visual fields. Eye chart is used to check visual acuity
3 Oculomotor 4 Trochlear 5 Abducens	Torch	Because of close association, these nerves are examined collectively. They innervate pupil and upper eyelid and are responsible for extraocular muscle movements
6 Trigeminal	Test tube of hot water Test tube of ice water Wisp of cotton wool Pin	*Sensory branch*—Vertex to chin tested for sensations of pain, touch and temperature. This includes reflex reaction of cornea to wisp of cotton *Motor branch*—Ability to bite is tested
7 Facial	Four small bottles with solutions which are salty, sweet, sour and bitter (Four wet cotton applicators)	Observe symmetry of face and ability to contract facial muscles. Instruct patient to taste and identify substance used. He should rinse his mouth well between each drop of solution. This is a test for the anterior two-thirds of the tongue
8 Acoustic	Tuning fork	Tests for hearing, air and bone conduction
9 Glossopharyngeal	Cotton applicator stick	Test posterior one-third of the tongue for taste and also check for gag reflex
10 Vagus	Tongue depressor	Checking voice sounds, observing symmetry of soft palate will give suggestion of function of vagus
11 Spinal accessory		Since this innervates the sterno-cleidomastoid and the trapezius muscles, the patient will be instructed to turn and to move his head and to elevate shoulders with and without resistance
12 Hypoglossal		Observe tongue movements

GUIDELINES: Assisting the Patient Undergoing a Lumbar Puncture

Purposes

1 To obtain cerebrospinal fluid for examination (microbiological, serological, cytological or chemical analysis).
2 To relieve cerebrospinal pressure.
3 To determine the presence or absence of blood in the spinal fluid.

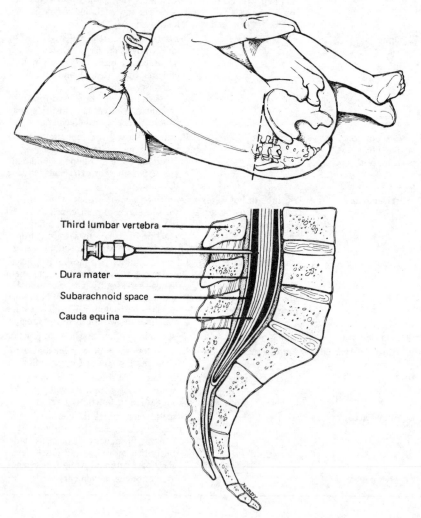

Figure 1.1. Technique of lumbar puncture.

Equipment

Sterile lumbar puncture set
Sterile gloves
Xylocaine 1–2%

Skin antiseptic
Band-Aid

Procedure

Nursing Action	Reason
Preparatory Phase	
1 Give a step-by-step résumé of the procedure.	1 Reassures patient and gains his co-operation.
For lying position (Fig. 1.1):	
2 Position the patient on his side with a pillow under his head. He should be lying on a firm surface.	
3 Instruct the patient to arch the lumbar segment of his back and draw his knees up to his abdomen, clasping his knees with his hands.	3 This posture offers maximal widening of the interspinous spaces and affords easier entry into the subarachnoid space.
4 Assist the patient in maintaining his position by supporting him behind the knees and neck. Assist the patient to maintain the posture throughout the examination.	4 Supporting the patient helps prevent sudden movements which can produce a traumatic (bloody) tap and thus impede correct diagnosis.
For sitting position:	
5 Have the patient straddle a straight-back chair (facing the back) and rest his head against his arms, which are folded on the back of the chair.	5 In obese patients and those who have difficulty in assuming an arched side-lying position, this posture may allow more accurate identification of the spinous processes and interspaces.
Performance Phase (by the doctor)	
1 The skin is prepared with antiseptic solution and the skin and subcutaneous spaces are infiltrated with local anaesthetic agent.	
2 A spinal puncture needle is introduced between L3–L4 or L4–L5 interspace. The needle is advanced until the 'give' of the ligamentum flavum is felt and the needle enters the subarachnoid space. The manometer is attached to the spinal puncture needle.	2 L3–L4 or L4–L5 interspace is *below* the level of the spinal cord.

Nursing Action	Reason

3 After the needle enters the subarachnoid space, the doctor may ask you to help the patient to slowly straighten his legs.

3 This manoeuvre prevents a false increase in intraspinal pressure. Muscle tension and compression of the abdomen give falsely high pressures.

4 Instruct the patient to breathe quietly (not to hold his breath or strain).

4 Hyperventilation may lower a truly elevated pressure.

5 The initial pressure reading is obtained by measuring the level of the fluid column after it comes to rest.

5 With respiration there is normally some fluctuation of spinal fluid in the manometer. Normal range of spinal fluid pressure with patient in the lateral position is 70–180 mm H_2O.

6 About 2–3 ml of spinal fluid is placed in each of three sterile test tubes for observation, comparison and laboratory analysis.

6 Spinal fluid should be clear and colourless. Blood spinal fluid may indicate subarachnoid haemorrhage, cerebral contusion or laceration.

QUECKENSTEDT TEST

1 The nurse is asked by the doctor to compress the jugular vein or veins for 10 s.
2 Pressure readings are made at 10-s intervals.
3 After the needle is withdrawn, a Band-Aid is applied to the puncture site.

This test is made when a spinal subarachnoid block is suspected (tumour; vertebral fracture or dislocation). In normal persons there is a rapid rise in pressure of cerebrospinal fluid in response to jugular compression with rapid return to normal when the compression is released. If the pressure rises and falls slowly, there is evidence of a block due to a lesion's compressing the spinal subarachnoid pathways. This test is not done if an intracranial lesion is suspected.

Follow-up Phase

1 Record (a) procedure (b) appearance of spinal fluid, (c) whether or not specimens were sent to laboratory, (d) spinal pressure readings and (e) condition and reaction of patients.
2 Keep the patient horizontal (prone, supine or on his side) for 4–12 hours. Encourage a liberal fluid intake.
3 Administer prescribed analgesia for headache if necessary.

Some patients suffer from postpuncture headache which is thought to be caused by the leakage of spinal fluid at the puncture site.

SPECIAL NEUROLOGICAL NURSING CONSIDERATIONS

Nursing Management of the Patient with a Head Injury

Clinical Manifestations

1 Unconsciousness or disturbance in consciousness.
2 Headache.
3 Vertigo.
4 Confusion or delirium.
5 Changes in body temperature.
6 Respiratory irregularities.
7 Symptoms of shock—coldness, pallor, perspiring, falling blood pressure.
8 Pupillary abnormalities.

Immediate Management in the Accident and Emergency Department

Nursing Alert: Regard every patient who has a head injury as having a potential spinal cord injury.

1 Maintain an open airway and ensure maximum respiratory function—oxygen deprivation and an excess of carbon dioxide may produce cerebral hypoxia and cause cerebral oedema with subsequent irreparable damage.
   a. Employ adequate suctioning procedures—patient may have aspirated blood and mucus from face and head injuries and the nasopharynx may be flooded with gastric contents—leads to pneumonitis which contributes to respiratory acidosis.
   b. Ensure adequate oxygenation and humidification.
   c. Assist with endotracheal intubation if patient is comatose.
   d. Place patient in a semiprone head-level position to transport him from the accident and emergency department to the ward.
2 Determine the baseline condition of the patient; start neurological observation records.
   a. Assess level of responsiveness.
   b. Determine presence of headache, double vision, nausea or vomiting.
   c. Evaluate pupil size and reaction to light.
   d. Measure blood pressure, pulse, respirations.
   e. Evaluate movement and strength of extremities.
   f. Assess for injuries to other organ systems.
3 Obtain as accurate a history as possible from patient or observer.
   a. What caused the injury? A high velocity missile? Object striking the head? A fall?
   b. What were the direction and force of the blow?
   c. *Was there loss of consciousness?* How long? Could the patient be aroused?
   d. Is there any amnesia?
   e. Was there any bleeding from eyes, ears, nose, mouth?
   f. Was there paralysis or flaccidity of the extremities?
   g. Are there any pupillary changes?
4 Be aware that convulsive seizures may occur.

Treatment and Nursing Management*

Objective

To observe the patient constantly for the development of focal or generalized deficits of function that indicate need for surgical intervention.

1   Support the airway—small degrees of anoxia rapidly increase cerebral dysfunction and brain swelling.

   a. Assist medical staff to carry out blood gas studies—to determine respiratory adequacy and assess effects of therapy.

   b. Prepare for endotracheal intubation or tracheostomy and ventilatory assistance if indicated.

   c. Position the patient in a semiprone, three-quarters prone or prone position with his head level—improves oxygen and carbon dioxide exchange and prevents aspiration of secretions or blood.

   d. Turn from side to side—to prevent stasis of secretions in lungs and pressure on skin.

2   Observe, evaluate and carry out repeated clinical examinations to determine minute-to-minute, hour-to-hour changes in patient's status.

Nursing Alert: A change in the level of responsiveness/consciousness is the most sensitive indicator of improvement or deterioration. The level of responsiveness may change from minute to minute.

   a. Observe and record:
       (1) Level of responsiveness/consciousness.
       (2) Changes in vital signs.
       (3) Motor strength.
       (4) Pupillary changes.

   b. See p. 142–The Patient with Increasing Intracranial Pressure.

3   Give fluids and electrolytes as prescribed by the medical staff. The patient may be kept slightly dehydrated to reduce extracellular fluid volume and cerebral oedema.

   a. Do not give fluids by mouth to an unconscious patient.

   b. Keep an accurate intake and output record.

   c. Give nasogastric feeds if patient is unable to swallow after several days.

   c. Be aware that patients with severe head injuries commonly develop stress ulcers which may produce severe gastrointestinal bleeding. This should be reported to medical staff at once.

   e. Give prescribed intravenous infusions slowly (except mannitol which is given quickly). Overhydration may lead to cerebral oedema.

   f. If the patient is unconscious it may be necessary to insert indwelling urinary catheter for assessment of urinary volume and to prevent restlessness from distended bladder.

NOTE: See also Management of an Unconscious Patient.

4   Control rising temperature with fans, tepid sponging and minimal amounts of bed clothing—to lower the metabolic requirements of the brain.

* See also nursing management of the unconscious patient, p. 18).

5 Give prescribed medication to combat brain oedema.
   a. Hyperosmolar solution (mannitol) given by intravenous infusion to dehydrate the brain and reduce cerebral oedema.
   b. Steroids (dexamethasone) may be given.
6 Observe ears and nose for leakage of cerebrospinal fluid—may indicate basilar skull fracture.

Nursing Alert: Cerebrospinal fluid leakage may mask the usual clinical signs of an expanding intracranial haematoma by preventing brain compression.

   a. Tape sterile cotton pad under nose or loosely against ear to collect drainage.
   b. Elevate head of bed approximately 30° as directed—to reduce intracranial pressure and promote spontaneous closure of leak (some neurosurgeons prefer that the bed be kept flat).
   c. Persistence of cerebrospinal fluid otorrhoea or rhinorrhoea usually requires surgical intervention.
7 Patient may need to be treated for shock—from associated injuries of chest, abdomen, pelvis, fractures.
   a. Medical staff may require intravenous fluids, plasma or dextran, until blood transfusions can be started; these should be given as prescribed.
   b. Hourly urinary volume measurements (via indwelling catheter).
8 Support the patient during periods of restlessness.
   a. Avoid restraints if at all possible; straining increases intracranial pressure.
   b. Medical staff may prescribe chloralhydrate, sparine. Narcotics and sedatives should not be given as these will mask levels of responsiveness.
   c. Maintain as quiet an environment as possible.
   d. Elevate head of bed 15° unless otherwise indicated to help reduce cerebral oedema (some neurosurgeons prefer that the bed be kept flat).
   e. Be aware that restlessness may be caused by cerebral hypoxia, respiratory obstruction, pain from fractured extremities, tight cast or bandages, extradural haematoma, or distended bladder.
9 Give phenytoin (Epanutin) or phenobarbitone as ordered—for control of seizures.
10 Protect the eyes from corneal irritation.
11 Carry out rehabilitation techniques.
   a. Put all extremities through range of motion exercises.
   b. Position the patient correctly to prevent contractures.
   c. Keep the skin dry, clean and free of pressure—to prevent pressure sores.
   d. Ensure a well-balanced diet.
   e. Gradually increase physical and mental activity (including resumption of increasingly difficult mental tasks).
12 Be aware of aftereffects of head injury—usually directly related to the severity of the injury.
   a. Headache.
   b. Dizziness and vertigo.
   c. Emotional instability or irritability.
   d. Brain damage.
   e. Post-traumatic epilepsy.
   f. Post-traumatic neuroses and psychoses.

Discharge Planning and Health Teaching

1 Encourage patient to continue his rehabilitation programme following discharge; improvement in status may continue up to 3 or more years following injury.
2 Headache may be the most reliable guide to recovery; use a second pillow/back-rest at night.
3 Encourage patient to return gradually to usual activities.
4 Family may need help in setting limits for injured patient's impulses (anger, etc.) and in realistically evaluating his capabilities. Family may have difficulty in understanding and accepting alterations in patient's behaviour.

Nursing Management of the Patient with Increasing Intracranial Pressure

Causes

1 Head injury.
2 Cerebral oedema.
3 Abscess or inflammation.
4 Haemorrhage.
5 Brain tumour.
6 Cranial surgery.

Nursing Alert: As intracranial pressure increases, the brain substance is compressed. A sudden increase may produce an emergency situation in a few minutes. This condition may lead rapidly to death or result in a vegetative existence for the patient.

Clinical Manifestations

1 Change in level of responsiveness (consciousness).
  a. *The level of responsiveness is the most important measure of the patient's condition.*
  b. Look for lethargy, delay in response to verbal suggestions, slowing of speech.
  c. Watch for sudden changes in condition—quietness to restlessness, orientation to confusion, increasing drowsiness, stupor, coma.
  d. *Progressive deterioration is a serious sign* that may require immediate surgical intervention.
2 Changes in vital signs.
  a. Pulse changes—slowing rate to 60 or below; increasing rate to 100 or above.
  b. Respiratory irregularities; slowing of rate with lengthening periods of apnoea; Cheyne–Stokes or Kussmaul breathing.
  c. Rising blood pressure or widening pulse pressure (the difference between systolic and diastolic blood pressure).
  d. Moderately elevated temperature.
3 Headache.
4 Vomiting.
5 Pupillary changes—increasing pressure or an expanding clot can displace the brain against the oculomotor or optic nerve.
  a. Observe size, reaction to light, deviation from midline.
  b. Look for dilating or nonreacting pupil(s), which may also be unequal.

Treatment and Nursing Management

Assessment of Patient's Level of Responsiveness

1   Response to commands:
   a. Answers questions readily and correctly.
   b. Can perform a complex manoeuvre.
   c. Responds to simple command.
   d. Gives delayed or unequal response.
   e. Reacts only to loud voice.
   f. Does not respond.
2   Assessment of spinal motor reflexes (pinch Achilles tendon, arm or other body site):
   a. Prompt, purposeful withdrawal.
   b. Sluggish or nonpurposeful movement of extremities.
   c. Facial grimace.
   d. Involuntary micturition.
   e. Extension of extremities.
3   Observation of patient's spontaneous activity:
   a. Verbal or other communication.
   b. Changes in posture (frequency).
   c. Breathing pattern.
   d. Retching, vomiting.
   e. Restlessness, twitching, tremors, convulsions.
4   Intracranial pressure monitoring may be used where available.
   a. Cannula (or catheter) is inserted into ventricle or subdural space and attached to a pressure transducer and recordings are then made.
   Normal level: 1–10 mmHg.
   Slight increase: 11–20 mmHg.
   Moderate increase: 21–40 mmHg
   Severely increased: More than 40 mmHg.*
   b. Effect of increased intracranial pressure on brain function varies; the cause of intracranial hypertension appears more important than the degree of pressure.
   c. A change in the position of the head (e.g., flattening of bed to give care), endotracheal aspiration, hyperventilation or compression of jugular veins (head falling to one side) may markedly increase intracranial pressure.
5   Keep a neurological observation record.
   Purpose: To provide a continuing assessment of the patient so that a *change* in condition may be noted immediately. All observations should be compared with and evaluated according to the *baseline* (initial) condition of the patient.
   a. Know the patient's baseline condition.
   b. Carry out *repeated* nursing assessments—to determine clinical improvement or deterioration.

Management of Intracranial Pressure

1   Osmotic diuretics (mannitol, glycerol)—given to dehydrate brain and reduce cerebral oedema (lowers intracranial pressure).

* Horton, J M (1975) The immediate care of head injuries, Anaesthesia, 30: 212–218

a. Observe for electrolyte disturbances (particularly hyponatremia) and dehydration.

b. Make sure that indwelling catheter is in bladder since dehydrating agents produce diuresis.

2 Steroids (dexamethasone).

Has dramatic effect in lowering cerebral oedema of brain tumour; appears less effective in head injury.

3 Controlled ventilation.

a. Hyperventilation with volume respirator—reduces blood volume in brain, causing vasoconstriction of cerebral vasculature which decreases intracranial pressure.

b. Avoid hypoxia.

4 Hypothermia to reduce cerebral metabolic need for oxygen and glucose.

5 Keep the head of the bed elevated 30–45° (some neurosurgeons prefer the patient kept flat).

6 Removal of cerebrospinal fluid—can be removed from lateral ventricle when the patient is being monitored.

7 Prepare for surgical intervention if patient's condition deteriorates.

GUIDELINES: Administering a Tepid Sponge for Fever

Fever is an abnormal elevation of body temperature.

A *tepid sponge* is the bathing of the body with tepid water (or alcohol and water) for a period of time to reduce fever. It is particularly effective in neurological conditions in which there is a disturbance of the temperature-regulating centre. Fever increases both intracranial pressure and the rate of development of cerebral oedema.

Causes

1 Infection.

2 Disturbance of temperature-regulating centre (trauma, central nervous system haemorrhage).

3 Tumours; diseases of blood-forming organs.

4 Heat stroke.

5 Drug toxicity; allergens.

6 Delirium tremens.

Purpose

To reduce body temperature when fever in itself may be deleterious.

Equipment

Basin of tepid water 21.1–29.1°C (70–85°F)

or

Basin of alcohol (25% saturated with tepid water)

Bath blanket

Towels

7 flannels/sponges/J cloths

Nursing Alert: Make certain that the patient is adequately hydrated; unrecognized dehydration can result in decreased circulating blood volume, causing peripheral vasoconstriction which prevents heat loss.

Procedure

Nursing Action	**Reason**

Preparatory Phase

1 Place bath blanket over patient.
2 Remove top bedding.

Performance Phase

Nursing Action	Reason
1 Take temperature, pulse and respiration before starting sponge.	1 This serves as a baseline for determining effectiveness of treatment.
2 Give antipyretic medication as directed 15–20 min before starting sponge. a. Acetylsalicylic acid or b. Chlorpromazine.	2 There is a more rapid reduction of fever when sponging is combined with administration of antipyretic medication. a. Has an anti-inflammatory, antipyretic or analgesic action. b. Controls shivering.
3 Place a wetted flannel on neck and in each groin and axilla.	3 The application of cold over superficial large blood vessels aids in lowering body temperature.
4 Expose the body area to be sponged. Place a towel under area. Sponge using circular movements.	4 Vaporization of water removes heat from the surface of the skin. Alcohol vaporizes at a lower temperature and removes heat from the skin more rapidly. Tepid water and alcohol are highly effective in producing vasodilation and evaporation of heat from skin.
5 If the patient's skin feels cold to the touch, apply skin friction to bring the blood to the surface.	
6 Bathe each extremity 5 min; bathe entire back and buttocks 5–10 min; bathe trunk and abdomen 5 min.	6 The fever sponge should not exceed 30 min.
7 Allow a fan to blow over the patient while sponging him if temperature is high.	7 Increased air movement augments heat loss.
8 Watch for extreme shivering. Cover the patient and wait a few minutes before proceeding with sponge.	8 Shivering may raise heat production.
9 Stop sponge if cyanosis, mottling, chilling do not stop when friction (rubbing) is applied to the skin.	9 These symptoms indicate a change in vasomotor tone.

Nursing Action	Reason

Follow-up Phase

1 Remove bath blanket and change sheet. Place a dry gown on patient.

2 Record temperature and pulse rate 10–15 min after sponge is finished.   2 Postsponge temperature indicates whether or not treatment has been effective.

Nursing Management of the Unconscious Patient

Clinical Problems

There are two major threats to the unconscious patient:

1 The disease or trauma that produced unconsciousness.
2 The threat of the unconscious state.

Objectives of Treatment and Nursing Management

Nursing Goal

To assume the protective reflexes for the patient until he is aware of himself and can function in his environment.

To Establish and Maintain An Adequate Airway (Fig. 1.2)

1 Place the patient in a three-quarter prone or semiprone position with his face dependent—prevents the tongue from obstructing the airway, encourages drainage of respiratory secretions and promotes oxygen and carbon dioxide exchange.

2 Insert oral airway if tongue is paralysed or is obstructing airway—an obstructed airway increases intracranial pressure. This is considered a short-term measure.

3 Prepare for insertion of cuffed endotracheal tube if patient's condition requires—endotracheal intubation is more effective in permitting positive pressure ventilation. The cuffed tube seals off the digestive tract, preventing aspiration and allowing efficient removal of tracheobronchial secretions.

4 The medical staff (usually anaethetist) may wish to use oxygen therapy, positive pressure assisted breathing techniques or mechanical ventilation with a ventilator when there is indication of impending respiratory failure.

5 Keep the airway free of secretions with efficient suctioning—in the absence of the cough and swallowing reflexes, secretions rapidly accumulate in the posterior pharynx and upper trachea and can pave the way to fatal respiratory complications.

   a. Attach open-end catheter to Y-tube.
   b. Keep one end of Y-tube open while inserting the catheter.
   c. When catheter is at desired level close the open end of Y with finger.
   d. Turn the suction on and slowly withdraw catheter with a twisting motion of the thumb and forefinger.

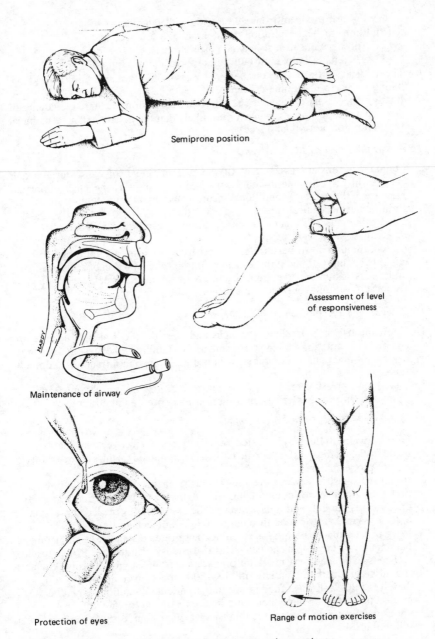

Semiprone position

Maintenance of airway

Assessment of level of responsiveness

Protection of eyes

Range of motion exercises

Figure 1.2. Nursing priorities in the care of the unconscious patient.

    e. Gently turn the head from side to side while suctioning.
    (1) Limit tracheal aspiration to intervals of a few seconds.
    (2) Allow patient to rest between aspirations.
    (3) Oxygenate the patient between aspirations as required.

6 The medical staff will carry out periodic measurements of arterial Po_2 and Pco_2 (blood gases) to determine efficiency of treatment.

7 It may be necessary for the patient to have a tracheostomy if there is evidence of inadequate respiratory exchange or it is likely that the patient will need artificial ventilation for more than a week.

To Assess the Level of Responsiveness

1 Maintain a constant assessment of the patient's level of consciousness and changes in responsiveness—the level of consciousness is the most important measure of the patient's condition. Unconscious patients may deteriorate rapidly from numerous clinical causes.

2 Record the patient's *exact reactions*, movements and quality of speech.
    a. Request the patient to speak.
    b. Ask the patient to perform some activity (raise arm, extend tongue, etc.).
    c. Apply painful stimuli if there is no response (pinching skin of arms or thighs) and assess patient's perception of pain. No response or a delayed or unequal response is an unfavourable clinical sign.

To Evaluate the Progression of Vital Signs

1 Know the patient's baseline vital signs and alert the medical staff if there are significant fluctuations of blood pressure and instability of the pulse and respiratory cycle—fluctuations of vital signs indicate a change in intracranial homoeostasis.

2 Take blood pressure readings, pulse and respiratory rates and temperature at frequently specified intervals until there is evidence of stabilization.

To Maintain Fluid and Electrolyte Balance

1 Give intravenous fluids as indicated. Serial laboratory electrolyte evaluations are made by the medical staff when the patient is maintained on intravenous fluids to ensure proper balance.

2 Initiate nasogastric feedings—feeding through a gastric tube ensures better nutrition than does intravenous feeding. Paralytic ileus is fairly frequent in the unconscious patient, and a nasogastric tube assists in gastric decompression.
    a. Insert small gastric tube through nose into stomach.
    b. Aspirate stomach before each feeding. If aspirated residual exceeds 50 ml, the patient may be developing an ileus. Gastric distension and vomiting may result.
    c. Feeds (Clinifeed or a made up preparation from the hospital diet kitchen) should be gradually increased until 400–500 ml are given at each feeding.
    d. Give 2000–2500 ml of fluid (according to patient's condition, remember head injured patients may have their fluid intake restricted to 1500 ml). An unconscious patient requires adequate fluid since high protein feedings can produce a solute diuresis.
    e. Rinse the tube with water after each feeding.

To Give Nursing Support as the Patient's Changing Condition Indicates

1 Be aware of the varying phases of restlessness—a certain degree of restlessness may be favourable, since it may indicate the patient is regaining consciousness. However, restlessness is quite common in cerebral anoxia or when there is a partially obstructed airway, distended bladder, overlooked bleeding, or fracture; it may be a manifestation of brain injury.

   a. Have adequate lighting in the room to prevent hallucinations as the patient regains consciousness.

   b. Pad side rails or use other devices to protect patient.

   c. Avoid oversedating the patient.

   d. Avoid restraints if at all possible.

   e. Speak softly to the patient, calling him by name.

   f. Touch him as gently as possible.

2 Keep the skin clean, dry and free of pressure—comatose patients are susceptible to formation of pressure sores.

3 Clip patient's nails to prevent excoriation of the skin.

4 Put all extremities through range of motion exercises four times daily—contracture deformities develop early in unconscious patients.

5 Turn the patient from side to side at regular intervals—turning relieves pressure areas and helps keep lungs clear by mobilizing secretions. Prolonged pressure on extremities produces nerve palsies.

6 Observe the patient for indication of an overdistended bladder.

   a. Utilize external sheath catheter (condom catheter) for male patient.

   b. If patient is unable to micturate, insert indwelling catheter with continuous drainage—infection invariably follows prolonged use of an indwelling catheter that is attached to straight drainage.

   c. Tape the catheter on the abdomen or horizontally to the side of the male patient and to the inner thigh of the female patient—to prevent urethral compression (male) and traction on the urethra.

7 Protect the eyes from corneal irritation—the cornea functions as a shield. If the eyes remain open for long periods, corneal drying, irritation and ulceration are apt to result.

   a. Make sure patient's eye is not rubbing against bedding if blinking and corneal reflexes are absent.

   b. Inspect the size of pupils and condition of eyes with a flashlight.

   c. Remove contact lenses if worn.

   d. Irrigate eyes with sterile prescribed solution and instil (usually normal sterile) artificial tear drops in each eye—prevents glazing and corneal ulceration.

   e. It may be necessary to carefully tape down the eyelids with a strip of hypoallergic tape or 'Steri-Strip'.

   f. Prepare for temporary tarsorrhaphy (suturing of eyelids in closed position) if unconscious state is prolonged.

8 Protect the patient during convulsive seizures (see below)—patient with head injury is a potential candidate for convulsive seizures.

   a. Protect the patient from self-injury.

   b. Observe the patient during the seizure and record observations.

   c. Give prescribed anticonvulsant medications through the nasogastric tube.
 9 Be alert for the development of complications.
   a. Respiratory complications (infections, aspiration, obstruction, atelectasis).
   b. Fluid and electrolyte imbalance.
   c. Infection (urinary, pressure sores, central nervous system).
   d. Bladder and gastrointestinal distension.
   e. Convulsive seizures.
10 Be aware that the patient will feel uneasy concerning his period of unconsciousness when he gains awareness of what has happened.

Nursing Management of the Patient Having a Convulsion

A *convulsion* is an involuntary contraction, or a series of contractions, of muscles resulting from abnormal cerebral stimulation (see treatment and nursing management of the epilepsies, p. 47).

Nursing Managment

Objective

To prevent injury to the patient.

1 Observe and record the progression of symptoms during the seizure.
   a. State whether or not the beginning of the attack was observed.
   b. Note the following:
      (1) The first thing the patient does in an attack—where the movements or stiffness starts; position of eyeballs and head.
      (2) The type of movements of the part involved.
      (3) The parts involved (turn back covers and expose patient).
      (4) Pupillary changes.
      (5) Incontinence of urine and faeces.
      (6) Duration of each phase of the attack.
      (7) Unconsciousness, if present, and its duration.
      (8) Any obvious paralysis or weakness of arms or legs after the attack.
      (9) Inability to speak after the attack.
      (10) Whether or not the patient sleeps after the attack.
2 Support the patient during the convulsive seizure.
   a. Ensure an adequate airway.
      (1) When jaws are clenched in spasm do not attempt to pry open to insert a mouth gag.
      (2) When respiration returns following the seizure and the patient becomes flaccid, turn his head to the side to facilitate drainage of mucus and saliva.
      (3) Try to hold the lower jaw forward when the patient is in flaccid stage.
   b. Try to protect the patient from injuring himself.
      (1) Protect his head with a folded blanket/pad to prevent head injury.
      (2) Loosen constrictive clothing.
   c. Give the patient privacy and protect him from curious onlookers.
   d. Stay with patient until he is fully conscious.
   e. Reorient him to his environment when he awakens.

f. Handle the patient with calm persuasion and gentle restraint when seizures are characterized by disturbed behaviour.

Family Health Teaching

Instruct the family as follows:

1 Summon medical assistance if a second convulsion follows before consciousness is regained. There is a risk of status epilepticus developing.
2 If the patient has severe postictal (following seizure) excitement, it may be necessary to bring him to the emergency department.

Nursing Management of the Patient Undergoing Intracranial Surgery

Craniotomy is the surgical opening of the skull to remove a tumour, relieve intracranial pressure, evacuate a blood clot or stop haemorrhage.
Craniectomy is excision of a portion of the skull.
Cranioplasty is repair of a cranial defect.

Treatment and Nursing Management

Preoperative Management

Objective

To determine the precise location of the lesion (clot, tumour, aneurysm).

1 Assist the patient undergoing diagnostic tests and frequent neurological examinations.
2 Evaluate and record patient's symptoms and signs (paralysis, aphasia) preoperatively in order to make postoperative comparisons.
3 Support the patient with neurological motor and sensory defects.
   a. Position paralysed extremities to prevent contracture deformities.
   b. Familiarize the blind patient with his environment.
      (1) Personnel entering room should announce themselves—helps patient understand incoming stimuli.
      (2) Help patient to assume an active role in his care.
   c. Assist the aphasic patient to communicate by means of picture cards, writing materials, etc.
   d. Protect the confused patient.
      (1) Remove disturbing environmental stimuli.
      (2) Keep patient oriented to time and place; place wall calendar and clock where patient can see them.
   e. Instruct and encourage the patient and family about the impending surgery—to relieve anxiety and tension.
4 Prepare the patient physically for surgery.
   a. Reassure patient about the fact that his head will be shaved (usually in the theatre), but a wig is made available on the NHS.
   b. The hair is often washed the night before surgery.
   c. Give enemas only as directed—straining upon defaecation raises intracranial pressure.

d. Give medications and treatment as indicated:
  (1) Steroids—to decrease cerebral oedema.
  (2) May be necessary to insert indwelling catheter—as dehydrating agents are usually given during operation.

Postoperative Management

Objectives

To watch for life-threatening complications, namely increasing intracranial pressure from oedema and bleeding.
To improve the functional status of the patient.

1 Establish proper respiratory exchange—to eliminate systemic hypercarbia and anoxia which increase cerebral oedema.
   a. Keep the patient in a lateral or a semiprone position—to facilitate respiratory exchange.
   b. Employ tracheopharyngeal aspiration—to remove secretions.
   c. Elevate the head of the bed 30 cm (12 in) after the patient is conscious—to aid venous drainage of the brain (some neurosurgeons prefer patient to be kept flat).
   d. See that the patient has nothing by mouth until an active coughing and swallowing reflex is demonstrated.
2 Assess patient's level of responsiveness.
   a. Response to commands:
     (1) Answers questions readily and correctly.
     (2) Can perform a complex manoeuvre.
     (3) Responds to simple command.
     (4) Gives delayed or unequal response.
     (5) Reacts only to loud voice.
     (6) Does not respond.
   b. Assessment of spinal motor reflexes (pinch Achilles tendon, arm or other body site):
     (1) Prompt, purposeful withdrawal.
     (2) Sluggish or nonpurposeful movement of extremities.
     (3) Facial grimace.
     (4) Involuntary micturition.
     (5) Extension of limbs.
     (6) No response.
   c. Observation of patient's spontaneous activity:
     (1) Verbal or other communication.
     (2) Changes in posture (frequency).
     (3) Breathing pattern.
     (4) Retching, vomiting.
     (5) Restlessness, twitching, tremors, convulsions.
3 Keep the patient normothermic during postoperative period—temperature control may be lost in certain neurologic states; a higher temperature increases the metabolic demands of the brain.
   a. Take rectal temperature at specified intervals.

Extremities may be cold and dry due to paralysis of heat-losing mechanisms (vasodilation and sweating).

b. Employ measures to reduce excessive fever when present.

(1) Remove blankets; place loin cloth over patient.

(2) Aspirin suppositories may be prescribed (High fever of central origin is less responsive to salicylates).

(3) Apply ice bags to axilla and groin—application of cold over large superficial vessel helps lower body temperature.

(4) Give tepid water or alcohol sponge (see p. 16).

(5) Use a fan blowing on patient—to increase surface cooling.

(6) Medical staff may prescribe chlorpromazine—prevents excessive shivering.

4   Evaluate for signs and symptoms of increasing intracranial pressure.

a. Assess patient (minute by minute, hour by hour) for:

(1) Diminished response to stimuli.

(2) Fluctuations of vital signs.

(3) Restlessness.

(4) Weakness and paralysis of extremities.

(5) Increasing headache.

(6) Changes or disturbances of vision; dilated pupils.

b. Control postoperative cerebral oedema.

(1) Keep patient *slightly* underhydrated—to combat cerebral oedema.

(2) Record urinary specific gravity at intervals—especially indicated for surgery of the pituitary and hypothalamus.

(3) Evaluate electrolyte status:

(a) Early postoperative weight gain indicates fluid retention; a greater than estimated loss of weight indicates negative water balance.

(b) Loss of sodium and chlorides will produce weakness, lethargy and coma.

(c) Low potassium will cause confusion and lower level of responsiveness.

(4) Give steroids, osmotic dehydrating agents and glycerol in selected cases, in postoperative period, according to doctor's instructions.

(5) Institute hypothermia procedures (see above) to decrease brain metabolism.

(6) Elevate head of bed 20–30° to reduce intracranial pressure and to facilitate respiration (some neurosurgeons prefer patient to be kept flat).

5   Perform supportive measures until the patient is able to care for himself.

a. Change position frequently since pain and pressure responses are variable.

b. Give analgesics that do not mask level of responsiveness—codeine, aspirin.

c. Support the patient if convulsive seizures occur (see p. 22).

d. Relieve signs of periorbital oedema.

(1) Bathe eyes frequently with normal saline.

(2) Watch for signs of keratitis if cornea has no sensation.

e. Put extremities through range of motion exercises.

f. Use aseptic measures in management of indwelling urethral catheter.

g. Evaluate and support patient during episodes of restlessness.

(1) Evaluate for airway obstruction, distended bladder, meningeal irritation from bloody cerebrospinal fluid.

(2) Pad patient's hands and bed rails—to protect from injury.

h. Watch for leakage of cerebrospinal fluid since there is ever present danger of meningitis.

(1) Differentiate between cerebrospinal fluid (CSF) and mucus.

(a) Collect fluid on Dextrostix—if CSF is present, indicator will have positive reaction since cerebrospinal fluid contains sugar.

(b) Assess for moderate elevation of temperature and mild neck rigidity.

(2) It may be necessary to keep cerebrospinal pressure low by periodic lumbar puncture—to reduce cerebrospinal fluid pressure and decrease its force against the wound. Following post fossa operations, frequent lumbar punctures are performed to remove blood stained cerebrospinal fluid and therefore decrease meningeal irritation.

i. Reinforce bloodstained dressings with sterile dressing; blood-soaked dressings act as a culture medium for bacteria.

j. Evaluate patient with hypophysectomy (surgery on pituitary) for diabetes insipidus.

(1) Weigh daily.

(2) Keep input and output record.

(3) Evaluate specific gravity of all urine passed.

6 Assess for complications.

a. Intracranial haemorrhage. (Postoperative bleeding may be intraventricular, intracerebral, intracerebellar, subdural or extradural.)

(1) Watch for progressive impairment of state of responsiveness, signs of increasing intracranial pressure.

(2) Prepare patient for CAT scanning.

(3) Prepare patient for reoperation and evacuation of haematoma.

b. Brain oedema.

c. Postoperative meningitis.

d. Wound infections (scalp, bone flap)—wound may have to be reopened.

e. Pulmonary complications.

f. Epilepsy. (There is a greater risk of epilepsy with supratentorial operations.)

(1) Give prescribed anticonvulsants on a long-term basis.

(2) Watch for status epilepticus which may occur after any intracranial operation.

g. Gastrointestinal ulceration (signs and symptoms of haemorrhage and perforation or both).

CRANIAL NERVE INVOLVEMENT

Bell's Palsy

Bell's palsy (facial paralysis) is due to peripheral involvement of the seventh cranial nerve (facial) on one side, producing weakness or paralysis of the facial muscles.

Clinical Manifestations

1 Distortion of face—from paralysis of facial muscles.
2 Feeling of numbness in face.
3 Eye problems:

a. Insensitive cornea (from denervation)—may be damaged without usual warning symptoms of pain.

b. Epiphora (overflow of tears down the cheek)—from keratitis caused by drying of cornea and lack of blink reflex; laxity of lower eyelid may alter proper drainage of tears.

c. Or decreased tear production—may lead to a dry eye which is predisposed to infection.

4 Speech difficulties.

5 Pain—behind ear or in face.

Clinical Features

1 The aetiology of Bell's palsy is unknown. The three theories of possible aetiologic causes (and combinations thereof) are vascular ischaemia, viral (herpes simplex; herpes zoster) and autoimmune disease.

2 It is more likely to occur in diabetic persons than in nondiabetics.

3 Bell's palsy can produce grotesque disfigurement with accompanying physical and emotional stress.

4 There is no clear method of determining the prognosis at the time of onset of paralysis.

Diagnosis

1 History of acute onset.

2 Tests of cranial nerve function.

3 Electrodiagnostic study of facial muscles through electromyography—electrodes placed over branches of facial nerve; facial muscles observed for movement.

Complications

1 Corneal ulceration; blindness.

2 Facial weakness.

3 Facial spasm with contracture and synkinesis (unintentional movement).

4 Crocodile tearing.

Treatment and Nursing Management

Objectives

To maintain muscle tone of the face.
To prevent or minimize denervation.

1 Give steroid therapy (prednisone)—may be helpful in reducing inflammation and oedema, which reduces vascular compression and permits restoration of blood circulation in the nerve; early administration appears to diminish severity of disease and mitigate pain.

2 Promote pain relief.
   a. Give salicylates or codeine as indicated.
   b. Apply heat to involved side of face—to provide comfort and to stimulate blood perfusion through facial muscles.

3 Protect the involved eye—facial paralysis may abolish the blinking reflex; eye is vulnerable to dust and foreign particles.

Nursing Alert: Keratitis is a major threat to a patient with Bell's palsy.

  a. Protect the cornea with preparation of artificial tears.
  b. Use mild eyewash several times a day during acute stage as directed.
  c. Use eye ointment at bedtime—helps to keep eyes closed during sleep by sticking the lashes together.
  d. See that patient wears a protective patch, particularly at night.
    (1) Patch may eventually abrade cornea as paretic (incompletely paralysed) eyelids are difficult to keep closed.
    (2) Eyelids may have to be sutured together.
  e. Instruct patient to use protective glasses (wraparound sunglasses or goggles) to decrease normal evaporation from eye.
4 Start facial massage (if no nerve tenderness present) several times daily to help maintain muscle tone.
  a. Teach patient to massage his face with gentle upward motion.
  b. Electrical stimulation to face (by physiotherapist) may or may not be prescribed.

Health Teaching

1 Reassure patient that spontaneous recovery occurs in majority of patients; recovery usually takes place in 3–5 weeks.
2 Keep the face warm.
3 Teach facial exercises—to prevent facial muscle atrophy and to improve strength of remaining innervated muscles. Do the following while looking in a mirror.
  a. Wrinkle forehead.
  b. Close eyes.
  c. Purse lips.
  d. Move mouth from side to side.
  e. Blow out cheeks.
  f. Whistle.
4 Reinforce teaching concerning eye care (see above).

Trigeminal Neuralgia (Tic Doloureux)

Trigeminal neuralgia (tic doloureux) is a condition of the fifth cranial nerve, characterized by sudden paroxysms of lancinating or burning pain (alternating with periods of complete comfort) in the distribution of one or more branches of the trigeminal nerve.

Aetiology

Unknown.

Clinical Manifestations

1 Sudden and severe pain appearing without warning—in distribution of one or more branches of trigeminal nerve (Fig. 1.3).
2 Numerous individual flashes of pain, ending abruptly; usually on one side.
3 Attacks precipitated by pressure on a trigger point, the terminals of the affected

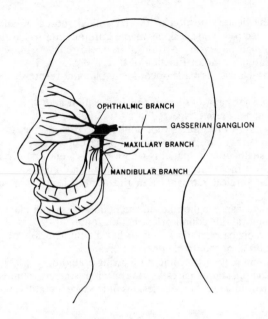

Figure 1.3. The main divisions of the trigeminal nerve are ophthalmic, maxillary and mandibular. Sensory root fibres arise in the Gasserian ganglion.

branches. (Movement of the face, talking, chewing, yawning, swallowing, shaving, cold wind, may precipitate an agonizing attack).

Treatment and Nursing Management

Objective

To give pain relief without loss of function.

1   Instruct patient to avoid exposing affected cheek to sudden cold if this is known to trigger the nerve—iced drinks, cold wind, swimming in cold water.

2   Drug therapy (antiepileptic drugs):
    a. Carbamazepine (Tegretol) or phenytoin (Epanutin)—relieves and prevents pain in some patients.
    b. Serum levels of drug monitored to avoid drug toxicity.
    c. Observe for evidences of haematological, hepatic, renal and skin reactions.

3   Surgical approach to treatment—used after medical treatment fails to give relief.
    a. Objective—to provide optimum pain relief with minimum impairment.
    b. Alcohol injection of ganglion of peripheral branches produces temporary chemical destruction of affected nerves.
       (1) Pain returns after nerve regeneration; usually 6–19 months.
       (2) Usually produces complete anaesthesia.
    c. Radiofrequency lesions—percutaneous electrocoagulation of the Gasserian ganglion and its rootlets—introduction of needle electrode through foramen

ovale to the desired portion of the trigeminal root; low voltage stimulation applied to electrode and a lesion is made. Carefully controlled electrical currents destroy enough of sensory portion of nerve to relieve pain without damaging touch sensation or motor function of face.

(1) Root selection is made by conscious patient's response to electrical stimulation.

(2) Abolishes pain, but leaves touch sensation intact.

(3) Permanent relief expected in most patients.

d. Open surgical procedures (not done in the first instance).

(1) Peripheral neurectomy (excision of part of a nerve).

  (a) Usually done in patients whose pain is from first division of nerve.

  (b) Gives more prolonged relief than alcohol injection.

(2) Open surgical retrogasserian rhizotomy (destruction of retrogasserian rootlets).

  (a) Gasserian ganglion lies in the middle fossa and may be reached by a subtemporal, intradural or extradural route.

  (b) Following operation, patient has a complete loss of sensation in the distribution of the divided nerve fibres.

  (c) See nursing management following craniotomy, p. 23.

  (d) Complications: paresthesias (burning, stinging, numbness, discomfort in and around eye, herpetic lesions of the face, keratitis and corneal ulceration).

CEREBROVASCULAR DISEASE

Cerebrovascular disease refers to any functional abnormality of the central nervous system caused by a pathological condition of the individual vessels or of the cerebral vascular system. It either causes haemorrhage from a tear in the vessel wall or impairs the cerebral circulation by a partial or complete occlusion of the lumen of the vessel.

Cerebrovascular Disease from Haemorrhage

1 *Extradural haemorrhage*—haemorrhage occurring outside the dura mater.
  a. This is considered a life-threatening emergency.
  b. See care of the patient with a head injury for principles of immediate care (p 11).

2 *Subdural haemorrhage*—haemorrhage occurring beneath the dura mater.
  See care of the patient with a head injury (p. 11).

3 *Subarachnoid haemorrhage*—haemorrhage occurring in the subarachnoid space.
  See nursing management of patient with cerebral haemorrhage (p. 43).

4 *Intracerebral haemorrhage*—haemorrhage occurring within the brain substance.
  See nursing management of patient with cerebral haemorrhage (p. 43).

Cerebrovascular Disease from Impairment of Cerebral Circulation

1 *Transient ischaemic attacks* (TIA)—transient attacks of dysfunction of central nervous system, lasting for several minutes with the absence of neurological disturbances between the attacks—may serve as a warning of impending stroke.
  a. Causes—transient impairment of the cerebral blood flow to a specific region

due to fall in cerebral perfusion pressure, atherosclerotic involvement of the vessels supplying the brain, cardiac arrhythmias, etc.

   b. Therapy—reconstructive vascular procedures (for extracranial lesions) if patient is a candidate for surgical intervention. Anticoagulant therapy.

2 *Cerebral thrombosis*—usually produces transient loss of speech, visual disturbance, hemiplegia, or paresthesia in one-half of the body which may precede severe paralysis. (See nursing management of the patient with a stroke.)

3 Cerebral embolism—caused by heart disease (infective endocarditis, rheumatic heart disease, prosthetic heart valves, myocardial infarction) or pulmonary emboli.

   a. Embolism usually lodges in middle cerebral artery or its branches where it disrupts circulation.

   b. Symptoms—sudden onset of hemiparesis or hemiplegia.

   c. See the nursing management of the patient with a stroke, in the discussion which follows.

STROKE OR CEREBRAL VASCULAR ACCIDENT (CVA)

A stroke (*cerebral vascular accident*) is a condition in which the blood supply to the brain is reduced as a result of transient ischaemic attacks, cerebral thrombosis, cerebral embolism, intracerebral or subarachnoid haemorrhage.

Clinical Manifestations of Impending Stroke

1 Memory impairment, vertigo, headache, syncope, blurring of vision, etc.

2 *Focal or neurological signs*—hemiparesis or hemiplegia, aphasia, homonymous hemianopia, ataxia, cranial nerve palsies, stupor, coma.

Persons at Risk for Stroke

Predisposing factors include the following:

1 Hypertension.
2 Elevated serum cholesterol.
3 Cardiac enlargement.
4 ECG changes indicating left ventricular hypertrophy.
5 Coronary artery disease.
6 Congestive heart failure, arrhythmia.
7 Abnormal glucose tolerance test (diabetes).
8 Cigarette smoking.

Treatment and Nursing Management

The Acute Phase: The Unconscious Patient

Objectives

To keep the patient alive.
To minimize cerebral damage by providing adequately oxygenated blood to the brain.

1   See the nursing management of the unconscious patient (p. 18).
2   Carry out a nursing assessment of the following:
   a. A change in the level of responsiveness as evidenced by movement, resistance to changes of position and response to stimulation.
   b. Presence or absence of voluntary or involuntary movements of the extremities; tone of the muscles; body posture and the position of the head.
   c. Stiffness or flaccidity of the neck.
   d. Comparison of pupils as to size, reaction to light and ocular position.
   e. Colour of the face and extremities; temperature and moisture of the skin.
   f. Quality and rates of pulse and respiration; body temperature and arterial pressure.
   g. Volume of fluids ingested or administered and volume of urine excreted each 24 hours.
3   Assure an adequate perfusion pressure so that oxygenated blood can reach the brain.
   a. Maintain blood pressure and cardiac output—to sustain cerebral blood flow.
   b. Watch for evidence of myocardial infarction, arrhythmias and congestive heart failure; arrhythmia may reduce cerebral blood flow and produce cardiac arrest.
   c. Ensure hydration; rehydration may reduce blood viscosity and thereby improve cerebral blood flow.
4   Reorient the patient when he begins to regain consciousness.
   a. Expect some dysphasia if patient has right-sided hemiplegia.
   b. Reassure patient that he has not lost his mind and that he will receive help with communication (speech therapist).
   c. *Talk* to the patient while caring for him.
   d. Make every effort to understand the patient.
   e. Maintain a calm and accepting manner during periods of emotional lability.
5   Remove indwelling catheter as soon as patient is conscious.
   a. Offer bedpan or urinal at scheduled short intervals.
   b. Lengthen time intervals as more bladder control is gained.
6   Prepare for surgical intervention if necessary—to halt potential occlusive lesions and restore circulation.
7   The following may be amenable to surgical intervention:
   a. Cerebral haemorrhage secondary to rupture of cerebral aneurysm.
   b. Ruptured berry-type aneurysm.
   c. Acute and chronic subdural haematomas.
   d. Arteriovenous malformation (angiomas).

Rehabilitation Phase

Objectives

To prevent deformities.
To retrain the affected arm and leg.
To help the patient gain independence in personal hygiene and in dressing and ambulation activities.

1   Position the patient in bed correctly—to prevent contractures, relieve pressure and maintain good body alignment. (These principles of positioning are also

carried out during the unconscious phase.) (See Fig. 1.4.) Nursing staff will be part of the rehabilitation team which includes physiotherapists, occupational therapists, speech therapists and clinical psychologists. It is important that at all times, the nursing staff reinforce the exercises and rehabilitation programmes designed by other members of the team.

2   Exercise the affected extremities passively and carry out range of motion exercises four to five times daily—to prevent contracture development in the paralysed extremity, to prevent further deterioration of neuromuscular system, to stretch soft tissues and to enhance circulation.

   a. Involve family in exercise programme since care of a stroke patient requires time and effort.

   b. Remind the patient to exercise unaffected limbs at intervals throughout the day—to prevent contracture development in the normal limbs.

   c. Teach patient to put his unaffected leg under the affected one in order to move and turn himself (Fig. 1.5).

   d. Instruct the patient to move his affected arm (and hand) with his good hand (Fig. 1.6).

3   Adjust nursing approach to the patient's condition.

   a. Test for hemianopia (defective vision in half of the visual field).

      (1) Show patient an object placed to one side and ask if he can identify it.

      (2) Hemianopia is evident if patient fails to see the object on the correct side, but responds by looking towards it on the other side. (Visual field is likely to be limited on the right if patient has right hemiplegia.)

   b. Place call light, bedside table, etc., on the side of his awareness.

   c. Approach the bed from the uninvolved side.

   d. Encourage the patient to turn his head from side to side to obtain the full view of a normal visual field.

   e. Have patient wear his spectacles.

   f. For patient with dysarthria (difficult speech) and dysphagia (difficulty in swallowing):

      (1) Give nasogastric tube feeding if indicated.

      (2) Give food and fluids from uninvolved side (if patient has droop of mouth).

      (3) Remind patient to chew on unaffected side.

      (4) Inspect patient's mouth for food collecting between cheek and gums on involved side; frequent oral hygiene is necessary.

   g. See p. 39 for nursing management of patient with aphasia.

4   Maintain bladder and bowel programme.

5   Assist the patient in getting out of bed as soon as permitted.

   a. *To develop sitting balance:*

      (1) Slowly assist patient to a sitting position.

      (2) Place patient's feet on floor (or on the seat of a chair).

      (3) Place the patient's unaffected hand behind him—to assist in maintaining balance.

      (4) Stand in front of patient—to help him maintain this posture. Watch for postural hypotension.

      (5) Assess for change in colour, shortness of breath, profuse perspiration—indications that patient should be placed back in dorsal position.

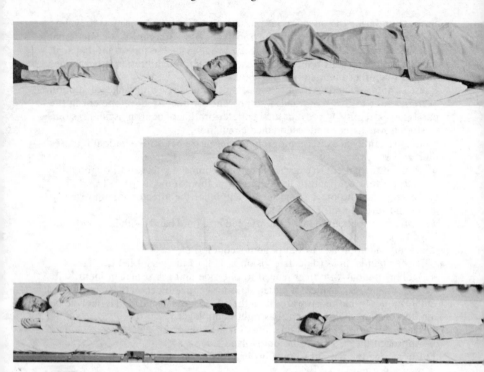

Figure 1.4. Positioning for a patient following stroke (dark side of pyjamas represents affected or hemiplegic side). a. A pillow is placed in the axilla to prevent adduction of the affected shoulder. Pillows are placed under the arm, which is in a slightly flexed position with each joint positioned higher than the preceding one. b. The trochanter role should extend from the crest of the ileum to the midthigh, since the hip joint lies between these two points. The trochanter role acts as a mechanical wedge under the protection of the greater trochanter and prevents the femur from rolling. c. A volar resting splint may be used to support the wrist and hand if the upper extremity is flaccid. d. Lateral or side lying position. The patient should be turned on his unaffected side. The upper thigh should not be acutely flexed. e. Prone position. A pillow is placed under the pelvis to promote hyperextension of the hip joints, which is essential from normal gait. Note position of arms.

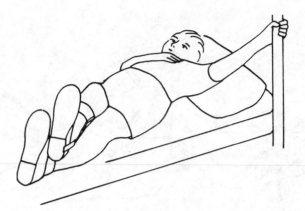

Figure 1.5. Bed exercise for the patient with hemiplegia: moving the legs over the side of the bed. The paralysed leg is carried by the uninvolved leg. (From: Hirschberg, G, Lewis, L and Vaughan, P (1976) Rehabilitation, 2nd edition, J B Lippincott.)

(6) Increase sitting time as rapidly as patient's condition permits.
b. *To develop standing balance:*
(1) Put walking shoes with strong shank on patient for all ambulation activities.
(2) Seat the patient on edge of bed and place a straight-back chair on each side of him (Fig.1.7a).
(a) Tie affected hand to the chair if patient lacks grasp strength.
(b) Assist the patient to a standing position, supporting (locking) his affected knee with the side of your knee (Figs. 1.7b and c).
(3) Stand behind patient and stabilize him at waist level.
(4) Assess for dizziness, pallor and increasing pulse rate.
(5) Assist patient to achieve standing balance at frequent intervals throughout the day.
(6) Help the patient begin walking as soon as standing balance is achieved (using parallel bars).
(7) Encourage patient to look at his feet occasionally—proprioceptive loss may accompany hemiplegia.
6   Encourage patient to perform his self-care activities as soon as possible.
a. Set realistic goals and add a new task daily if possible.
b. Have the patient immediately transfer all self-care activities to the unaffected side. Teach one-handed methods.
c. Encourage him to brush his teeth, comb his hair and bathe and feed himself.
d. Help the patient to dress himself for ambulatory activities.
(1) Instruct family to bring clothing that is one size larger than usually worn.
(2) Have patient dress himself (with assistance if necessary) while seated—to achieve better balance.
(3) Use clothing with front fasteners; stretch fabrics are preferable.
(4) Teach only one activity at a time.

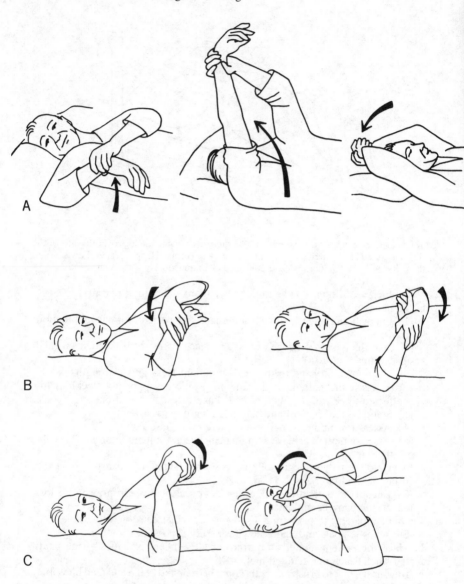

Figure 1.6. a. Exercise to maintain range of motion of the involved shoulder and the elbow in hemiplegia. b. Exercise to maintain range of motion of pronation and supination in affected hand. c. Exercise to maintain range of motion of the wrist and the finger in hemiplegia. (From: Hirschberg, G, Lewis, L and Vaughan, P (1976) Rehabilitation, 2nd edition, J B Lippincott.) Lippincott.)

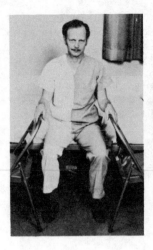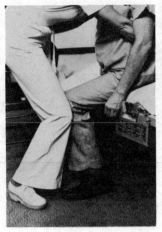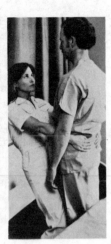

Figure 1.7 a. Getting the patient out of bed following a stroke. Place the bed in a low position so that the feet are resting on the floor. The affected hand may be tied to a chair for stabilization. Observe the patient's reaction and increase sitting time as rapidly as the patients condition permits. b. Rising to a standing position. Help the patient to come to a standing position while supporting his affected knee with the nurse's knees. This support will prevent the patient's affected knee from buckling. c. Stabilizing the patient as he assumes a standing position.

7 Assist in securing supportive devices if needed—most patients develop spasticity of lower extremity and will lack motor control.
   a. The physiotherapist may secure posterior knee splint if patient has a weakened or absent quadriceps muscle—gives better balance and helps prevent loss of position sense.
   b. The physiotherapist may secure an adjustable aluminium tripod when patient is able to walk alone.
8 The physiotherapist may advise the use of a sling on the paralysed arm when patient is in upright position, if arm is flaccid or if patient complains of arm pain and heaviness.
   a. Remove sling frequently and exercise arm.
   b. Instruct patient to interlace his fingers, placing the palms together. With elbows extended, lift both arms above head repeatedly throughout day.
   c. When seated, keep the affected arm and hand elevated with a pillow.
   d. Instruct patient to flex and extend his wrist and fingers with unaffected hand at frequent intervals.
9 Secure a wheelchair of the correct size, with brakes that the patient can manage if he is unable to ambulate (physiotherapist will advice on this).
   a. Place wheelchair on patient's unaffected side; allows him to see wheelchair and lead with the stronger leg.

    b. Lock wheelchair brake and remove pedals. Instruct the patient as follows:
        (1) Lean forward, placing weight over strong leg. Push up with strong arm and foot.
        (2) Place most of the weight on the strong leg while keeping weak knee locked.
        (3) Pivot in the direction of the stronger leg; bring weak leg over to stronger leg. Maintain standing position a few moments.
        (4) Lower body into chair gradually, using strong arm and leg.
        (5) Push wheelchair with uninvolved leg.

10 Prepare the patient for discharge.
    a. Some patients will have to be transferred to rehabilitation centres for further therapy.
    b. Encourage patient to keep active, adhere to his exercise programme and remain as self-sufficient as possible.

Family Health Teaching

Instruct the family as follows; with the help and advice of other members of the health care team.

1 Expect some emotional lability and some degree of brain damage if the patient has had a more severe stroke.
    a. Patient may cry easily; this does not necessarily imply unhappiness.
    b. Hemiplegic patients may be easily confused, forgetful, discouraged, hostile, unco-operative, withdrawn and dependent.
    c. Support him psychologically; hemiplegia has a tremendous psychological impact on the patient (and his family).
2 Avoid doing those things for the patient that he can do for himself.
3 Be supportive and sympathetic but firm and direct.
4 Install handrails by the toilet and bath or shower and put safety rails on the bed.
5 Obtain self-help devices to assist in activities of daily living; modify and adapt devices and 'gadgets' to meet individual patient's needs.
    a. A brush with suction cups may be applied to washbasin—patient can rub hands against it to wash.
    b. Long-handled brush and comb.
    c. Flexible hose with shower head; bar stool for bath or shower.
    d. Knife–fork combination—to cut food.
    e. Nonslip mat under plate; plate guard to keep food from being pushed off plate.
6 See that patient has rest periods.
7 Set realistic goals.
8 The patient will need to attend outpatient clinics.
9 Take advantage of community service agencies.

APHASIA

Aphasia is a conceptual disturbance of language resulting from cerebral dysfunction. It may involve impairment of the ability to read and write as well as to speak, listen and comprehend.

Causes

1 Traumatic head injury.
2 Cerebral vascular accident.
3 Tumour.
4 Cerebral abscess.

Types of Aphasia

1 Motor aphasia or expressive aphasia—loss of ability to express one's thoughts in speech and writing; person understands what is said to him but he cannot produce sequence of movements necessary to utter words.
2 Sensory aphasia or receptive aphasia—inability to comprehend spoken or written language.
3 Central or global aphasia—a combination of both motor and sensory aphasia. The terms aphasia strictly indicate a complete loss of function whereas dysphasia implies partial loss; however, the prefixes a- and dys- are often used interchangeably.

Nursing Management

Principle

There are a variety of symptoms and disorders underlying aphasia. Therefore, the treatment is individualized.

Objective

To stimulate attempts at communication.

1 Determine the communication abilities of the patient—usually done by speech therapist.
2 Give the patient as much psychological security as possible.
3 Give the patient plenty of *time* to speak and respond; he cannot sort out incoming messages and formulate a response under pressure.
   a. Speak slowly while making eye contact with the patient.
   b. Face the patient.
   c. Avoid talking too fast, too loudly or too much.
   d. Use short sentences; pause; see if he indicates that he understands.
   e. Supplement speech with gestures when indicated.
   f. Talk to him while caring for him. Know his former interests.
   g. Be consistent—by using the same wording each time instructions are given and questions are asked.
4 Keep the environment relaxed.
5 Keep distractions at a minimum—damaged input pathways cannot sort out distracting stimuli in the environment.
6 Use as many sensory channels as possible.
   a. Supplement auditory stimulation with visual stimulation.
   b. Use visual aids (pictures); ask patient to point to and name what he sees.
   c. Use games, television, tape-recorders, cassettes, etc., to stimulate his interest.

d. Encourage patient to use any form of communication—gestures, writing, drawing, etc., until his speech begins to return.

e. Elicit responses from patient, e.g. "Please nod your head if you understand." Reinforce every correct response.

7   Give support by assuring the patient that there is nothing wrong with his intelligence.

a. Treat him as an intelligent adult.

b. Accept the patient as he is now; avoid artificial praise.

c. Maintain a calm, accepting and deliberate manner especially during periods of emotional lability.

8   Encourage the patient to socialize with his family and friends.

a. Seek the help of other people to read aloud, play games, do puzzles.

b. Have his grandchildren visit and talk with him.

c. Keep him in the social world.

9   Watch the patient for clues and gestures if his speech is unintelligible or jargon-like.

a. Continue to listen to him.

b. Nod and make neutral statements occasionally.

c. Shift the topic when appropriate to provide another point of interest and frame of reference.

10 Observe the patient during the course of his daily schedule for clues to evaluate and assess his progress.

Family Health Teaching

1   See items 1–10 above.

2   The patient's ability to speak may vary from day to day. Fatigue has an adverse effect on speech.

3   The patient is likely to become terribly frustrated by his inability to communicate; ignore swearing and abusive language.

4   Aphasia can also involve the patient's understanding. Some persons cannot express themselves but can comprehend the spoken or written word; others can speak but do not understand; while some who do neither may respond to gesture and actions.

SUBARACHNOID HAEMORRHAGE

Subarachnoid haemorrhage is bleeding into the subarachnoid space.

Causes

1   Ruptured aneurysm.

2   Head injury.

3   Arteriovenous malformation.

4   Primary or metastatic brain tumours.

5   Haemorrhagic disorders—leukaemia, aplastic anaemia, anticoagulant therapy, etc.

6   Hypertensive vascular disease.

Clinical Manifestations

May occur with or without premonitory signs; related to location, site and rate of development of haemorrhage.

1 Abrupt onset of intense headache.
2 Dizziness and vomiting.
3 Unconsciousness (unfavourable prognosis).
4 Convulsions.
5 Varying abnormalities in vital signs; neurological impairment—depending on severity of haemorrhage; site of bleeding usually determines neurological signs.
6 Hemiplegia.
7 Stiff neck; back pain.
8 Photophobia.

Treatment and Nursing Management

Objectives

To determine cause of bleeding.
To survive effects of bleeding.
To prevent immediate and long term rebleeding.

1 Place patient on strict bed rest for approximately 6 weeks.
2 Support patient undergoing lumbar puncture to confirm diagnosis (see p. 8).
3 Support patient undergoing cerebral angiography (to identify source of bleeding (see p. 2).
4 Give prescribed medications, usually dexamethasone and transensamic acid if haemorrhage from an aneurysm or arteriovenous malformation.

CEREBRAL ANEURYSM (INTRACRANIAL ANEURYSM)

A *cerebral aneurysm* is a sac formed by dilation of the walls of an artery within the head.

Aetiology

1 Congenital defect of vessel wall (most common).
2 Arteriosclerosis—reflects an acquired defect in vessel wall with subsequent weakness of wall.
3 Mycosis (rare).
4 Syphilis (rare).
5 Trauma.
6 Vasculitis secondary to drug addiction (heroin).

Clinical Manifestations

1 Due to compression of cranial nerve or brain substance.
2 Due to leakage from or rupture of aneurysm.
   a. Headache—usually severe and of sudden onset, usually frontal; disturbances of consciousness.

b. Pain and rigidity in back of neck and spine.
c. Visual disturbances—visual loss, diplopia (double vision), ptosis (drooping of upper eyelid).
d. Tinnitus (ringing in the ears).
e. Dizziness; nausea and vomiting.
f. Hemiparesis (muscular weakness affecting one side of body) or hemiplegia (paralysis of one side of body).

Underlying Principles

1   Early recognition of warning signs should prompt early surgical intervention before any further haemorrhage develops.
2   An aneurysm may cause pressure on the third cranial nerve, producing dilatation of the pupil on the same side.
3   Rupture of an aneurysm leads to subarachnoid haemorrhage.
4   Spontaneous subarachnoid haemorrhage is confirmed by lumbar puncture.

Treatment

Objective

To stop or diminish flow of blood in the aneurysmal sac.

Surgical

Patients with no or only minor neurological deficit (cranial nerve palsy) are usually referred for surgery. Patients should be on strict bed rest prior to surgery.

1   Intracranial procedures.
  a. Clipping the aneurysm across its neck to isolate aneurysm from blood vessel.
  b. Clip-wrap procedure—patching and reinforcing the defect in the media of the vessel wall as well as positioning a clip across the neck of the aneurysm.
  c. Wrapping aneurysms that have no clearly defined neck with single butter muslin, gauze, muscel or plastic material.
  d. See nursing management of patient following craniotomy (p. 23).
2   Extracranial procedure.
  Ligation of carotid artery in neck—to reduce pressure in the aneurysm and reduce the danger of rupture and haemorrhage.

Medical

Patients not suitable for surgery.

1   Bed rest—place on strict bed rest for approximately 6 weeks; high incidence of recurrence 10–14 days following first bleed.
2   Avoid overexertion, straining. Many neurosurgeons allow patients out of bed to use commode as this is less stressful than using a bedpan.
3   Drugs—dexamethasone and transensamic acid (an antifibrinolytic) and hypertensive agents may be given, but hypertension should be reduced gradually.

BRAIN ABSCESS

A *brain abscess* is a localized collection of pus within the brain substance.

Aetiology

1 By direct invasion of the brain.
  a. Cerebral trauma or surgery.
  b. Spread of infection from otitis media, mastoiditis, osteomyelitis of skull.
2 By spread of infection from other organs (remote from the brain) by haematogenous or metastatic spread.
  a. From the lung—pneumonia, bronchiectasis, lung abscess, tuberculosis.
  b. From the heart—infective endocarditis, congenital heart disease.
  c. From other organs—septicaemia, pelvic abscess.

Nursing Alert: Have a high degree of suspicion of brain abscess when neurological signs and symptoms develop in a person with a recent history of sinus or ear infection.

Clinical Manifestations

Caused by major alterations of intracranial mass dynamics (oedema, brain shift), by infection or by location of the abscess.

1 Headache—may be from increased intracranial pressure; worse in a.m.
2 Focal neurologic signs (depending on site of abscess)—weakness of arm or leg, visual impairment, focal epileptic seizures, papilloedema.
3 Fever and leucocytosis; temperature may by subnormal when there is a thick-walled abscess.
4 Change in patient's mental alertness.

Treatment and Nursing Management

Objective

To eliminate the abscess.

1 Observe patient for increased intracranial pressure (p. 14)—cerebral oedema surrounds an acute brain abscess and may produce sudden increase of intracranial pressure.
  a. Secondary midbrain and brain stem compression can lead to rapid coma and death.
  b. Patient may be given dexamethasone for cerebral oedema.
  c. Keep neurological observation record.
2 Give prescribed antibiotic therapy—to reduce the virulence of or to eliminate organism. Large doses of the appropriate antibiotic may be given to penetrate the abscess cavity until the lesion becomes encapsulated and ready for surgical intervention.
3 Assist in diagnostic studies for determining accurate localization of abscess; laboratory studies, computerized axial tomography and repeated neurological examinations.
4 Record seizures if they occur (see p.   ). Patient may receive anticonvulsant medication as a prophylactic measure.

5 Prepare for surgical intervention (the definitive treatment).
   a. Drainage of abscess through burr holes.
   b. Craniotomy with elevation of bone flap and removal of abscess. (See nursing management of patient undergoing intracranial surgery, p. 23.)
6 Support the patient during repeated x-ray studies following treatment to ascertain if infection has been eradicated.
   a. Relapse is common.
   b. Mortality rate is fairly high.
   c. Neurological defects following treatment of brain abscess include hemiparesis, seizures, visual defects, cranial nerve palsies and learning problems in children.
   d. Prognosis is related to the neurological status of the patient when therapy is begun.

Health Teaching

1 It is important that the anticonvulsant medication be taken on a daily basis as prescribed.
2 *Prevention:* Treat otitis media, mastoiditis, sinusitis and other systemic infections to prevent brain abscess.

BRAIN TUMOUR

A *brain tumour* is a localized intracranial lesion which occupies space within the skull and tends to cause a rise in intracranial pressure.

Incidence

1 Tumours of the brain originate in the brain (including the roots of the cranial nerves and the meninges) in about 95% of all patients with this problem.
2 Tumours may be benign or malignant; however any mass within closed cranial vault may be lethal.
3 The greatest incidence of brain tumours occurs between the ages of 30 and 50 years.

Classification

1 *Tumours arising from covering of brain:*
   Meningioma—encapsulated, well-defined, growing outside the brain tissue; compresses rather than invades brain.
2 *Tumours developing in or on the cranial nerves:*
   a. Acoustic neuroma—derived from sheath of acoustic nerve.
   b. Optic nerve spongioblastoma polare.
3 *Tumours originating in the brain connective tissue:*
   Gliomas—infiltrating tumours that may invade any portion of brain. Most common type of brain tumour.
   Astrocytoma
   Oligodendroglioma   Subclassified according to predominating
   Microglioma   cells (histology).
   Medullablastoma

4 *Metastatic lesions*—most common primary site is lung or breast.
5 *Tumours of the ductless glands:*
   a. Pituitary.   **b.** Pineal.
6 *Blood vessel tumours:*
   Haemangioblastoma.
7 *Tumours in children.*

Clinical Manifestations

General Symptoms

1 Brain tumour is usually characterized by a *progressive* course of symptoms over a period of time.
2 Brain tumours manifest themselves by:
   a. *Symptoms due to increased intracranial pressure:*
      (1) Headache—intensified by activity that increases intracranial pressure (stooping, straining).
      (2) Vomiting, unrelated to food intake—usually due to irritation of vagal centres in medulla.
      (3) Papilloedema—oedema of optic nerve disc.
      (4) Mental clouding, lethargy.
   b. *Symptoms due to local effects of tumour's interference with specific regions of the brain:*
      (1) Motor abnormalities—rigidity, lack of co-ordination, weakness, convulsive seizures.
      (2) Sensory abnormalities—aberrations in smell, vision, hearing.

Manifestations According to Site

1 *Frontal lobe tumour.*
   a. Mental changes (memory loss, euphoria, personality changes, loss of interest, moral laxity).
   b. Headache.
   c. Focal seizures.
   d. Hemiparesis or aphasia.
   e. Failing or blurring vision.
   f. Impairment of sphincter control.
2 *Temporal lobe* (may be relatively silent).
   a. Focal epileptic seizures.
   b. Dysphasia or aphasia.
   c. Papilloedema.
   d. Headache.
   e. Behaviour disorders.
3 *Parietal lobe tumours.*
   a. Motor seizures.
   b. Sensory loss or visual impairment.
   c. Jacksonian convulsions.
4 *Occipital tumours.*
   a. Visual impairment and visual hallucinations.
   b. Focal seizures.

5 *Cerebellar tumours* (common brain tumours of childhood).
  a. Disturbances of equilibrium and co-ordination.
  b. Early development of increasing intracranial pressure and papilloedema.
6 *Tumours of brain stem.*
  Symptoms of cranial nerve palsies (dysphagia, dysphonia, nystagmus, ataxia in extremities).
7 *Tumours of the third ventricle.*
  Symptoms arise from increasing intracranial pressure.

Diagnosis

Objective

To determine the precise location of the tumour.

1 X-ray of skull—to demonstrate intracranial calcification, displacement of calcified pineal gland, signs of increased intracranial pressure, bone destruction.
2 X-ray of chest—metastatic brain tumours are associated with many primary or metastatic lung tumours.
3 Brain scan—abnormal amount of radioactive material will be present in area of tumour and can be localized with scintillation counter.
4 Computed tomography—gives information concerning number, size, density of lesion(s) and extent of secondary cerebral oedema; provides information about ventricular system.
5 Neurological examination—to determine area(s) of involvement.
6 Audiometry or vestibular function studies—performed when acoustic neuroma is suspected.

Treatment

Objectives

To remove the tumour and cure the patient (if possible).
To achieve palliation by partial tumour removal and by decompression, radiation or chemotherapy or combinations of these.

Problems Affecting Treatment

1 Effectiveness of treatment depends on type and site of tumour; many tumours are in vital or inaccessible areas (brain stem tumours); even biopsies in such locations can produce unacceptable disabilities.
2 Nonencapsulated and infiltrating tumours make complete removal almost impossible; resulting neurologic defects (blindness, paralysis) would be too severe.
3 Cures may be obtained in certain tumours (meningiomas, acoustic neuromas, pituitary adenomas, dermoids, astrocytomas) if they are treated early.

Principles of Treatment

1 Brain tumours require different therapeutic approaches depending on cell type and location and on age and condition of the patient. Each patient (and his lesion) is evaluated individually and the therapeutic programme designed accordingly.
2 Treatment usually involves a multidisciplinary approach including surgery, radiation and chemotherapy.

3   Surgical approaches include total tumour excision, decompression, cerebrospinal fluid-vascular shunt. (See p. 23 for nursing management of patient undergoing intracranial surgery.)
4   Support the patient undergoing radiation.
    a. Give steroids (dexamethasone) as directed—to reduce cerebral oedema associated with brain tumours.
    b. Steroids may be introduced prior to therapy and withdrawn gradually as soon as definitive local treatment (surgery/radiation) has demonstrated clinical results.
    c. Local radiation to tumour is usually carried out, except in cases of medulla-blastoma, when total CNS radiation is carried out.
    d. Observe for headache, nausea and vomiting occurring during course of radiation therapy.
    e. Loss of hair may be expected; regrowth may be expected after several weeks.
    f. See Nursing Management of Patient Undergoing Radiation Therapy.
5   Encourage the patient undergoing chemotherapy.
    a. Chemotherapeutic drugs may be given singly or in combination (BCNU, vincristine, mithramycin, methotrexate, etc.).
    b. Dosages of chemotherapeutic drugs may be limited by their toxicity.
    c. Assess patient for signs and symptoms of drug toxicity; bone marrow depression, liver function abnormality, etc.
    d. See Nursing Management of Patient Undergoing Chemotherapy (Volume 1, Chapter 7).
    e. See Nursing Management of Patient With Cancer (Volume 1, Chapter 7).
6   Management of patient with brain metastases from systemic cancer (lung, breast, malignant melanoma, leukaemia).
    a. Patients with systemic tumours may function well until tumour metastasizes to nervous system and rapidly produces frightening and disabling symptoms (motor loss, cranial neuropathies, intellectual impairment, convulsive seizures).
    b. Metastases to brain are commonly multiple and often unresectable.
    c. Therapeutic approach includes surgery, radiation and chemotherapy; palliation more effective if treatment is started before major neurological deficits develop.
    d. See Nursing Management of Patient with Cancer (Volume 1, Chapter 7).

THE EPILEPSIES

The epilepsies are paroxysmal transient disturbances of brain function that may be manifested as episodic impairment or loss of consciousness that may or may not be associated with convulsions, sensory phenomena, erratic behaviour or a combination of all of these.

The basic problem is thought to be due to an electrical disturbance in the nerve cells in one section of the brain that causes them to give off abnormal, recurrent, uncontrolled electrical discharges.

Causes

The underlying disorder of the brain may be structural, chemical or physiological or a combination of all three.

1   Head/brain injury.

2 Congenital anomalies; inherited metabolic errors.
3 Infectious disorders (meningitis, encephalitis).
4 Vascular disturbances.
5 Metabolic or nutritional disturbances.
6 Brain tumour.
7 Degenerative disorders.
8 Genetic disorders.
9 Idiopathic (cause unknown).

Clinical Manifestations

1 Loss of consciousness.
2 Disturbances of the mind.
3 Excess or loss of muscle tone or movement.
4 Disorders of sensation or special senses.
5 Disturbances of the autonomic functions of the body.

Diagnosis

1 History of seizures (as noted by patient and observers).
2 Electroencephalograph (EEG)—finds and measures brain electrical discharge pattern; useful in locating the site where epileptic discharge begins, its spread, intensity, duration; helps classify seizure type.

International Classification of Epileptic Seizures*

Partial Seizures (seizures beginning locally)

1 Partial seizures with elementary symptomatology (generally without impairment of consciousness).
   a. With motor symptoms (includes Jacksonian seizures).
   b. With special sensory or somatosensory symptoms.
   c. With autonomic symptoms.
   d. Compound forms.
2 Partial seizures with complex symptomatology (generally with impairment of consciousness).
   (*temporal lobe or psychomotor seizures*)
   a. With impairment of consciousness only.
   b. With cognitive symptomatology.
   c. With affective symptomatology.
   d. With 'psychosensory' symptomatology.
   e. With 'psychomotor' symptomatology (automatisms).
   f. Compound forms.

Generalized Seizures (bilaterally symmetrical and without local onset)

1 Absences (*petit mal*).
2 Bilateral massive epileptic myoclonus.
3 Infantile spasms.

* Abstracted from: Gastaut, H (1970) Clinical and electroencephalographical classification of epileptic seizures, Epilepsia, 11: 102–113

4   Clonic seizures.
5   Tonic seizures.
6   Tonic–clonic seizures (*grand mal*).
7   Atonic seizures.
8   Akinetic seizures.

Unilateral Seizures (or predominantly unilateral)

Unclassified Epileptic Seizures (due to incomplete data).

Treatment and Nursing Management (see nursing management of patient having a convulsion, p. 22)

Objectives

To determine and treat (if possible) the primary underlying cause of the seizures.
To prevent a recurrence of seizures and therefore allow the patient to live a normal life.
To gain an understanding of the patient and his relationship to his environment.

1   Emphasize the importance of *regularity* in taking the prescribed antiepileptic medication to reduce number and/or severity of seizures.
    a. Objective of drug therapy: to suppress seizure activity with minimum dosage of medication and without side-effects.
    b. Drug therapy is regarded as a form of control; not a cure.
      (1) The choice of drug(s) is determined by the type of seizure.
      (2) The dosage is adjusted according to patient's clinical response and plasma drug concentration.
      (3) See Table 1.2 for list of drugs in current use.
    c. Treatment is usually started with one drug; the dose is increased slowly until seizures are controlled or toxic symptoms develop. A second (or rarely a third) drug is added in the same manner if one drug fails to give control.
    d. Serum plasma concentration of antiepileptic drug is measured to serve as a guide to drug therapy; helps to individualize drug regimen and to detect patient noncompliance.
      (1) Gas–liquid chromatography is the laboratory technique used for measuring antiepileptic drug blood levels.
      (2) Helpful in monitoring drug levels of growing children.

Nursing Alert: The patient should not stop taking his antiepileptic medication without medical supervision since sudden withdrawal can cause an increase in seizure frequency or precipitate the development of status epilepticus.

    e. Patient should watch for toxic effects of antiepileptic medication—drowsiness, gingival hyperplasia, nervousness, visual difficulties, motor inco-ordination, staggering, ataxia, bone marrow depression leading to blood dyscrasias.
      (1) Advise patient to avoid taking medication on an empty stomach; gastritis is apt to occur, especially with phenytoin (Epanutin).
      (2) Instruct patient to brush teeth frequently and massage gums to prevent gingival infection.
2   See nursing management of patient with convulsive seizures, p. 22.
3   Neurosurgical management of the epilepsies.

Table 1.2. Primary Antiepileptic Drugs

Chemical Class	Indications	Drugs		Company
		Generic Name	Trade Name	
Hydantoins	Generalized convulsive seizures; all forms of partial seizures	Phenytoin Mephenytoin Ethotoin	Dilantin Mesantoin Peganone	Parke-Davis Sandoz Abbott
Barbiturates	Generalized convulsive seizures; all forms of partial seizures	Phenobarbitone Primidone	Luminal Mysoline	Winthrop I.C.I.
Oxazolidinediones	Generalized non-convulsive seizures (absences)	Troxidone Paramethadione	Tridione Paradione	Abbott Abbott
Succinimides	Generalized non-convulsive seizures (absences)	Ethosuximide	Zarontin	Parke-Davis
Dibenzoazepine	Partial seizures with complex symptomatology; generalized convulsive seizures	Carbamazepine	Tegretol	Geigy
Benzodiazepines	Generalized non-convulsive seizures Generalized convulsive seizures; all forms of partial seizures	Diazepam Clonazepam Sodium valproate	Valium Rivofril Epilim	Roche Roche Reckitt-Labaz

Surgical procedures performed when attacks are frontal in origin, in an area that can be excised without producing unacceptable neurological deficits (or increasing deficits already present) and when treatment with drugs is ineffective.

(1) Cortical resection—excision of affected area of cortex (based on cortical EEG findings, preoperative studies and pattern of seizures).

(a) Temporal lobectomy (temporal lobe most frequently involved).

(b) Excision of epileptogenic foci in other lobe carried out less frequently.

(c) Postoperative care is similar to that of other neurosurgical patients (see p. 23); in addition, patient is continued on antiepileptic drug until time proves that seizure tendency has been removed.

(d) Postoperative rehabilitation will be required to help patient attain psychosocial independence and a meaningful life-style.

(2) Stereotactic procedures—technique of placing a discrete lesion in a particular brain site to destroy epileptogenic foci.

Discharge Planning and Health Teaching

1   Encourage the patient to study himself and his environment to determine what specific factors precipitate his seizures—illness, emotional stress, physical stress, hyperventilation, altered sleep patterns, photosensitivity or other sensory stimuli, etc.

2 The medication must be taken daily to prevent seizures; medication may have to be adjusted due to recurrent illness, weight gain, increase in stress, etc.
3 Practice *regularity* and *moderation* in daily activities; diet, exercise, rest, avoidance of certain stimulating stresses.
   a. Have regular hours for sleep.
   b. Avoid emotional overstimulation (watching late TV, etc.).
   c. Avoid alcohol when seizures are known to follow alcoholic intake.
   d. Seek help (if necessary) during periods of crisis—death in family, divorce, etc.).
4 Report any changes in health status—easy bruising, purpura, bleeding gums, jaundice, fever, recurrent infections or dermatosis.
5 Have follow-up urinalysis and blood studies.
6 Stress the importance of activity, both physical and mental. Activity tends to inhibit, not stimulate, epileptic seizures.
7 Reorient the attitude of patient and family to the disease.
   a. Help the family to understand that the patient has experienced rejection, anxiety (due to unpredictable seizure activity), feelings of being 'different'.
   b. Encourage patient or family to discuss feelings and attitudes about epilepsy.
   c. Epilepsy can be *controlled*; it is not insanity or a supernatural condition.
8 Have a wallet card and wear a medical-alert bracelet indicating that the wearer has epilepsy.
9 Learn of the services and publications of:

> British Epilepsy Association
> 3–6 Alfred Place
> London WC1E 7ED.

Status Epilepticus

Status epilepticus (acute prolonged repetitive seizure activity) is a series of generalized convulsions without return to consciousness between attacks.

Underlying Considerations

1 Status epilepticus is considered a serious medical emergency. It has a high mortality and morbidity rate (subsequent mental retardation or neurological defects).
2 Common factors that precipitate status epilepticus include withdrawal of anti-epileptic medication, fever and intercurrent infection.
3 Convulsive status epilepticus may be brought on by other conditions (cerebrovascular disease, head trauma, anoxic factors, metabolic abnormalities).

Medical and Nursing Treatment

Objectives

To stop the seizures as quickly as possible.
To ensure adequate cerebral oxygenation.
To maintain the patient in a seizure-free state.

1   Maintain an adequate airway.
2   Adequate oxygenation should be ensured—there is some respiratory arrest at height of each seizure which produces venous congestion and hypoxia of the brain.
3   Antiepileptic drugs may be given by continuous intravenous infusion.

NOTE: Epanutin (phenytoin) must never be given via intravenous infusion as it precipitates in all solutions. It must be given directly into a vein.

4   It may be necessary to paralyse and ventilate patients in status epilepticus.
5   Monitor vital and neurological signs at regular periods.
6   Assist with electroencephalographic monitoring—this may have to be done in the patient's room with a portable machine.

PARKINSON'S DISEASE

Parkinson's disease is a progressive neurological disorder affecting the brain centres responsible for control of movement. It is characterized by bradykinesia (slowness of movement), tremor and muscle stiffness or rigidity.

Pathophysiology

The major lesion appears to be loss of melanin pigment and degeneration of neurones in the substantia nigra of the brain.

Aetiology

1   Unknown.
2   Viruses, encephalitis, cerebrovascular disease and certain metallic poisons have been suspected.
3   Theory advanced that there is an imbalance of two neurochemical systems, cholinergic and dopaminergic, and that the symptoms of parkinsonism are caused by overactivity or underactivity of one or the other of these systems.
4   Genetic susceptibility (positive family history).

Clinical Manifestations

1   Bradykinesia (dyskinesia, hypokinesia)—usually becomes the most disabling symptom.
2   Tremor—tends to decrease or disappear on purposeful movement.
3   Rigidity, particularly of large joints.
4   Muscle weakness—affecting eating, chewing, swallowing, speaking, writing.
5   Mask-like facial expression; unblinking eyes.
6   Depression.
7   Dementia.

Treatment and Nursing Management

Treatment is based on a combination of drug therapy, physical therapy and rehabilitation techniques, and patient and family education.

Objective

To keep the patient functionally useful and productive as long as possible.

Drug Therapy

1 *Levodopa (L-Dopa) Therapy*
   a. Levodopa (an amino acid which is depleted in the substance of the brain involved in nerve transmission in patients with Parkinsonism) is given in increasing doses until patient's tolerance is reached; it relieves rigidity in majority of patients and usually improves tremor.
   b. Levodopa must be given in large enough doses and for a long enough time to build up an effective and stable blood level.
   c. Dosage is increased gradually until maximum therapeutic effect is achieved and side-effects appear—nausea, vomiting, anorexia, postural hypotension, mental changes (confusion, agitation, mood alterations), cardiac arrhythmias, twitching.
   d. Give levodopa after meals.
   e. Beneficial effects most pronounced in first few years of treatment; adverse effects may increase with continued use.
      (1) Abnormal involuntary movements—typically choreoathetoid in nature, affecting face and mouth initially, and then involving body and extremities.
      (2) On–off phenomena—sudden episodes of immobility.
   f. Levodopa is not a cure for Parkinsonism but is effective in controlling patient's symptoms, particularly bradykinesia and rigidity.
2 *Levodopa in combination with carbidopa:* Carbidopa (a selective dopa decarboxylase inhibitor) reduces the peripheral metabolism of dopa; administration of carbidopa with levodopa makes more levodopa available for transport to the brain.
      Sinemet (combination of carbidopa and levodopa)—potentiates therapeutic effects of levodopa; appears to achieve a therapeutic effect with much lower dose of levodopa and thus reduces incidence of side-effects.
      Madopar—a combination of levodopa and beseride.
3 *Anticholinergic agents*—counteract the action of acetylcholine in the central nervous system.
   a. Anticholinergics are given for patients with mild disability, who have poor response or sensitivity to levodopa; or they may be used in combination with levodopa.
   b. Frequently used anticholinergics include:
      (1) Benhexol hydrochloride (Artane).
      (2) Orphenadrine hydrochloride (Disipal).
      (3) Procyclidine hydrochloride (Kenadrin).
      (4) Benztropine (Cogentin).
   c. Assess for side-effects of anticholinergic agents—dryness of mouth, blurred vision, urinary retention, constipation, mental confusion.
4 *Antihistaminic compounds*—may be effective for tremor.
5 *Antidepressants*—may be given to reduce depression which frequently accompanies Parkinsonism and the drug therapy.
6 *Tranquillizers*—may be given for nervousness and irritability.

Physiotherapy (supervised by physiotherapist)

1   Encourage patient to continue on an exercise and physiotherapy programme to increase muscle strength, improve co-ordination and dexterity, treat muscular rigidity and prevent contractures.
2   Emphasize the importance of a *daily* exercise programme (walk, ride stationary bike, swim, garden)—to maintain joint mobility.
     Instruct patient to:
     a. Exercise each joint daily.
     b. Lengthen stride when walking; swing arms while walking—loosens arms and shoulders and lessens fatigue.
     c. Practice breathing exercises—to mobilize rib cage.
3   Advise patient to do stretching exercises (stretch–hold–relax) to loosen the joint structures.
4   Encourage patient to take warm baths, massage and passive and active exercises—to help relax muscles and relieve painful muscle spasms that accompany rigidity.
5   Advise patient to have frequent rest periods—patient becomes fatigued and frustrated by his symptoms.
6   Try to have patient seen by a physiotherapist on a regular basis—reinforces his programme, introduces new programme of exercises.

Psychological Support

1   Help patient establish achievable goals (improvement of health and mobility, lessening of tremors).
2   Encourage patient to be an *active* participant in his therapy and in social and recreational events—Parkinsonism tends to lead to depression and withdrawal.
3   Have a planned programme of activity throughout day—prevents daytime sleeping, disinterest and apathy.
4   Re-emphasize that disability can be prevented or delayed; offer realistic reassurance.
5   Try to dispel anxiety and fears of patient that may be as disabling to him as his disease.

Surgical Intervention

1   Thalamotomy—stereotaxic placement of a lesion in the small area of the brain where the tremors originate; area is inactivated by heat, freezing or other methods—relieves contra-lateral tremor and rigidity of extremity.
2   Does not alter course of progressive Parkinson's disease, but can help some patients with the unilateral syndrome (tremor and rigidity on one side of body).
3   See p. 23 for the nursing management of the patient undergoing intracranial surgery.

Health Teaching

1   See drug therapy, physiotherapy and psychological support given above.
2   Avoid a high protein diet when taking levodopa since a high protein meal can block the effects of levodopa in some patients.
3   Try the following routine when feet and legs seem to the 'glued' to the floor.

a. Raise head.
b. Raise toes (eliminates muscle spasm).
c. Rock from side to side while bending knees slightly.
d. Or raise arms in a sudden, short motion.
4 Attempt to get out of a chair quickly, placing feet well apart, to overcome pull of gravity.

MULTIPLE SCLEROSIS

Multiple sclerosis is a chronic, progressive disease of the central nervous system characterized by a patchy loss of myelin (fatty sheath) in the brain and spinal cord. There are numerous hypotheses concerning the aetiology of MS; namely, infection by a slow virus, autoimmune process, epidemiologic factors, etc.

Clinical Manifestations

The signs and symptoms reflect the location and areas of demyelinization within the central nervous system. Patients with MS have a wide range of clinical symptoms; there is great variability in the course of the disease, with many remissions and exacerbations.

1 Weakness and sensory disturbances.
2 Abnormal reflexes, either absent or hyper.
3 Visual disturbances; impaired vision, diplopia.
4 Tremor, ataxia, inco-ordination.
5 Paresthesias.
6 Sphincter impairment.
7 Impaired vibration and position sense.
8 Emotional lability; euphoria, depression.

Incidence

Multiple sclerosis is one of the commonest neurological diseases and primarily affects young adults (20–40 years of age). It occurs in temperate climates, particularly in the northern hemisphere and is rare in the tropics. However, a number of these patients have little or no disability for many years after diagnosis.

Objectives of Treatment and Nursing Management

Objectives

To keep the patient as active and functional as possible in order to lead a purposeful life.
To relieve the patient's symptoms and provide him with continuing support.

To Strengthen Muscles and to Prevent and Treat Muscle Spasticity

Spasticity interferes with normal function

1 Patient should do muscle stretching exercises daily—to minimize joint contractures. The opinions of neurologists differ as to the extent and value of physiotherapy to prevent muscle spasticity.

2   Drugs: muscle relaxants (diazepam); antispasmodic agents (lioresal).
3   Advise patient to avoid muscle fatigue.
4   Utilize braces, crutches, Zimmer frames to keep patient ambulant for as long as possible.

To Avoid Skin Pressure and Immobility

Since there is usually sensory loss, pressure sores accompany severe spasticity in an immobile patient.

1   Relieve pressure.
   a. Change position at least every 2 hours if patient is in bed.
   b. Change position every 30 min if in wheelchair.
   c. Use flotation pad, sheepskin, ripple mattress and other aids to distribute pressure away from bony points and over a wider area.
   d. Teach patient to inspect pressure areas (using a long-handled mirror for posterior sites) for evidences of redness and heat.
2   Avoid skin trauma, heat, cold and pressure.
3   Give careful attention to sacral and perineal hygiene.
4   See p. 73 for discussion of prevention and treatment of pressure sores.

To Assist patient to Overcome Effects of Inco-ordination (caused by motor dysfunction)

1   Teach patient to walk with feet wider apart—to widen his base of support and increase his walking stability.
2   Have patient use a stick or Zimmer frame.
3   Utilize wrist cuffs, eating utensils—to help overcome inco-ordination of upper extremities.

To Support the Patient With Bladder Disturbances

Bladder dysfunction may lead to progressive renal failure.

1   See Management of Patient with a Neurogenic Bladder.
2   Assess for urinary retention.
   a. Catheterize patient; insert indwelling catheter only if absolutely necessary.
   b. Give urinary antiseptics—to reduce incidence of infection.
3   Ensure adequate fluid intake (3–5 l daily)—to reduce urinary bacterial count, minimize precipitation of urinary crystals and stone formation and encrustation of the lumen of the indwelling urethral catheter.
4   Support the patient who has urinary incontinence (or frequency and urgency).
   Female patient
   a. Set up a micturition time schedule; every $1\frac{1}{2}$–2 hours initially with lengthening time intervals if regimen is successful.
   b. Encourage the patient to drink a measured amount of fluid every 2 hours.
   c. Have the patient try to micturate 30 min after drinking.
   d. Use slipper bedpan at night; set alarm clock for patient with diminished warning sensation.
   e. For permanent urinary incontinence, urine may have to be diverted by means of ileal conduit.

Male patient
a. See a, b and c, under female patient, above.
b. Use urinal at night.
c. For permanent incontinence, patient may wear external sheath or condom appliance for urine collection.

To Place the Patient on a Bowel Programme if He Has Bowel Incontinence

1 Establish a programme of *regularity*.
   a. Have patient eat regularly scheduled meals.
   b. Establish bowel evacuation at *same time each day*.
2 Insert a glycerine suppository into the rectum 30 min before scheduled bowel evacuation time—*after* eating a meal (preferably after breakfast).
3 Advise patient to attempt to have a bowel movement within 30 min of eating, using as normal a position for defaecation as possible.
   a. Instruct patient to bear down and contract abdominal muscles.
   b. Teach patient to apply pressure to abdomen with hands—to assist with defaecation.
4 After this routine is established, mechanical stimulation with the suppository may not be necessary.

To Treat the Patient With Appropriate Therapy During Periods of Exacerbation

The residual effects of the disease may increase with each exacerbation. Neurologists differ in their approach to treatment during periods of exacerbation—some of the following may be used.

1 ACTH may be given for short periods during acute exacerbations—may reduce severity of episode.
2 Encourage bed rest for a few days during acute exacerbation—continued activity appears to worsen attack.
3 Try to have patient avoid any known factor that causes exacerbation—allergy, infection, cold, etc.
4 Aim to prevent permanent damage; continue with range of motion exercises, specific muscle exercises, etc., as physical strength permits.
5 Take corrective action for each new problem as it rises.
6 Invent, adapt and modify equipment that can be used for self-help devices so that patient will not lose ground.

To Help Patient with Optic and Speech Defects

Cranial nerves affecting sight and speech are affected by multiple sclerosis.

1 Utilize eye patch, frosted lens—to block visual impulses of one eye when patient has diplopia (double vision).
2 Secure services of speech therapist—to strength the muscles of speech.
3 Prism glasses may be useful for bedridden person.
4 For person who has impaired eyesight or who is unable to hold book, turn pages, or read regular print, secure books and magazines recorded on discs, tape cassettes, page turning machines, usually provided by the occupational therapy department.

To Train Patients in Activities of Daily Living and To Keep Patient as Independent as Possible

1 Physiotherapist will teach transfer activities and these should be reinforced by nursing staff.
2 Selection of correct sized wheelchair.
3 Use assistive and self-help devices.
   a. Toilet facilities—raised toilet seat or bedside commode.
   b. Bathing facilities—use stool in shower or bath and hand rails.
   c. Self-care aids—prism glasses, telephone modications, long-handled combs, tongs, modified clothing.

Discharge Planning and Health Teaching

1 Review objectives of treatment and nursing management given above.
2 Help the family (and patient) understand the stresses imposed by multiple sclerosis.
   a. There are embarrassing and humiliating symptoms to which the person may respond 'inappropriately'.
   b. Patient may have brain damage with resultant denial of his disease, euphoria or depressive and paranoid behaviour.
   c. MS patients are often forgetful and easily distracted.
3 Understand that patients adapt to illness in many ways—denial, depression, withdrawal, inactivity, resentment, etc.
4 Patient may have feelings of alienation from family, others, work and social life; he feels that his personal worth is lessened.
   a. Try to keep him in the mainstream of life as much as possible.
   b. Contact local branch of Multiple Sclerosis Society, 286 Munster Road, London SW6 6AP, for services, publications and contact with other MS patients.
   c. Encourage patient to keep up social interests and activities.
5 Try to keep up the activities (physical, social, etc.) that patient is able to do; once lost, certain abilities are almost impossible to regain.
   a. Physical abilities may vary from day to day.
   b. Devise modifications that will allow continuance of certain activities; obtain gadgets and adaptive devices for self-help (mail-order gift companies, medical supply catalogues, rehabilitation literature).
6 Try to avoid physical and emotional stresses—may worsen symptoms and impair performance.
7 Assist the patient to accept his new identity as a handicapped person and cope with the disruption in his life.
8 Keep channels of communication open.
9 Offer meaningful and realistic short-term goals—to achieve a sense of purpose.
10 Patient should try to avoid hot weather or hot baths as this often makes disabilities worse.

MYASTHENIA GRAVIS

Myasthenia gravis is a disorder of neuromuscular transmission in the voluntary muscles of the body characterized by excessive fatigability of muscle function.

Altered Physiology

Defect in transmission of impulses from nerve to muscle cells which may be due to inadequate synthesis or release of acetylcholine at the neuromuscular junction.

Clinical Manifestations

1   Diplopia (double vision), ptosis (drooping of one or both eyelids)—from involvement of ocular muscles.
2   Sleepy, mask-like expression—from involvement of facial muscles.
3   Speech weakness, choking, aspiration of food—from weakness of laryngeal and pharyngeal muscles.
4   Muscle weakness characteristically worse after effort and improved by rest; may involve any striated muscle.

Diagnosis

1   Pharmacological test:
    a. Endrophonium (Tensilon) test—intravenous injection of endrophonium may relieve weakness markedly in 30 s; useful for patients with ocular, facial or oropharygeal weakness.
    b. Neostigmine methysulfate (Prostigmin) test—given to evaluate extremity strength; positive result evidenced by increase in muscular strength about 30 min after injection; permits measurement of changes in strength of all muscles.
2   Electromyographic testing (EMG) to check muscle fatigability.
3   Chest x-ray—to rule out thymoma (tumour of the thymus).

Treatment and Nursing Management

Objective

To increase muscle strength.

Primary Drug Therapy

1   Anticholinesterase drugs—will increase response of muscles to nerve impulses and improve strength; by temporarily inhibiting acetylcholinesterase at the neuromuscular junction, they enhance the action of acetylcholine there.
    a. Neostigmine bromide (Prostigmin).
    b. Neostigmine methylsulphate (Prostigmin) (injectable).
    c. Pyridostigmine bromide (Mestinon).
2   Drug given exactly on time to control symptoms; a delay in drug administration may result in patient's losing his ability to swallow.
3   Toxicity and side-effects of anticholinesterase:
    a. Gastrointestinal—abdominal cramps, nausea, vomiting, diarrhoea.
        (1) Drug may be taken with small amount of milk, crackers or other buffering substance or after meals.
        (2) Side-effects may be ameliorated or prevented by addition of atropine or atropine-like drugs to regimen.
        (3) Give diphenoxylate hydrochloride (Lomotil) for diarrhoea.
    b. Skeletal—fasciculations (fine twitching), spasm, weakness.

    c. Central nervous system—irritability, anxiety, insomnia, headache, dysarthria, syncope, coma, convulsions.

    d. Other—increased salivation and lacrimation, increased bronchial secretions, moist skin.

Nursing Alert: Watch for increase in muscle weakness within 1 hour after taking anticholinesterase drug; be alert for signs of respiratory embarrassment.

4   After medication adjustment has been made, patient learns to take his medication when necessary. Individual doses may vary with physical or emotional stress, intercurrent infection, etc.

5   Timespan Mestinon may be taken at bedtime for its prolonged effect.

6   Sedatives and tranquillizing drugs are given with caution; may aggravate hypoxia and hypercapnia and cause respiratory and cardiac depression.

7   Anticholinesterase drugs are not to be taken with morphine, ether, quinine (commercial cold preparations), procainamide and certain antibiotics.

8   Corticosteroid therapy may be of benefit to patient with severe, generalized myasthenia; patient may exhibit a marked further decrease in strength during course of ACTH therapy, but will generally develop a remission.

Surgical Intervention (Thymectomy)

May give improvement or remission of the disease, especially in patients with follicular hyperplasia of the thymus gland who are under 40 and have had myasthenia for less than 5 years.

1   May be carried out by transcervical or sternal-splitting procedure.

2   Preoperative evaluation includes assessment of respiratory status (tidal volume, vital capacity), muscular strength and patient's chewing, swallowing and ocular movements.

3   Postoperative nursing management (in intensive care unit) includes:

    a. Monitoring and caring for patient on mechanical ventilator, if needed.

    b. Continuing assessment of ventilatory function.

    c. Temporary cessation of anticholinesterase medications.

Crises in Myasthenia Gravis

Sudden exacerbation of weakness that may endanger life.

1   Sudden respiratory distress combined with varying signs of dysphagia (difficulty in swallowing), dysarthria (difficulty in speaking), eyelid ptosis and diplopia are indications of impending crisis.

2   Types of crises in myasthenia gravis.

    a. Myasthenic crisis—may result from natural deterioration of disease, emotional upset, upper respiratory infection, surgery or trauma; or may be brought about by ACTH therapy.

    Patient may be temporarily resistant to anticholinesterase drugs or may need increased dosage.

    b. Cholinergic crisis—from overmedication with anticholinergic drugs.

    c. Brittle crisis—occurs with an unpredictable response to drugs and is not controlled by increasing or decreasing anticholinesterase therapy.

3   Nursing and medical management during crisis.

a. Place patient in intensive care unit for constant monitoring—myasthenia gravis is a disease of rapidly fluctuating intensity and patient is on verge of respiratory arrest.

b. Provide ventilatory assistance when muscles of respiration and swallowing become involved.

(1) Suction patient as indicated—*aspiration is a common problem.*

(2) Prepare patient for tracheostomy.

(3) Appropriate antibiotic therapy will be prescribed if respiratory infection is a contributing factor.

c. Determine the time of onset of symptoms in relation to the last dose of anticholinesterase—may show whether patient is undermedicated or having a cholinergic reaction.

Tensilon may be given to differentiate type of crisis; Tensilon (intravenous) improves patient in myasthenic crisis, temporarily worsens patient in cholinergic crisis and is unpredictable in brittle crisis.

d. Appropriate drugs as determined by patient's status:

(1) For myasthenic crisis: Neostigmin methylsulphate (Prostigmin) administered parenterally if patient is in true myasthenic crisis.

(2) For cholinergic crisis: Atropine may be given to reduce excessive secretions; all anticholinesterase drugs are withdrawn.

e. Administer fluids, medication and food via nasogastric tube if patient is unable to swallow.

f. Avoid giving enemas—may cause sudden collapse.

g. Develop a communication system for patient on ventilator (or if he is too weak to speak).

(1) Try to read lips of patient.

(2) Use picture cards, hand signals, etc.

(3) Give hand bell to patient.

h. Give continuing psychological support since patient is usually alert and anxious. Reassure him that the crisis will pass and that he will not be left alone.

Health Teaching

Instruct the patient as follows:

1 Know the basic facts about anticholinergic drugs: action, reason for and importance of timing, dosage adjustment, symptoms of overdose and toxic effects. Know the drugs that interact with anticholinesterase drugs.

2 Try to prevent factors (emotional upset, infections) which may increase weakness and precipitate myasthenic crisis.

3 Wear an identification bracelet signifying that you have myasthenia gravis.

4 Have mealtimes coincide with peak of anticholinesterase effect (when swallowing ability is best); have standby suction available in home if swallowing difficulties occur. (Use a blender when necessary.)

5 Wear an eyepatch over one eye (alternating from side to side) if diplopia occurs.

6 Avoid vigorous physical activity and other factors leading to fatigue.

7 Avoid contracting colds and influenza—respiratory infections are extremely dangerous to the myasthenic individual.

8   Avoid excessive heat and cold (lying in sun for long period); weak spells may follow long exposure to excessive heat/cold.
9   Advise the dentist that you are myasthenic since Novocain is usually not well tolerated.
10   Rest when fatigue sets in; do not force yourself to continue with an activity.

ACUTE INFECTIOUS POLYNEURITIS
(LANDRY–GUILLAIN–BARRE SYNDROME)

Acute infectious polyneuritis is a clinical syndrome of unknown cause involving the nervous system and characterized by paresthesias of the extremities and by muscle weakness or paralysis. It may be due to an allergic or immunological reaction and is frequently preceded by an infection.

Clinical Manifestations

1   Muscle weakness of legs—may progress to rapidly ascending paralysis involving the trunk, upper extremities and facial muscles (complete paralysis).
2   Paresthesia (tingling and numbness) of lower extremities.
3   Difficulty in chewing, swallowing and talking—from cranial nerve involvement.
4   Absence of deep tendon reflexes.

Treatment and Nursing Management

Objective

To support respiration when rapidly ascending paralysis develops.

1   Monitor vital capacity since respiratory failure is a common cause of death.
    a. Watch for breathlessness while talking, shallow and irregular breathing, increasing pulse rate and *change* in the respiratory pattern.
    b. Patient may need to be placed on a mechanical ventilator when respiratory insufficiency occurs.
    c. The heart may need to be monitored for arrhythmias.
2   Feed patient via nasogastric tube if he is unable to swallow.
3   Watch for urinary retention—thought to be due to involvement of autonomic fibres passing through the sacral nerve roots.
4   Give corticosteroids and/or immunosuppressive therapy according to therapeutic plan; may be of value if given early in course of disease; relapse may occur after corticosteroids are withdrawn.
5   Put extremities through range of motion; use nursing support to prevent contractures, pressure sores. (See Rehabilitation Nursing, Volume 1, Chapter 2.)

Health Teaching

There may be a rather lengthy convalescence; patients usually recover in 3–6 months; a few have sequelae up to several years. Some patients remain severely disabled.

FRACTURES AND DISLOCATIONS OF THE SPINE

Underlying Considerations

1 Fractures of the spine are serious because of danger of injury to the spinal cord.
2 Fractures appear most frequently in fifth, sixth and seventh cervical vertebrae, the twelfth thoracic and the first lumbar vertebrae—there is a greater range of mobility of the vertebral column in these areas.
3 Spinal cord injury may follow an injury without vertebral interruption (e.g., hyperflexion neck injury).

Causes

1 Trauma—automobile and motorcycle accidents, falls, diving and surfing injuries, trampoline injuries—may cause compression, contusion or laceration of the cord, haemorrhage into its substance, or compression of its vascular supply.
2 Infections or inflammatory arthritis—producing spontaneous dislocations of cervical spine.
3 Prior laminectomy.

Clinical Manifestations

1 Severe pain in back, especially on movement.
2 Tenderness directly over localized area of injury.

Nursing Alert: Injury to the spinal cord may produce paralysis of the body below the level of the lesion.

Treatment and Nursing Management

Objectives

To reduce the fracture and obtain immobilization of the spine as soon as possible to prevent cord damage.
To observe for symptoms of progressive neurological damage.

1 See Moving the Patient From the Scene of the Accident on a Transfer Board (Volume 1, Chapter 5).
2 Maintain the airway and ventilate the patient.
   a. Respiratory problems are frequently seen in quadriplegic patient.
   b. Patients with cervical spinal cord injuries may have paralysis of intercostal and abdominal muscles.
   c. Assess strength of cough.
   d. Measure vital capacity.
3 Evaluate the patient constantly for motor and sensory changes—motor and sensory loss occurs from cord oedema, transection of cord.
   a. Direct the patient to move his toes or turn his feet.
   b. Pinch the skin, starting at shoulder level and progressing down the sides of both extremities.
      (1) Ascertain when patient feels pinching sensation.
      (2) Record findings—for subsequent comparison.
      (3) Note presence or absence of a level of sweating.

      (4) Note that any evidence of neurological deterioration raises suspicion of cord oedema or postoperative haematoma (in operative patients)—indicates need for immediate surgical intervention.

4   Transfer the patient to a Stryker frame. (If none is available, place on a firm mattress with a bedboard under the mattress.)

      a. Keep patient in an extended position—do not allow body to be twisted or turned.

      b. Place patient (who is strapped to a transfer board) directly on the posterior frame of a Stryker frame.

      c. Place a blanket roll between the patient's legs.

      d. Place anterior frame in position. Secure frame straps.

      e. Turn the patient to the prone position.

      f. Remove frame straps, head bandage and posterior frame. Remove transfer board.

5   *For patient with fracture or injury of cervical vertebrae:*

      a. To manage a cervical spine injury there must be immediate immobilization, early reduction and stabilization.

      b. Immobility of vertebral column may be obtained by plaster cast, cervical collar, traction or skeletal traction with skull tongs (Crutchfield, Gardner–Wells) or halo skeletal fixation.

      c. Use of Crutchfield tongs—achieves both reduction and immobilization of fracture or dislocation.

Objective: To obtain a steady pull along the long axis of the cervical spine while the head is in a neutral position.

      (1) Tongs inserted in outer table of the cranium; under local anaesthesia.

      (2) Initially 4.5–9 kg (10–20 lb or more) of traction is applied, depending on patient's size and the degree of displacement.

      (3) The traction is gradually increased by addition of weights—as the amount of traction is increased, the spaces between the intervertebral discs widen and the vertebrae slip back into position. Reduction will take place after correct alignment has been regained.

      (4) X-rays are made every few hours until the fracture is reduced.

      (5) When reduction is obtained the weights are gradually removed and x-rays are taken again to verify reduction.

      (6) Elevate head of bed (if patient is on regular bed)—patient's body serves as a counterweight to that applied by traction weight.

        (a) Keep traction tongs several inches from top of bed and allow weights to hang free—to prevent interference with traction.

        (b) Give tranquillizers for apprehension and restlessness.

      (7) Watch for signs of infection, including drainage from stab wounds.

      (8) Check back of head periodically for signs of pressure; massage back of head periodically.

      (9) Give back care by pressing down on the mattress with one hand and washing and massaging with the other.

      (10) If possible, turn patient on his side while he is being fed to minimize possibility of aspiration.

(11) Duration of cervical traction depends on severity and mechanism of injury; usually a minimum of 6 weeks.

(12) Fitted moulded collar usually applied when patient is mobilized after traction is removed.

d. Halo skeletal traction—consists of a skeletal traction device attached to the skull by pins that penetrate the skin and external table and are connected to a plaster body cast by an adjustable steel frame.

(1) Anticipate some inflammation and drainage around the pin sites; patient may experience a slight headache or minor pain around the skull pins for several days following application.

(2) Cleanse around the pin sites daily and shorten patient's hair periodically.

e. Patient may require open reduction (surgery); measures will still have to be taken to maintain reduction.

6   Report immediately any decrease in neurological function.

a. Keep a neurological assessment record.

b. Observe for symptoms of progressive neurological damage—symptoms of cord compression depend on level at which compression occurs. Clinical symptoms of cord compression are indistinguishable from those of cord oedema.

(1) Loss of sensation.

(2) Inability to move extremities.

7   Prepare for laminectomy if progressive symptoms of cord compression occur permits direct exploration and decompression of cord. Surgeons differ in their opinions about the value of direct exploration.

8   Evaluate for presence of spinal shock—spinal shock represents a sudden loss of continuity between spinal cord and higher nerve centres. There is a complete loss of all reflex, motor, sensory and autonomic activity below the level of the lesion.

a. Falling blood pressure.

b. Paralysis of body below level of cord injury.

c. Bladder distension—from paralysis of bladder.

d. Bowel distension—caused by depression of reflexes; retroperitoneal haemorrhage may occur with fracture of low back, producing paralytic ileus.

9   Maintain the patient's body defences until shock remits and the system has recovered from the traumatic insult. (Spinal shock is temporary, but may last several weeks.)

a. Support the airway, especially in cervical cord injury.

b. Support circulation—give blood transfusions as indicated.

c. Avoid overdistension of bladder—after spinal injury the bladder may lack functional nerve supply; overstretching of bladder may produce permanent damage. (Urinary tract infection is common cause of death after spinal injury.)

(1) Insert indwelling catheter early in acute phase.

(2) Remove catheter as soon as possible.

(3) Initiate bladder training regimen.

d. Treat for acute gastric dilatation and ileus.

(1) Observe for abdominal distension and listen with stethoscope for presence or absence of peristaltic sounds.

(2) Initiate gastric suction to reduce distension and prevent vomiting and aspiration.

(3) Give neostigmine methylsulphate—for severe bowel distension.
(4) Administer rectal tube to relieve gaseous distension.
(5) Give intravenous infusions for fluid replacement.
(6) Place patient on bowel training regimen as required.

10 Prevent pressure sores—inadequate peripheral circulation from spinal shock can cause pressure ulcer to develop within 6 hours.

a. Patients with initial vasovagal instability as well as associated injury may not be able to tolerate positional changes because of episodes of cardiopulmonary arrest.

b. Pressure on the denervated skin will sooner or later result in tissue breakdown.

c. *Objective:* to avoid ischaemia of the skin.
Turn every 2 hours using turning frame, if patient can be turned.
(1) Use electric turning bed (Stoke–Egerton).
(2) Inspect vulnerable skin areas.

11 Maintain patient in proper alignment to prevent contracture deformities.
Dorsal or supine position.

a. Position feet against padded footboard—to prevent footdrop.

b. Be sure there is a space between end of mattress and foot of bed—to allow for free suspension of the heels.

c. Apply trochanter rolls from crest of ilium to midthigh of both extremities—to prevent external rotation of the hip joints.

d. Initiate passive range of motion exercises for affected extremities within 48–72 hours *upon order*—to preserve joint motion.

e. Ambulate only upon order—if patient has partial cord function, activity may produce further cord injury.

12 Assess for complications.

a. Vein thrombosis or pulmonary embolism—from immobilization, muscular and vasomotor paralysis, factors affecting blood coagulation (hypoproteinaemia, infection, etc.).

b. Hyperthermia—during period of spinal shock, patient does not perspire on the paralysed portions of his body since sympathetic activity is blocked. (See p. 13 for treatment of hyperthermia.)

c. Autonomic hyper-reflexia or autonomic dysreflexia—from exaggerated autonomic responses to stimuli (distended bladder or bowel, stimulation of skin by pressure sore, catheter manipulation); may be accompanied by immediate and dangerous elevation of arterial blood pressure.
(1) Syndrome characterized by severe headache, profuse sweating, flushing of skin above level of lesion, bradycardia, severe hypertension.
(2) Treatment.

Nursing Alert: Hyper-reflexia is considered an emergency.

Objective: to remove the triggering stimulus.
(a) Place patient in 45° or sitting position—to help lower the blood pressure.
(b) Drain the bladder. (Do not irrigate catheter with more than 30 ml of irrigating solution.)

(c) Remove any other stimuli that may be triggering episodes; cold air, object on skin, etc.

(d) Make a note of what caused the attack, patient is apt to have another episode of hyper-reflexia.

d. Contractures.

e. Kidney and bladder infections.

f. Depression.

13 See paraplegia for psychological support, p. 72.

14 Employ active rehabilitation procedures when patient's spine is stable enough to assume upright position.

    a. Programme is designed according to neurological deficit.

    b. *Objective:* to strengthen muscles still innervated or when return of function is evident.

        (1) Muscle strengthening exercises for shoulder depressors, maintenance of sitting balance, getting up and down from wheelchair, or whatever is possible for individual patient.

        (2) Period of immobilization determined by patient's condition (usually 6 weeks on a turning frame and 6 weeks of gradual mobilization with brace or cast, depending on level of lesion, etc.).

PROLAPSED INTRAVERTEBRAL DISC (SLIPPED DISC)

Prolapse or herniation of the intravertebral disc is a protrusion of the nucleus pulposus into the annulus fibrosus, with subsequent nerve compression.

Types of Disc Herniation

1 Cervical.
2 Thoracic (rare).
3 Lumbar.

Causes

1 Degeneration.
2 Trauma (accidents, strain, repeated minor stresses).
3 Congenital predisposition.

Clinical Manifestations

Depend on location, size, rate of development (acute or chronic) and effect on surrounding structures.

Cervical Disc

1 Pain and stiffness in neck, top of shoulders and in region of scapulae.
2 Pain in upper extremities and head.
3 Paresthesia and numbness of upper extremities.

Lumbar Disc

1 Low back pain accompanied by varying degrees of sensory and motor impairment.

2   Pain in buttock and thigh radiating to calf and ankle—aggravated by actions that increase intraspinal pressure (sneezing, straining).
3   Postural deformity of lumbar spine.
4   Pain induced by stretching sciatic nerve.
   a. Place patient on his back with his knees straight.
   b. Raise the unflexed leg (one at a time).
   c. This manoeuvre causes stretching of sciatic nerve that is transmitted to nerve roots, producing pain that radiates into the leg.
   d. Patient will experience little or no pain if leg is raised while bent at the knee since this relaxes tension on sciatic nerve.
   e. Lasègue sign—pain with straight-leg raising and absence of pain with bent-leg raising.
5   Muscle weakness.
6   Alterations in tendon reflexes.
7   Sensory loss.

Diagnosis

1   X-ray of spine—to rule out other lesions that cause similar signs and symptoms.
2   Myelogram—demonstrates area of pressure and localizes herniation of disc; disc protrusion is seen as indentation of dye.

Treatment and Nursing Management

Cervical Disc (usually occurs at C5–6 or C6–7)

Objectives

To rest and immobilize the cervical spine to allow for healing of soft tissues.
To reduce inflammation in supporting tissues and affected nerve roots in the cervical spine.

1   Immobilize and rest the cervical spine by one of the following methods:
   a. Cervical collar—allows maximal opening of intervertebral foramina.
     (1) Collar should hold the head in a neutral or slightly flexed position.
     (2) Inspect under the collar at intervals for skin rash or friction.
     (3) In acute herniation the collar may have to be worn night and day until pain subsides (2–3 weeks).
     (4) Cervical isometric exercises are started when patient is pain-free—to strengthen neck musculature in preparation for 'weaning' from collar.
   b. Cervical traction—increases vertebral separation and thus relieves pressure on nerve (Fig. 1.8).
     (1) Cervical traction should be comfortable.
     (2) Patient must be relaxed.
     (3) Keep head of bed elevated and make sure that traction is in alignment.
     (4) Inspect for skin burns from cervical halter; pad under the halter as necessary.
     (5) Encourage male patient not to shave since beard offers a form of padding; shaving may cause irritation.
   c. Bed rest—reduces inflammation and oedema in soft tissues around disc,

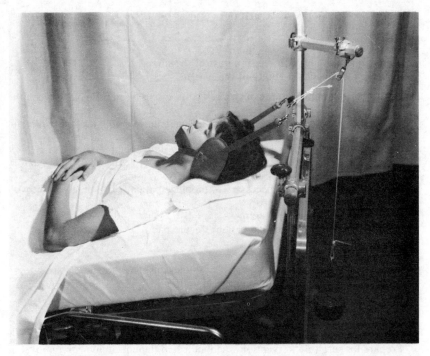

Figure 1.8. Cervical traction. The patient should be assessed for pressure sores developing under chin or occiput. The head of the bed is elevated to provide countertraction.

relieving pressure on nerve roots; relieves cervical spine of supporting weight of head.

2 Muscle relaxants may be prescribed to control muscle spasm and allow for patient comfort.

3 Give analgesics and sedatives to control discomfort and anxiety often associated with a cervical disc lesion.

4 Prepare for surgical intervention if significant neurological deficit from nerve root compression occurs, for unremitting and recurrent pain or for signs of cord compression.

5 *Discharge planning and health teaching* (cervical disc). It may take 6 weeks to recuperate from significant disc lesions. Instruct the patient as follows:

a. Avoid extreme flexion, extension and rotation of the cervical spine while working.

b. Keep head in a neutral position while sleeping.

(1) Pillow should be filled with feathers or down.

(2) Sleep on side or back; do not sleep prone.

(3) Avoid excessive neck flexion—do not prop up in bed with several pillows.

c. Avoid excessive automobile riding during acute phase—vibration has adverse effect on spine.

Lumbar Disc—(majority of herniations occur at L4–L5 or L5–S1 interspace)

Objectives

To relieve the pain and slow the progress of the disease.
To increase the functional ability of the patient.

1   Encourage the patient to remain on bed rest—disc is freed from stress when the patient is horizontal.
   a. Place patient in position of comfort—usually upright with moderate hip and knee flexion.
   b. Place hinged bedboard under mattress—to limit spinal flexion.
   c. Help patient to ambulate (usually after 2 weeks bed rest) when inflammatory reaction and oedema from disc herniation have subsided.
   d. Use corset or brace if necessary to mobilize patient (for obese patient with poor abdominal musculature).
2   Use of appropriate drug therapy.
   a. Analgesic agents to relieve patient's acute pain.
   b. Anti-inflammatory agents.
      Systemic steroids (dexamethasone).
3   Utilization of heat and massage by physiotherapist to relax muscle spasm.
4   Watch for development of neurological deficit.
   a. Muscle weakness and atrophy.
   b. Loss of sensory and motor function.
   c. Unrelieved acute pain.
5   Have the patient increase his activities gradually if his symptoms abate.
6   Prepare for surgical intervention when indicated (laminectomy with removal of ruptured disc). Indications for operative intervention include compression of cauda equina (motor and sensory paresis, loss of sphincter control), nerve root compression and lack of response to conservative therapy.
   a. Patients with multilevel involvement may have recurrences of pain and disability and may require reoperation(s).
   b. Spinal fusion may be required on reoperation.
7   *Discharge planning and health teaching.*
   a. Encourage patient to do lumbar flexion exercises after acute symptoms subside—to strengthen abdominal muscles and flexors of the spine.
      (1) Start exercises gently and gradually.
      (2) Discontinue exercises if pain worsens.
   b. Advise patient to sleep on side with knees and hips in position of flexion (pillow between knees).
      (1) Do not sleep in prone position—hyperextends the spine.
      (2) Pick up loads correctly (bend knees, keep back straight, avoid lifting anything above the elbows).
      (3) Avoid lifting while back is in a flexed or rotated position.
   c. Encourage proper posture while standing, sitting, walking and working.
   d. A lumbar sacral support (corset) may be necessary for persons with poor abdominal musculature—serves to pull in abdomen and alter lumbar-sacral curve, which relieves strain on ligaments.

MANAGEMENT OF THE PATIENT FOLLOWING A LAMINECTOMY

Laminectomy is the removal of the lamina to expose the neural elements in the spinal canal. It allows inspection of the spinal canal and identification and removal of pathology and compression from the cord and roots.

Indications for a Laminectomy

1 As an emergency procedure to prevent irreversible neurological damage.
2 For progressive central nervous system involvement with muscular weakness and atrophy.
3 For recurring episodes of pain or unrelieved acute pain (intervertebral disc).

Postoperative Nursing Management

Objective

To provide a stable spine to meet the functional demands of the body. (See also the preoperative principles for patient undergoing orthopaedic surgery.)

Cervical Disc

1 Check neurological and vital signs at frequent intervals—there is always the possibility of respiratory difficulty, paralysis and urinary retention following operation on the cervical spine.
2 Assess for signs of urinary retention—may be the first indication of a haematoma at the operative site.
3 Be aware that a sore throat will be a major complaint of patient.
   a. Do not give any spray or throat lozenges that numb the throat since this may cause choking.
   b. Observe for pulmonary secretions since patient may be afraid to cough because of pain from sore throat.

Lumbar Disc

1 Position the patient effectively.
   a. Use pillow under head and elevate the knee rest slightly—slight knee flexion relaxes muscles of the back.
   b. Encourage the patient to move and turn from side to side to relieve pressure.
      (1) Turn patient as a unit (log rolling); place pillow between his legs while turning.
      (2) Place pillow between legs when patient is lying on his side.
      (3) Avoid extreme knee flexion when patient is on side.
2 Encourage early ambulation as soon as patient is able. To get patient out of bed:
   a. Raise head of bed as patient lies on his side.
   b. Encourage patient to move to the edge of the bed.
   c. Help patient to raise himself (with feet hanging over side of bed) to a full sitting position.
   d. Caution him to sit and stand with one smooth motion.
3 Give analgesics and sedatives to relieve pain and anxiety; discomfort in immediate postoperative period may vary from mild to severe pain.

4   Explain to the patient that there may be varying degrees of pain and sensory manifestations in the legs (sciatica type pain) due to temporary inflammatory changes, oedema and swelling of compressed nerve.
5   Be alert for postoperative complications of infection.

Discharge Planning and Health Teaching

1   It may take 6 weeks for ligamentous attachments of the muscles and skin to heal.
2   Instruct the patient as follows:
   a. Increase activities as tolerated—move up to the point of individual tolerance.
   b. Avoid activities that produce flexion strain on the spine—stair climbing, automobile riding.
   c. Have scheduled rest periods.
   d. Apply heat to back when indicated—helps absorb exudates in the tissues; warm bathing is helpful.
   e. Avoid heavy work for 2–3 months after surgery.
   f. Resume exercises to strengthen abdominal and erector spinae muscles as directed.
   g. A brace or corset may have to be worn if back pain persists.
3   See health teaching for herniation of intervertebral disc, p. 70.

PARAPLEGIA

Paraplegia is loss of movement and sensation in the lower extremities.
   Quadriplegia is loss of movement and sensation involving both upper and lower extremities and the whole trunk.

Causes

1   Trauma—accidents, gunshot wounds.
2   Spinal cord lesions (intervertebral disc, tumour, vascular lesions).
3   Multiple sclerosis.
4   Infections and abscesses of spinal cord.
5   Congenital defects.

Nursing Management

1   See the nursing management of patient with spinal cord injuries for immediate management principles, p. 63.
2   Understand the psychological significance of the disability.
   a. Support the patient through his stages of adjustment to injury—shock and disbelief, denial, depression, grief, etc.
   b. Allow the patient to work through his feelings about his disability at his own pace (unless his responses continue to be exaggerated or maladaptive).
      (1) Realization of the finality of paraplegia or quadriplegia may prolong the grief process.
      (2) Patient experiences a loss of self-esteem in areas of self-identity, sexual identity and social and emotional roles.
   c. Be aware that the patient may take one of two courses:

(1) Acceptance of disability leading to development of realistic goals for the future.

(2) Rejection of disability—may exhibit self-destructive neglect, noncompliance with therapeutic programme.

Patient may require supportive psychotherapy and additional recreational therapy to prevent social and intellectual isolation.

3   Prepare for weight-bearing activities—patient with complete cord severance should start early weight bearing to decrease osteoporotic changes in long bones and to reduce incidence of urinary infections and the formation of renal calculi.

a. Antiembolic or elastic stockings may be applied to prevent pooling of blood. A patient with a spinal cord paralysis lacks vasomotor tone in the lower extremities and will become hypotensive in the upright position.

b. A tilt-table may be used—to help patient overcome vasomotor instability and tolerate upright posture.

(1) Start with elevation of 45° and gradually increase angle of elevation over a period of days.

(2) Take blood pressure immediately before and as soon as patient is positioned on tilt-table.

(3) Observe for nausea and excessive perspiration.

c. *Or* use high-back reclining wheelchair with extension leg rests; raise backrest slowly and lower leg rest gradually over a period of 7–10 days.

4   Initiate bladder training programme.

a. Give meticulous attention to indwelling catheter.

b. See Principles of Bladder Training (Volume 1, Chapter 2).

5   Start bowel training programme.

a. Objective is to obtain reflex bowel evacuation by conditioning.

b. See Bowel Training process (Volume 1, Chapter 2).

6   The physiotherapy programme will aim towards building the unaffected part of body to optimal strength—to prepare for ambulation with braces and crutches.

Encourage patient to continue with muscle strengthening exercises for hands, arms, shoulders, chest, spine, abdomen and neck—patient must bear full weight on these muscles.

7   Prevent the complications of paraplegic disorders.

a. Infection of urinary tract; urinary calculi; urethrocutaneous fistula.

(1) Prevent overdistension of the bladder.

(2) Maintain continuous urinary drainage using a three-way system or as some centres prefer carry out intermittent catheterization as instructed.

(3) Frequent specimens of urine should be sent for culture and sensitivity analysis.

(4) Encourage fluid intake of at least 4000 ml/24 hours; urinary output should be 2000 ml/24 hours.

(5) Prevent periurethral abscess formation and urethrocutaneous fistula—in male patient tape the penis horizontally to the side to prevent pressure and kinking of the urethra on the catheter at the penoscrotal angle.

b. Development of pressure sores.

(1) Some surgeons prefer patient to be nursed on a Stryker frame—prevents pressure on heels and other bony prominences and facilitates turning. If not on Stryker frame, patient is turned manually preferably by three or four nurses, so

that the patient maybe turned in 'one piece', maintaining proper alignment of the vertebral column.

(2) Turn every 2 hours; give skin care immediately after turning.

(3) Give special attention to the perineal area.

(4) Prevent development of hypoproteinaemia.

    (a) Give high vitamin, high protein, high calorie diet.

    (b) Give high protein formula as in-between-meal feedings.

(5) It is important that the patient maintains a normal haemoglobin and normal red blood cell count.

  c. Abdominal distension; reflex ileus; faecal impaction.

(1) Use rectal tube and intestinal decompression for patients with high cervical and thoracic cord lesions.

    Omit gas-forming foods and liquids.

(2) Ensure total evacuation of faecal material from lower bowel every day.

    (a) Give enemas or colonic irrigation.

    (b) Employ regular digital examination of rectum—to determine presence of impacted faecal material.

    (c) Keep patient on bowel training programme.

  d. Ankylosis of joints; contractures; spasticity.

(1) Start passive exercises and range of motion early in course of treatment.

(2) Position patient in functional positions.

(3) Use splints and supports for spastic joints as indicated by patient's condition and on the advice of the physiotherapist and medical staff.

  e. Autonomic dysreflexia (see p. 66).

8 Support the counselling services provided for the patient.

  a. Rehabilitation engineering services—provide a greater range of self-help and mobility devices.

  b. Occupational therapy—selects and utilizes devices which can aid patient in mealtime, dressing and other activities.

  c. Vocational assessment and rehabilitation counselling.

  d. Sexual counselling.

(1) Most cord-injured persons can have some form of meaningful sexual relationship; patient may want and require counselling on positions, techniques, etc.

(2) Female patient may experience little sensation during intercourse, but fertility and ability to bear children are usually not affected.

  e. Family may require counselling and social services to help them cope with burden of spinal cord injury on their life-style and socioeconomic status.

INTRACTABLE PAIN

Intractable pain is pain that causes incapacitation of function and that cannot be relieved satisfactorily by drugs short of drug addiction or large doses of sedation.

Causes

1 Malignant disease (especially of cervix, bladder, prostate, lower bowel).

2 Trigeminal neuralgia.

3 Postherpes zoster (shingles).
4 Uncontrollable ischaemia or other forms of tissue destruction.

Neurosurgical Procedures for Management of Intractable Pain

Objective

To interrupt the pathways by which the painful sensations are perceived.

Posterior Spinal Rhizotomy

Surgical interruption of selected posterior spinal nerve roots between the ganglion and the cord. This results in sensory deficit (loss of sensation).

Sensation may gradually return after 1–2 years, and even more distressingly severe paresthesias or dysesthesias (pain induced by touch) may appear later.

Chemical Rhizotomy

Injection of alcohol (phenol) into the subarachnoid space; medication is manoeuvred over affected nerve roots by tilting the patient to achieve desired level. The patient's perception of pain is absent but motor nerve root sensations are not.

Cordotomy

Surgical interruption of the anterolateral quadrant of the spinal cord for the relief of intractable pain.

1 Obliterates pain and temperature sense but leaves motor function intact.
2 May be done by (a) open operation (via laminectomy) or by (b) percutaneous needle insertion. An electrode is introduced through the spinal needle and a lesion produced by a radio frequency current at the desired level. This is useful for patient who cannot tolerate a laminectomy.
3 Cordotomy is helpful for patients with unilateral pain of malignant origin, especially of thorax, abdomen or lower extremities.
4 *Nursing management following cordotomy*
   a. See management of the patient following a laminectomy, p. 71 , for principles of care also relevant to these operations.
   b. Watch for complications:
      (1) Respiratory.
      (a) Observe for loss of volume of voice and fatigue.
      (b) Medical staff should monitor arterial blood gases. Patients with reduced oxygen levels may require oxygen at night until blood gas levels return to normal. (Patient may ventilate adequately while awake but may experience progressive hypercarbia and hypoxia while asleep.)
      (c) Assisted mechanical ventilation may be required.
      (2) Urinary retention (usually transient).
      (3) Ipsilateral (on the same side) leg weakness—usually disappears in a few days.
      (4) Haemorrhage—may produce motor and sensory loss; immediate surgical intervention is indicated.
      Test motion, strength and sensation of each extremity every few hours during the first 48 hours.

    c. Feel patient's skin temperature at intervals to ascertain skin temperature changes.

    d. Watch for development of pressure sores.

      (1) Teach patient to inspect his skin using a hand mirror to view hard-to-see areas.

      (2) Place patient on bladder training programme if high cervical procedure has caused loss of bladder control.

5 *Family and patient health teaching.*

    a. Protect patient against external temperature changes and extremes of weather; he may not be aware of sunburn/frostbite.

    b. Test bath water before getting in tub.

    c. Avoid constricting clothing that impairs circulation.

    d. Sexual function is usually impaired in males.

Sympathectomy

Interrupts afferent pathways in the sympathetic division of the autonomic nervous system, used to control pain from causalgia and peripheral vascular disorders (eliminates vasospasm and improves peripheral blood supply).

Procedures Altering Patient's Response to Pain

1 *Thalamotomy*—destruction (unilaterally or bilaterally) of specific cell groups within thalamus. It is accomplished through burr holes—a lesion is produced by radio frequency current, cryosurgery, etc. This technique is useful for pain of central origin.

Suppression of Pain by Electrical Stimulation (pain modulation; neuromodulation)

Neuromodulation is the suppression of pain by the application of an electronic device to modify nervous system function. It is accomplished by (1) transcutaneous electrical nerve stimulation or (2) dorsal column stimulation.

1 *Underlying principles.*

    a. This therapy is based on the theory (gate control theory) that nondestructive stimuli can interfere with the transmission of pain within the central nervous system. It is thought to relieve pain by preventing pain messages from reaching the brain. The exact mechanics are not yet fully known.

    b. It is nondestructive in nature and does not carry the potential risks of weakness, numbness, dysesthesia, bladder/bowel incontinence, impotence or irreversibility as do destructive surgical procedures for pain relief.

    c. The system consists of a pulse generator (containing the power source and electronics of the system), a pair of electric cables and two flexible electrodes which transfer the stimulating signal.

    d. *Objective:* to help the patient live with his pain without permitting it to affect his life adversely.

2 *Transcutaneous electrical nerve stimulation*—passage of small electrical currents through the skin for the purpose of relieving pain.

    a. Electrodes are placed over or around patient's pain area or on any peripheral nerve pathway.

    b. Procedure:

(1) The skin is washed with mild soap and water and dried thoroughly to reduce skin resistance.

(2) Electrode gel is applied to the electrodes, which are then placed over the nerves that serve the painful area.

(3) The patient operates the amplitude control until stimulation is felt (buzzing or tingling feeling). The amplitude is increased until the sensation is strong but not uncomfortable. Patient then adjusts the rate and pulse width control.

(4) The patient is taught to control the amplitude, frequency and duration of stimulation.

c. *Health teaching.*

(1) Give the patient the instruction booklet provided by the manufacturing company.

(2) Batteries must be replaced whenever levels of stimulation cannot be achieved.

(3) The electrodes are washed with alcohol and water after each use. The pulse generator and cables are wiped clean with a damp cloth moistened with alcohol/water solution.

(4) Apply talcum powder to the cables periodically to prevent tangling.

(5) Avoid getting the pulse generator wet; avoid pulling or kinking of the cable wire.

3 *Dorsal column stimulation*—is a method for the relief of chronic intractable pain that uses an implanted device that allows the patient to apply pulsed electrical stimulation to the dorsal aspect of the spinal cord.

a. The unit consists of a radio-frequency stimulation transmitter, a transmitter antenna, a radio-frequency receiver and a stimulation lead.

b. The battery-powered transmitter and antenna are worn externally while the receiver and lead are implanted.

A laminectomy is performed above the highest level of pain input for the placement of the electrode in the subdural space. A small subcutaneous pocket is developed over the clavicular area (site may vary) for placement of receiver. The two are connected by a subcutaneous tunnel.

c. A careful preoperative evaluation is performed to select patient who will benefit from dorsal column stimulation—history, physical examination, pain questionnaire, examination to determine areas of pain involvement, psychological and psychiatric evaluation and a trial of transcutaneous stimulation.

(1) Trial of transcutaneous stimulation (see above) gives opportunity for patient to receive stimulation sensation—to test his tolerance of the sensation, his ability to operate the system and the efficacy of the system.

(2) It is essential that the patient understand that the stimulator will replace drugs and that it is installed for a lifetime.

d. Postoperative nursing management.

(1) See p. 71 for the nursing management following a laminectomy.

(2) Assess for paraplegia, quadriplegia and urinary incontinence.

(3) Evaluate extremities for leg movement hourly. Report any decrease in movement immediately.

(4) Look for leakage of cerebrospinal fluid at laminectomy site—dura is opened in surgery.

(5) Give medication as prescribed for relief of incisional pain.

(6) Medical staff will withdraw narcotics as rapidly as possible.

(7) Help patient to become independently involved with his activities of daily living as rapidly as possible—inactivity serves to compound his problems.

(8) Look for signs of infection at implantation site—dorsal column stimulator is a foreign body within the patient.

(9) The dorsal column stimulation system may be tested when the patient is fully alert; initial testing may not be accurate because of overlying bandage at receiver site.

e. *Health teaching.*

(1) Give the patient the manufacturer's instruction booklet to acquaint him with his system.

The stimulation transmitter has four basic controls: two for the patient to use during operation of the system and two for the doctor to use when determining the voltage the patient will receive.

(2) The patient is taught the method of attaching the antenna to the skin (and proper skin care), use of battery pack and how to make and modify dorsal column stimulation settings.

(a) Antenna is secured in place by an adhesive disc centred over the implanted receiver. (The antenna site is cleansed daily and the adhesive discs are changed daily.)

(b) Connect transmitter to antenna and adjust settings slowly to the point at which the patient first feels a definite sensation and the stimulation results in the desired effect.

(c) Encourage patient to try different stimulation frequencies to determine which frequency gives best pain relief.

(d) Have the patient keep a record of stimulation use.

(e) Instruct the patient that postural changes will cause changes in stimulation intensity.

(f) Warn patient not to adjust doctor's controls.

(g) Instruct patient to keep several batteries in reserve; battery life depends on extent of use. Patient should be instructed in battery changing procedure.

(h) Clean transmitter and antenna with gauze pad moistened with equal amounts of water and alcohol. (See instruction booklet.)

FURTHER READING

Books

Bannister, R (1980) Brains Clinical Neurology, 5th edition, Oxford University Press

Barr, M L (1979) The Human Nervous System—An Anatomical Viewpoint, 3rd edition, Harper & Row

Bickerton, J and Small, J C (1981) Neurology for Nurses, Heinemann

Carini, E and Owens, G (1980) Neurological and Neurosurgical Nursing, 7th edition, C V Mosby

Forsythe, E (1979) Living with Multiple Sclerosis, Faber & Faber

Jennett, B (   ) An Introduction to Neurosurgery, 3rd edition, Heinemann

Jennett, B and Teasdale, G T (1980) Management of Head Injuries, Davis

Marshall, M (1979) Current Topics in Anaesthesia, Series 3—Neuroanaesthesia, Edward Arnold
Martin, G (   ) A Manual of Head Injuries in General Surgery, Heinemann
Pierce, D S and Nickel, V H (1977) The Total Care of Spinal Cord Injuries, Little, Brown & Co
Sutherland, J M and Eadie, M J (1980) The Epilepsies—Modern Diagnosis and Treatment, 3rd edition, Churchill Livingstone
The Back Pain Association and the Royal College of Nursing (1981) The Handling of Patients—A Guide for Nurse Managers

Articles

Bartlett, J (19   ) Aneurysms and arteriovenous malformations, Medicine, 38: 1681
Maggs, A (1981) Multiple sclerosis I, Nursing Times
Maggs, A (1981) Multiple sclerosis II, Nursing Times
Mathews, B (19   ) Multiple sclerosis, Medicine, 32: 1664
Mathews, B (1981) Clinical forum—Epilepsy, Nursing Mirror
Mathews, B (1975) A symposium of spinal injuries, Nursing Mirror
Utley, D (19   ) Subarachnoid haemorrhage, British Journal of Hospital Medicine
Young, J A (1981) Head Injuries I—Advances in care during the past decade, Nursing Times
Young, J A (1981) Head Injuries II—Advances in diagnostic equipment, Nursing Times

Chapter 2

EAR DISORDERS

Terminology   81
Examinations and Diagnostic Procedures   82
Ear Hygiene   83
Problems Affecting the External Ear   85
  Guidelines: Irrigating the External Auditory Canal   86
Acute Otitis Media   87
Serous Otitis Media   89
Chronic Otitis Media and Mastoiditis   90
Perforation of Eardrum   91
  Tympanoplasty   92
Otosclerosis   94
  Stapedectomy   95
Ménière's Disease (Endolymphatic Hydrops)   96
Communicating With a Person who has a Hearing Impairment   97
Further Reading   98

TERMINOLOGY

Ear Care Specialists

1 *Otolaryngologist*—a doctor who specializes in problems related to the ear, nose and throat.
2 *Audiologist*—an individual who specializes in nonmedical evaluation and rehabilitation of hearing disorders (usually not a doctor).

Classification of Hearing Loss

1 *Conductive loss*—a hearing loss due to an impairment of the outer or middle ear or both. If causative problem cannot be corrected, a hearing aid may help.
2 *Sensorineural (perceptive) loss*—a hearing loss due to disease of the inner ear or

nerve pathways; sensitivity to and discrimination of sounds are impaired. Hearing aids usually are helpful.

3 *Combined hearing loss*—a combination of the above.

4 *Psychogenic hearing loss*—usually a manifestation of an emotional disturbance and unrelated to evident structural changes in the hearing mechanisms. Loss is often total, but without physical basis; thus patient may suddenly recover.

EXAMINATIONS AND DIAGNOSTIC PROCEDURES

Tuning Fork (nonquantitative)

1 A unique and inexpensive instrument that can differentiate between conductive and perceptive deafness.

2 A 512 cps (cycles per second) tuning fork is preferred; when a low frequency fork of 128–256 cps is used, the patient finds it difficult to determine whether the vibration is felt or heard.

3 By striking the fork on your knees rather than on the heel of a shoe or on a hard object, a better patient response will be obtained. (Striking fork on a hard surface will result in overtones.)

4 Types of deafness
   a. *Conductive deafness*—caused by a disorder of the auditory canal, eardrum or middle ear (e.g., disruption of ossicles or fluid).
   b. *Perceptive (sensorineural) deafness*—caused by a disorder of the organ of Corti or the auditory nerve.

Weber Test (valuable when hearing loss is unilateral)

1 Place tuning fork on the forehead so that hearing in the two ears may be compared.

2 Some examiners prefer to have the patient keep his lips open and hold the vibrating fork in his clenched teeth or against the bridge of the nose. (Nasal and dental areas are more sensitive to vibration.)

3 If patient indicates he hears vibrations in the middle of his head:
   a. This may be normal.
   b. This may be deafness of equal quality in both ears.

4 Variations imply hearing inequality.
   a. In conductive hearing loss, bone-conducted sounds shift to poorer ear.
   b. In sensorineural hearing loss, sounds are louder in the better ear (because patient cannot hear any better than the nerve will allow, and the nerve in the poorer ear is damaged).

*Rinne Test**

1 After the fork is struck to set it in vibration, the handle is placed against the mastoid process at the level of the upper portion of the ear canal.

2 Then the prongs are placed beside the ear, in front of the auditory canal.

3 The patient is asked to tell where he heard the sound better or longer.

4 'Rinne positive'—tone was heard longer by air conduction, which may be normal or may indicate a perceptive loss.

* Of limited value unless physician is certain clinically that the patient has a hearing loss.

5   'Rinne negative'—tone was heard longer by bone conduction, which indicates
    conduction loss.
6   'Rinne equal'—tone heard the same by air and bone conduction and may indicate
    a loss, probably conductive.

Ear Condition	Weber Test	Rinne Test
Normal, no hearing loss	No shifting of sounds laterally	Sound perceived longer by *air* conduction
Conductive loss	Shifting of sounds to poorer ear	Sound perceived as long or longer by *bone* conduction
Sensorineural loss	Shifting of sounds to better ear	Sound perceived longer by *air* conduction

Audiogram (Fig. 2.1).

Types

1   Pure-tone audiometry.
    a. Sound stimulus consists of a pure (musical) tone.
    b. The louder the tone required before patient hears it, the greater the hearing
    loss.
    c. Decibel—unit of measuring loudness or intensity of sound.
2   Speech audiometry.
    The spoken word is used to evaluate ability to understand and discriminate
    sounds.

Procedure

1   Test is performed in a soundproof room.
2   Patient is instructed to don earphones and to signal (1) when he hears the tone,
    and (2) when the tone disappears.
3   Air conduction is measured by applying tone directly to external auditory open-
    ing.
4   Nerve conduction is measured when stimulus is applied directly to the mastoid
    process.

Evaluation

1   Normal human ear perception—20 cps or 20–20 000 Hz (Hertz).
2   Frequencies significant for speech range—500–2000 Hz.
3   Clinical level of loudness—30 decibels over threshold, i.e., the level at which
    speech discrimination is tested using phonetically balanced spoken words.

EAR HYGIENE

Hygienic Measures

1   Avoid putting matches, toothpicks, etc., into the external auditory canal (danger

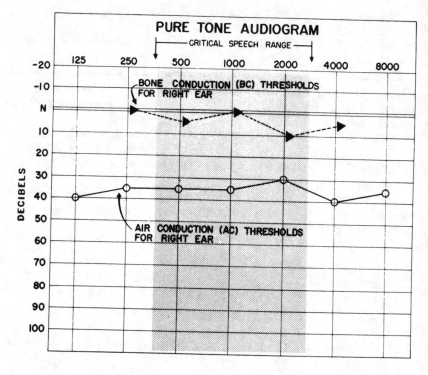

Figure 2.1. An audiogram presents a graphic outline of the individual's hearing as measured by tones of different pitches ranging from 125 through 8000 cycles per second (cps or Hz). Thresholds for these different tones as heard by air and bone conduction are plotted on this graph. The information is important for determining the type of hearing loss. Also, by testing through the critical speech range (approximately 300 to 3000 cps), one can predict how much difficulty there may be in hearing and understanding speech. (From: Nilo, E R Hearing Impairment. In Saunders, W H et al. Nursing Care in Eye, Ear, Nose and Throat Disorders, 2nd edition, C V Mosby.)

of possible infection and damage to the eardrum). Many doctors even object to the use of Q-tips.

2   If it becomes necessary to remove wax deposits, the most effective and least harmful ways are to use sodium bicarbonate ear drops, warm olive oil and glycerol. Dioctyl sodium sulphosuccinate (Waxsol) is used but more expensive. These preparations should be introduced into the meatus on a cotton wool plug and left for several hours or overnight. After three nights of treatment the ear is gently syringed with warm water.

3   The use of organic solvent preparations should be avoided. They are rarely effective and may cause irritation.

4   During an upper respiratory infection, avoid vigorous blowing of the nose, since middle ear infection can result.

5   In the presence of an ear infection, take precautions when swimming—either avoid this sport or insert a sheepskin plug into the ear canal. It is preferable not to get the head wet.

Noise

1   Excess noise is detrimental to health and decreases work efficiency; conversely, elimination of noise or substitution of pleasant soft music increases work efficiency.
2   The decibel (db) is the unit of measurement of sound intensity.
    a. Leaves rustling in a breeze—10 db.
    b. Ordinary conversation—50 db.
    c. Noisy subway—80 db.
    d. Jet plane (100 ft away)—140 db.
3   Frequency—number of sound waves emanating from a source per second. This is described as cycles per second (cps or Hz).
4   Pitch is related to frequency.
    a. For example—100 cps or Hz is low pitch, 10 000 cps or Hz is high pitch.
    b. A healthy young adult can distinguish frequencies from 16 to 20 000 cps.
5   Health implications.
    a. Individuals react differently to noise.
    b. The noise level in the home should not exceed 35–40 db.
    c. Very loud electrical music can damage hearing.
    d. Protective muffs are recommended in work areas where the noise level exceeds 80–85 db.

PROBLEMS AFFECTING THE EXTERNAL EAR

External Otitis

1   *Cause:*
    Bacterial or fungal infections due to
    (1) Abrasion of ear canal.
    (2) Swimming in contaminated water.
2   *Clinical manifestations:*
    a. Pain—moving or even touching the auricle intensifies pain.
    b. Tissues may be oedematous.
3   *Treatments:*
    a. Administer codeine or soluble aspirin for pain.
    b. Apply heat for comfort.
    c. Instil ear drops (antibiotic) for anti-inflammatory and anti-infection effect if prescribed.
    d. Caution patient to avoid showering or swimming until infection is cleared.

Cerumen in Ear Canal

1   Accumulated earwax does *not* have to be removed unless it becomes impacted and interferes with hearing.
2   To irrigate ear canal, see Guidelines, p. 86

Foreign Bodies in External Canal

1   Inserted by young children or handicapped persons.
2   Insects.
    Treat by instilling olive oil drops to smother insect, which then will float out.
3   Vegetable foreign bodies (peas).
    a. Irrigation is contraindicated because vegetable matter absorbs water, which would further wedge foreign body in ear canal.
    b. Unskilled persons should not attempt to remove foreign body because:
        (1) It may be forced into bony portion of the canal.
        (2) The canal skin may be perforated.
        (3) The eardrum may be perforated.
    c. Removal should be done skilfully with instruments by a medical officer; if the victim is very young, general anaesthesia is required.

GUIDELINES: Irrigating the External Auditory Canal

Purposes

1   To remove discharge from the canal.
2   To facilitate removal of cerumen or foreign bodies.
3   To apply heat to the tissues of the ear canal.

Nursing Alert: Ask the patient if he has a history of draining ears, or if he has ever had a perforation or other complications from a previous ear irrigation. If the reply is affirmative, check with the physician before proceeding with the irrigation.

Equipment and solutions

Kind and amount of solution required, e.g., soluble sodium bicarbonate (4—5 g/ 100 ml), normal saline or tapwater.
Tray containing
    Protective towels.
    Cotton balls and cotton applicators.
    Bowl containing solution.
    Metal ear syringe or irrigating container with rubber syringe, e.g., Higginson's.
    Paperbag for disposable cotton.
    Kidney dish or container to catch the return flow of solution.

Procedure

Preparatory Phase

1   After explaining procedure to patient, place him in appropriate position, i.e., sitting or lying with head tilted towards affected ear.
2   Place protective towelling over shoulder.

Nursing Action	Reason

Performance Phase

1 Use a cotton applicator to remove any discharge on outer ear.	1 To prevent carrying discharge deeper into canal.

Nursing Action	Reason
2 Place kidney dish close to the patient's head and under the ear.	2 To provide a receptacle to receive irrigating solution.
3 Test temperature of solution by allowing some to run on inner aspect of wrist. Should be 35–40.6°C (95–105°F).	3 More comfortable for patient; solutions that are hot or cold are most uncomfortable and may initiate a feeling of dizziness.
4 Ascertain whether impaction is due to a foreign hygroscopic (attracts or absorbs moisture) body before proceeding.	4 If water contacts such a substance, it may cause it to swell and produce intense pain.
5 Gently pull the outer ear upwards and backwards (adult); downwards and backwards (child).	5 To straighten ear canal.
6 Place tip of syringe or irrigating catheter at opening of ear; gently direct stream of fluid against sides of the canal (Fig. 2.2).	6 To permit direction for inflow and outflow; if stream is directed forcefully against eardrum, it is possible to rupture it.
7 Observe for signs of pain or dizziness.	7 If they occur, discontinue treatment.
8 If irrigating does not dislodge the wax, instil several drops saturated solution of sodium bicarbonate, two or three times daily for 2–3 days.	8 To soften and loosen impaction.

Follow-up Phase

1 Dry external ear with cotton wool mops.
2 Remove soiled towels, etc. and make patient comfortable.
3 Record: Time of irrigation, kind and amount of solution used, nature of return flow, effect of treatment.

ACUTE OTITIS MEDIA

Acute otitis media is an inflammation of the middle ear caused by the entrance of pathogenic organisms. Normally the middle ear is sterile in its environs.

Aetiology

Haemolytic streptococcus, pneumococcus, staphylococcus, influenza bacillus.

Mode of Entry

1 Auditory canal—if drum is perforated.
2 Eustachian tube—during indiscriminate use of nasal drops or nasal douching or as a result of forcibly sneezing or blowing the nose.
3 Rarely, following a fracture of the skull.

Clinical Manifestations

1   Variable—may be mild or severe.
2   Pain is usually the first symptom—may be in and about the ear and it may be intense.
    May be relieved by spontaneous perforation of the drum or by myringotomy.
3   Fever—may be caused by a virus; in some patients temperature may rise to 40.0–40.6°C (104°–105°F).

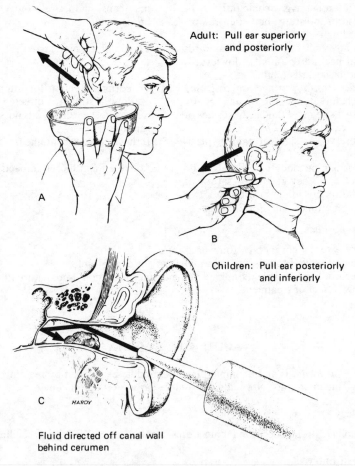

Adult: Pull ear superiorly and posteriorly

A

B

Children: Pull ear posteriorly and inferiorly

C   HARDY

Fluid directed off canal wall behind cerumen

Figure 2.2.   Ear irrigation. a. The external auditory canal in the adult can best be exposed by pulling the earlobe upwards and backwards. b. The same exposure can be achieved in the child by gently pulling the auricle of the ear downwards and backwards. c. An enlarged diagram showing the direction of irrigating fluid against the side of the canal. NOTE: This is more effective in dislodging cerumen than if the flow of solution were directed straight into the canal.

4   Headache, difficulty hearing, ear and head noises, anorexia, nausea and vomiting.

Treatment and Nursing Management
1   Varies with virulence of bacteria, efficiency of therapy and resistance of patient.
2   Usually the drug of choice is penicillin unless patient is allergic to it, in which case erythromycin is used. Ampicillin is used for infants and small children.
3   Aspirin and local heat are comfort measures which may permit patient to rest more comfortably if pain is a problem. (Sedation is usually avoided, for it may interfere with the early detection of intracranial complications.)
4   Some doctors believe the most effective therapy is to administer decongestants along with self-inflation of the ear by the Valsalva manoeuvre.
    a. This is accomplished by having the patient try to exhale forcefully while holding his nose and mouth tightly—this forces air along the eustachian tube into middle ear.
    b. When successful, the patient will experience a 'pop' and an immediate (perhaps temporary) improvement.
    c. It should be performed 10–12 times daily.
5   Employ wide-spectrum antibiotic therapy.

Nursing Alert:
1   With wide-spectrum antibiotic therapy, acute otitis media may be become subacute with continued purulent discharge.
2   Healing may take place, but the patient may be left with a residual deafness.
3   Recognize that such symptoms as headache, slow pulse, vomiting and vertigo are significant and should be reported.
4   Secondary complications may involve the mastoid or even the brain, producing meningitis or brain abscess.

6   *Myringotomy*—an incision made into the posterior inferior aspect of the tympanic membrane for draining purposes (to relieve pressure and drain pus from middle ear infection).
    a. The incision heals rapidly.
    b. Hearing is not adversely affected.
    c. This procedure is done less frequently now because antibiotic therapy usually makes it unnecessary. However, it may be done because of failure to respond to antibiotic therapy, for severe persistent pain and for persistent conductive hearing loss.

SEROUS OTITIS MEDIA

Serous otitis media (also known as 'glue ear') is the result of the treatment of recurrent nasopharyngeal infections with antibiotics. When this treatment is given the mucous membrane of the walls of the infected middle ear and Eustachian tube undergo change when the number of the mucosal cells producing serous fluid increases. This fluid produces deafness of the middle ear which untreated may cause permanent impairment of hearing.

Treatment and Nursing Management

1 Incision under general anaesthetic and aspiration of fluid.
2 Drainage by using a small plastic grommet inserted into the tympanic membrane. This remains patent and preserves the necessary aeration of the middle ear.
3 The grommet is eventually extended into the external auditory meatus after which the tympanic membrane heals, or it is removed surgically.
4 Postoperatively instil ear drops as directed.
5 Leave cotton wool in the external auditory meatus if required.
6 Remove ear bandage as directed.

CHRONIC OTITIS MEDIA AND MASTOIDITIS

Chronic otitis media occurs as a result of repeated bouts of otitis media which cause perforation of the eardrum. This condition often begins in childhood and continues into adult life.

Causes

1 A strain of organism which is resistent to the antibiotic used.
2 A particularly virulent strain of organism.
3 Poor management of acute suppurative otitis media.

Altered Physiology

1 Marginal perforation of drum membrane.
2 Presence of cholesteatoma (soft ball of dead skin) which erodes vital structures.
   a. Caused by an ingrowth of skin from the perforated drum.
   b. Fills areas in the mastoid and middle ear.
   c. May encroach upon vital structures—facial nerve, labyrinth and brain.

Clinical Manifestations

Symptoms are minimal: mild deafness, foul-smelling discharge.

Diagnosis

1 Presence of above symptoms.
2 X-rays to note mastoid pathology.

Treatment and Nursing Management

Antibiotic Therapy

1 Often effective in simple chronic otitis media.
2 Sometimes disappointing when certain resistant organisms are involved.

Surgery

1 Indicated when cholesteatoma is present.
2 Indicated when there is pain or complications—profound deafness, dizziness, sudden facial paralysis, stiff neck (may lead to meningitis or brain abscess).

3 *Cortical Mastoidectomy*—removal of mastoid cells—indicated when there is persistent tenderness, fever, discharge from ear or headache.
4 *Radical mastoidectomy*—removal of all diseased tissue from mastoid area and middle ear.
5 *Posteroanterior mastoidectomy*—combines simple mastoidectomy with tympanoplasty.

Nursing Concern

1 Shaving depends upon nature of the incision.
  a. Postaural—(incision behind the ear). Clip hair and shave scalp for 3–4 cm around ear (only if desired by surgeon).
  b. Endaural—(incision through the ear canal). Shave is unnecessary.
2 Provide for relief of pain preoperatively.
   Give acetylsalicylic acid or codeine.
3 Postoperatively, administer sedatives for pain and restlessness.
4 Assist with dressing change since area is packed with gauze for drainage; this may be done daily or every other day on the doctor's instruction.
5 Observe for possible complications:
  a. Facial paralysis may be indicative of facial nerve injury.
    (1) Immobility on side of face affected.
    (2) Eye cannot close, mouth droops.
    (3) Patient unable to whistle.
    (4) Patient unable to drink without dripping from mouth.
    (5) When patient speaks or smiles, immobility of affected side is noticeable.
  b. Infection.
    (1) Observe for clinical signs of inflammation.
    (2) Administer antibiotics as prescribed.
  c. Vertigo—may be apparent following radical mastoidectomy due to inner ear disturbance.
  d. Spread of infection to brain.
    Unusual rise in temperature, chills, stiff neck, nausea and vomiting.
6 Note status of hearing.
  a. If stapes has been removed or dislodged, then hearing is lost.
  b. If stapes or cochlea have not been removed or disturbed, then hearing is regained; a hearing aid may be required.

PERFORATION OF EARDRUM

Aetiology and Altered Physiology

1 Infection is the most frequent cause of permanent perforation of the tympanic membrane; often this is due to acute or chronic suppurative otitis media.
2 Trauma is the next cause of permanent perforation; may be due to:
  a. A severe blow on the ear.   **d.** Force of a stream of water.
  b. Blast effect of high explosives.   **e.** Burns of face and head.
  c. Foreign objects.   **f.** Postmyringotomy defects.

Treatment

Medical

Most accidental perforations of the eardrum heal spontaneously.

Surgical

Myringoplasty or Tympanoplasty, Type I–IV.

Tympanoplasty

Tympanoplasty is a reconstructive operation on the diseased or deformed components of the middle ear.

1 Objective is to improve or preserve the conductive mechanisms in an effort to salvage or improve hearing.
2 Impetus for tympanoplasty has been aided by:
   a. Illuminated binocular microscope.
   b. Use of antibiotics to prevent or control infection.

Physiological Principles of Hearing

Why an intact drum is needed to hear.

1 Sound waves are transformed from airborne vibrations to mechanical stimulation of endolymphatic lymph; this is accomplished by the conductive ability of the eardrum and ossicles.
2 The ratio of the small oval window to the large tympanic membrane is 1:22; this, combined with the vibratory action of the ossicles, means a great increase in force from the air to the inner ear fluids.
3 When there is a disturbance in the above relationships, the result is a loss of hearing.
4 From the oval window, bordered by the annular ligament, impulses are received by the stapes footplate from the incus, malleus and drum membrane.
5 A lag phase is normal after sound waves stimulate the oval window and before the final effect of the stimulus reaches the round window.

Altered Physiology

1 When there is a perforation of the eardrum, the lag phase (described above) disappears, with the result that sound waves hit the oval and round windows at the same time, causing diminished effect of labyrinth fluid motility → lessened stimulation of hair cells in the organ of Corti → diminished hearing.
2 Infections often produce fibrosis or necrosis of all or part of the ossicular chain.
3 Granuloma, polyps and fibrous or bony plaques may resist normal function of the oval and round windows.
4 In addition to sequelae from otitis media, otosclerosis may exist.
5 Obstruction of tympanic orifice of the eustachian tube may produce dysfunction.

Types of Tympanoplasty (Table 2.1)

Myringoplasty

1 *Purpose*—to close perforation by placing a graft over it, in order to create a closed middle ear section which in turn will improve hearing.

2 *Indications.*
   To avoid risk of contamination when patient bathes, swims or dives—this in turn prevents recurrence of chronic otitis media or mastoiditis.

3 *Contraindications.*
   a. Ossicular involvement.
   Prediction of surgical results can be made preoperatively by testing for improvement of hearing levels by placing a temporary patch over the defect. If no improvement noticed in audiometric testing, the ossicular chain may be involved.
   b. Presence of active infection.
   c. Presence of chronic middle ear infection, impairing or preventing drainage via eustachian tube.
   d. Sinusitis or allergy which produces a chronic infectious discharge via nasopharynx.
   e. History of acute exacerbations of otitis media.

Table 2.1. Types of Tympanoplasty

Type	Middle Ear Damage		Repair Process
	Tympanic Membrane	Ossicles	
I	Perforated	Erosion of malleus and/ or incus	Close perforation; graft against incus or whatever remains of malleus
II	Tympanic membrane destroyed or widely perforated	Rest of ossicular chain destroyed *but* stapes are intact and mobile	Grafts implanted to contact the normal stapes
III	Tympanic membrane destroyed or widely perforated	Ossicular chain destroyed. Head, neck and crura of stapes destroyed. Stapes footplate mobile	Expose mobile stapes footplate—graft implanted. Air pocket between graft and round window provides protection
IV	Tympanic membrane destroyed or widely perforated	Ossicular chain destroyed. Head, neck and crura of stapes destroyed. Stapes footplate fixed	Make opening in horizontal semicircular canal; graft seals off middle ear to give sound protection for round window Tympanoplasty and fenestration of lateral semicircular canal

4 *Surgical repair.*
>   Perforation is closed using one of the following:
>   **a.** Fascia from temporal muscle (in almost all cases).
>   **b.** Vein grafts from hand or forearm (occasionally).

5 *Postoperative management.*
>   **a.** Administer antibiotics for several days postoperatively as directed to ensure freedom from infection.
>   **b.** Reinforce external dressings if they become soiled; otherwise leave dressings intact.
>   **c.** Remove gauze packing in canal at end of week; do not apply suction or probe canal.

6 *Patient instruction.*
>   **a.** Avoid shampooing or showering, which could cause contamination of ear canal, until permission is obtained from doctor.
>   **b.** Continue with antibiotics beyond first week if there is evidence of infection.
>   **c.** Use antihistamine with an ephedrine derivative for at least 1 month postoperatively.
>   **d.** Continue using an antihistamine if the patient experiences rhinologic allergy.

Types I–IV

1 *Purpose* (see Table 2.1). These procedures are modifications used to correct various middle ear problems.

2 *Preoperative and operative treatment.*
>   **a.** Topical and systemic antibiotics are administered when infection is present.
>   **b.** Suitable replacement (polyethylene tubing, stainless steel wire, bone, cartilage) is used to maintain continuity of conduction sound pathway.
>   **c.** The necessity of a two-stage procedure should be determined.
>   (1) First stage—eradication of all diseased tissues; area is cleaned out to achieve a dry, healed middle ear.
>   (2) Second stage—(performed 2–3 months after first stage) reconstruction, using grafts.

3 *Postoperative nursing management.*
>   **a.** Reinforce outer dressings as necessary but keep inner dressings intact.
>   **b.** Assist patient in getting out of bed for the first time because he may become dizzy.
>   **c.** Notify doctor of any dizziness; medication will be prescribed as needed for vertigo and nausea.
>   **d.** Caution patient not to blow his nose with force and to avoid wetting dressings during bathing.
>   **e.** Note that hearing improvement is achieved in inverse proportion to the amount of surgery required; the simpler the surgery, the better the chance for hearing to improve.

OTOSCLEROSIS

Otosclerosis is a form of deafness caused by the formation of new spongy bone in the labyrinth, fixation of the stapes and prevention of sound transmission through the ossicles to the inner fluids.

Incidence and Clinical Manifestations

1 Cause is unknown.
2 Occurs more commonly in women than men; rare in the black race.
3 Has a hereditary basis.
4 Patient presents a history of slow, progressive hearing loss with no middle ear infection.
5 A frequent complaint is buzzing or ringing noises in the ears; both ears are usually affected equally.

Diagnosis

1 Audiometry findings substantiate hearing loss.
2 Bone conduction is much better than air condition. Reduced tuning fork transmission by air, whereas there is intensification of bone conduction sound when tuning fork handle is placed over the mastoid bone.

Stapedectomy

A *stapedectomy* involves removal of otosclerotic lesions at the footplate of stapes and the creation of a tissue implant with prosthesis to maintain suitable conduction. To perform such delicate surgery, the otologic binocular microscope is used.

Types of Prostheses

1 Steel wire and fat implant.
2 Gelfoam and stainless steel wire.
3 Metal or teflon 'piston'.
4 Vein graft and polyethylene tubing (least frequent).

Nursing Management

1 Observe for unusual symptoms, such as:
   a. Fever—may indicate infection, external otitis, otitis media.
   b. Headache—may indicate infection, nerve encroachment.
   c. Vertigo—may indicate labyrinthitis or inner ear reaction.
   d. Ear pain—may indicate infection or irritation of auditory nerve.
2 Position patient postoperatively as desired by doctor.
   a. Some surgeons prefer that the patient be positioned with operated ear uppermost to maintain position of graft and stability.
   b. Others prefer that patient be lying on operated ear to permit drainage.
   c. Still others advocate that the patient assume the most comfortable position.
3 Administer antimotion medications and sedatives if patient experiences vertigo, nystagmus or nausea.
4 Assist patient when he first tries to walk; he may feel dizzy for the first few days.
5 Instruct patient not to blow his nose for a week; air may be forced up the Eustachian tube and disturb the operative site.
6 Encourage a restricted head position if the surgeon fears a misplacement of the prosthesis.
7 No water must get into the ear until healing has taken place.

8   Administer analgesics as prescribed for first several hours.
9   Advise patient that it may be weeks before full effect of surgery is determined as far as hearing is concerned. At first, hearing may be impaired because of tissue oedema, packing, etc.
10   Note that while patient may be ready for discharge in 4 or 5 days, packing is not removed until the sixth or seventh day, in the doctor's office.
11   Instruct patient as follows:
   a. Do not play football or box (but flying, tennis and squash are permissible).
   b. Do not blow nose.
   c. Protect ears when going outdoors for the first week and avoid loud noises.
   d. Avoid crowds or exposure to colds so that upper respiratory infection is prevented.

MÉNIÈRE'S DISEASE (ENDOLYMPHATIC HYDROPS)

Ménière's disease involves the inner ear and causes a triad of symptoms: vertigo, hearing loss and tinnitus.

Aetiology

1   Ménière's syndrome stems from labyrinthine dysfunction.
2   Suggested theories as to the cause of this syndrome:
   a. Increase in pressure of endolymph.
   b. Emotional or endocrine disturbance.
   c. Vasomotor changes causing a spasm of the internal auditory artery.
   d. Allergic manifestation.

Clinical Manifestations

During Attack

1   Dizziness, tinnitus and reduced hearing occur on involved side.
2   Patient complains somewhat of headache, nausea, vomiting, inco-ordination.
3   Sudden attacks occur in which patient complains that room appears to spin around.
4   Sudden motion of the head may precipitate vomiting.
5   Patient often presents a history of ear trouble, vasomotor rhinitis and allergies.
6   The most comfortable position for the patient is lying down.
7   Personality changes manifest themselves in irritability, depression, withdrawal and refusal to eat.
8   Vertigo attacks may last several hours or all day.

After or Between Attacks

1   Patient behaves normally; may continue his work.
2   Only complaint may be tinnitus or impaired hearing.

Diagnosis

Caloric Test.

1   Useful in differentiating Ménière's syndrome from intracranial lesion.
2   Fluid, which is above or below body temperature, is instilled into auditory canal.

3 Reactions:
   a. Normal patient—complains of dizziness.
   b. Patient with acoustic neuroma—no reaction.
   c. Patient with Ménière's syndrome—severe attack (as described above).
4 Nursing management:
   a. Anticipate possibility of patient vomiting; have emesis basin and protective draping.
   b. Support patient as he walks after the test, since he may be dizzy.

Medical Therapy

1 Initial treatment incorporates a low-salt diet and fluid restriction with supplementary diuretics when needed.
2 Low salt diet—about 800–1000 mg/sodium per day; if symptoms persist, lower sodium content (even down to 500 mg/day).
3 Administer vasodilating drugs, such as nicotinic acid (25–100 mg 6 hourly) cyclandelate (Cyclospasmol, 200 mg 6 hourly) or beta-pyridyl carbinol (Ronicol, 25 mg 6 hourly).
4 During the attacks, if vomiting present, dimenhydrinate (Dramamine) 50 mg 4 hourly) or prochlorperazine (Stemetil) 5 mg 6 hourly, may be prescribed.

Surgical Treatment

1 *Destruction of the labyrinth*—recommended if the patient experiences progressive hearing loss and severe vertigo attacks and cannot assume normal tasks.
2 *Ultrasonic surgery*—semicircular canal reached through a mastoid incision; ultrasonic energy applied directly via a probe to the bone in the canal (may cause transient facial paralysis).

Nursing Management

1 Recognize the need for encouragement and understanding; this is particularly true when the patient experiences symptoms of a subjective nature.
2 Remind the patient to slow down his bodily movements since jerking or making sudden movement may precipitate an attack.
3 Protect the patient who has an attack by placing him in a bed with bed sides in position; if he is standing, help lower him to the floor to avoid injury.
4 Postoperatively, patient may experience vertigo; therefore, he may be more comfortable in bed for the first 2 days.
5 Assist patient when he gets out of bed since he may be unsteady; remind him to change his movements easily.
6 Inform him that dizziness may persist as long as 4–6 weeks.
7 Note that a possible complication is Bell's palsy (a peripheral facial weakness with noticeable pain near the angle of the jaw or behind the ear. This will clear up eventually.

COMMUNICATING WITH A PERSON WHO HAS A HEARING IMPAIRMENT

When the Person is Able to Lip-Read

1 Face the person as directly as possible when speaking.
2 Place yourself in good light so that he can see your mouth.

3   Do not chew, smoke or have anything in your mouth when speaking.
4   Speak slowly and enunciate distinctly.
5   Provide contextual clues that will assist him in following your speech. For example, point to a tray if you are talking about the food on it.
6   To verify that he understands your message, write it for him to read. (That is, if you doubt that he is understanding you.)

When it is Difficult to Understand the Person when He Speaks

1   Pay attention when the person speaks; his facial and physical gestures may help you understand what he is saying.
2   Exchange conversation with him where it is possible to anticipate his replies—this is particularly helpful in your initial contact with him and may help you become familiar with his speech peculiarities.
3   Anticipate context of his speech to assist in interpreting what he is saying.
4   If unable to understand him, resort to writing or include in your conversation someone who does understand him; request that he repeat that which is not understood.

FURTHER READING

Books

Birrell, J F (Ed) (1977) Logan Turner's Diseases of the Nose, Throat and Ear, 8th edition, Wright
Ludman, H (1981) A B C of Ear, Nose and Throat, British Medical Journal
Miles Foxan, E H (1980) Lecture Notes on Diseases of the Ear, Nose and Throat, 5th edition, Blackwell Scientific Publications
Pracy, Siegler and Stell (Eds) (1980) A Short Textbook: Ear, Nose and Throat, 2nd edition, Hodder & Stoughton
Singh, R (1980) Anatomy of Hearing and Speech, Oxford University Press

Articles

Callery, P (1981) Nursing care study—tonsillectomy, adenoidectomy and bilateral myringoctomy, Nursing Times, 77: 1201–1204
Dickinson, T (1981) Dealing with the disadvantaged. Communicating with deaf patients, British Medical Journal, 282: 544
Honeysett, J (1981) Swimming aids for laryngectomies, Nursing Times, 77: 1045–1046
Journal of Community Nursing (1981) Special report on laryngectomy, Journal of Community Nursing, 5: 4–6 and 9–10
Ross, T (1981) Breaking through the sound barrier, Nursing Mirror, 152: 20–23
The Symposium (1981) Ear, Nose and Throat, The Practitioner, 225: 1545–1585
World Health (1981) Issue on oral Health, World Health, June

Chapter 3

EYE PROBLEMS

Eye Care Specialists   99
Normal Vision and Refractive Errors   100
Examination and Diagnostic Procedures   101
  Guidelines: Assisting the Patient Undergoing Schiøtz Tonometry   104
  Guidelines: Instillation of Eyedrops   106
  Guidelines: Irrigating the Eye (Conjunctival Irrigation)   107
Eye Injuries (Trauma to the Eye)   108
  Guidelines: Removing a Particle from the Eye   110
  Guidelines: Removing Contact Lenses   111
Inflammatory Conditions of the Eye   114
  Superficial Lid Infections   114
  Conjunctivitis   114
  Uveitis   115
  Sympathetic Ophthalmia   115
Corneal Ulcer   116
Eye Conditions Possibly Requiring Surgery   117
  Caring for the Patient Having Eye Surgery   117
  Corneal Transplantation (Keratoplasy)   119
  Detached Retina   121
  Cataracts   123
  Glaucoma   130
  Acute (Angle-closure) Glaucoma   131
  Chronic (Open-angle) Glaucoma   133
Further Reading   135

EYE CARE SPECIALISTS

Definitions

Ophthalmologist or *Oculist* is a doctor who specializes in the investigations and treatment of eye diseases and defects, performing surgery when necessary, or prescribing other types of treatment including spectacles.

Optician

1 *Dispensing optician* is a maker or seller of spectacles or optical instruments; one who makes and adjusts spectacles in accordance with the prescription of the oculist.
2 An *ophthalmic optician* specializes in sight testing and eye examination. He can prescribe glasses and recognize, but not treat, eye disease.

NORMAL VISION AND REFRACTIVE ERRORS

Vision

Vision is the passage of rays of light from an object through the cornea, aqueous fluid, crystalline lens and vitreous body to the retina and its appreciation in the cerebral cortex.

Normal Vision—Emmetropia

Rays coming from an object at a distance of 6 m (20 ft) or more are brought to focus on the retina by the cornea and lens, without the use of accommodation.

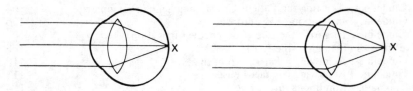

Abnormal—Ametropia

Errors of Refraction

Myopia—Nearsightedness

Rays of light coming from an object at a distance of 6 m (20 ft) or more are brought to focus in front of the retina.

Correction—Concave lenses.

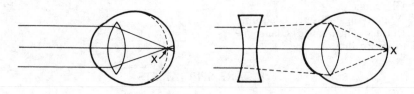

Hypermetropia—Farsightedness

Rays of light coming from an object at a distance of 6 m (20 ft) or more brought to focus on the back of the retina.

Correction—Convex lenses.

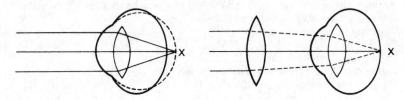

Astigmatism

Uneven curvature of the cornea. Causing the patient to be unable to focus horizontal and vertical rays of light on the retina at the same time.

Correction—Cylindrical lenses.

Accommodation

In accommodation, the focusing apparatus of the eye adjusts to objects at different distances by means of increasing and decreasing the convexity of the lens—the lens has the power of accommodation, the ciliary muscle is the muscle of accommodation.

Presbyopia

Near vision is impaired. Lens loses it elasticity with advancing years. Subject cannot focus near objects on the retina (will read at arm's length).

Correction—Convex lenses for reading and close work.

EXAMINATION AND DIAGNOSTIC PROCEDURES

External Examination

Includes examination of eye and adnexa.

Visual Acuity

Visual acuity is tested (using Snellen's Test Type) in all cases of eye emergency and on admission to hospital.

1   Each eye is tested separately, if patient wears glasses for distance vision, he is asked to keep them on. Note if patient is wearing contact lenses when testing vision.
2   Other eye covered by occluder.
3   Letters or objects are of a size that can be seen by normal eye at a distance of 6 m (20 ft) from the chart.
4   Letters appear in rows and are arranged from above down, so that the normal eye can see them at distances of 60, 36, 24, 18, 12, 9, 6, 5 m.
5   When a person can identify letters of the size 6 line at 6 m, his eye is said to have 6/6 vision.
6   If the letters of the size 60 cannot be read at 6 m, the patient is moved towards the chart 1 m at a time.

7 If the patient can read the size 6 line at 3 m, record as 3/60.
8 Additionally, if vision is less than 3/60, test may be taken with patient standing or sitting 1 ft from nurse/doctor as follows:
   Counting fingers—recorded as C.F.
   Hand movement—recorded as H.M.
   Light projection—recorded as L. Projection
   Light perception—recorded as L. Perception
   No light perception—recorded as N.L.P.

Visual Fields

To determine function of retina, optic nerve and optic pathways.

1 Equipment—Perimeter, tangent screen, light source and test objects.
2 Fields.
   a. Peripheral—useful in detecting disorders that cause constriction of peripheral vision in one or both eyes.
   (1) Patient is seated at a perimeter with chin supported on a rest.
   (2) Each eye is examined in turn, the other being covered by a spring occluder. The patient focuses with the unoccluded eye on a spot in the central portion of the perimeter.
   (3) A test object (white spot) is brought in from the side at 12–15° intervals throughout 360°.
   (4) The patient is asked to signal when he sees the test object.
   (5) The object is passed along the same meridian from the seeing to the nonseeing segment and the patient is asked to signal when it disappears.
   b. Central.
   (1) Patient is seated 1 m from a black tangent screen mounted on a wall.
   (2) Each eye is tested in turn for central vision, including the determination of blind spot and scotoma (visual field defect).

Colour Vision Test

Performed to determine a person's ability to perceive primary colours and shades of colour; it is particularly significant for individuals whose occupation requires colour perception: transportation workers, nurses, doctors, artists, interior decorators, etc.

1 Equipment.
   Ishihara colour test plates—32 plates in book form consisting of dots of primary colours printed on a background of similar dots in a confusion of colours.
2 Procedure:
   a. Various plates are presented to the patient at reading distance under specified illumination (usually daylight).
   b. The patterns may be numbers or a winding line which the normal eye can perceive instantly, but which are confusing to the person with a colour perception defect.
3 Outcome:
   a. Colour blindness—person unable to perceive numbers or winding lines.
   b. Red–green blindness—8% males; 0.4% females.
   c. Blue–yellow blindness—rare.

Refraction

A clinical measurement of the error of focus in an eye. In children.

1   Usually accomplished by instilling a mydriatic drop with cycloplegic effect (atropine or cyclopentolate) into the lower conjunctival sac.
2   The ciliary muscle is relaxed.
3   Accommodative power is lowered (cycloplegia).
4   The pupil is dilated (mydriasis), which facilitates the examination. In adults—no mydriatic/cycloplegic required.
5   The refractive state of the eye can be determined as follows:
    a. Objectively—via retinoscopy.
    b. Subjectively—trial of lenses to arrive at the best visual image.

Internal Examination

Ophthalmoscopic Examination

The interior of the eye is examined where a beam of light is reflected through the pupil, which is usually dilated with drops, but if undesirable, examination can be made through the small aperture. The examiner uses either a direct or indirect ophthalmoscope.

1   Defects that may be detected:
    a. Media—cataracts, vitreous opacities.
    b. Choroid—tumours, inflammation.
    c. Retinal blood vessels—pathological changes as in diabetics mellitus, hypertension, degeneration.
    d. Retina—detachment, scars.
    e. Optic disc (blindspot)—glaucous cupping.

Gonioscopy

Direct visualization of the function of the iris and cornea (angle of the anterior chamber).

1   Equipment—Local anaesthetic drops, gonioscope (goniolens), slit lamp (biomicroscope). Methylcellulose (artificial tears) drops.
2   Procedure:
    a. Local anaesthetic drop instilled into the eye.
    b. The gonioscope (goniolens) is placed over the cornea, methylcellulose drops instilled between the cornea and goniolens.
    c. The patient fixes his gaze as the examiner views the anterior chamber through the slit lamp.

Tonometry

The measurement of intraocular pressure.

1   Applanation tonometry.
    a. This is the most effective measuring method for determining intraocular pressure and used in combination with the slip lamp. A hand-held type is available for the patient confined to bed or domiciliary work.

   b. After instillation of local anaesthetic drops—amethocaine 1%—the cornea is
   stained with fluorescein.
   c. Record the intraocular pressure by registering the force required to flatten an
   area of the cornea. 'Normal' pressure of the eye using this method is between
   11–18 mmHg.
2 Schiøtz tonometry.
   a. After instillation of amethocaine drops 1% the Schøtz tonometer is gently
   rested on the cornea, the intraocular pressure is measured by indentation of area
   of cornea.
   b. The indicator measures the pressure in mmHg.
   c. 'Normal' pressure using this instrument is between 18–22 mmHg.

GUIDELINES: Assisting the Patient Undergoing Schiøtz Tonometry

Schiøtz tonometry is the measuring of intraocular pressure by means of placing a
sensitive instrument (Schiøtz tonometer, Fig. 3.1) on the centre of the cornea.
Normal reading: 18–22 mmHg. This procedure can be performed by a doctor or
nurse.

Purpose

To measure one of the diagnostic criteria of glaucoma.

Procedure

Preparatory Phase

The patient sits either in a tilt-type chair (tilted back) or lying down on examination
couch, and is asked to look upward.

Action	Reason
Performance Phase	
1 Amethocaine drops 1% instilled in both eyes.	1 This will produce corneal anaesthesia within a minute.
2 Place the sterile plunger of the tonometer gently on the centre of the cornea.	2 Pressure from the eye will be transferred to the sensitive measuring indicators.
3 Repeat for other eye.	
4 Ask patient to keep both eyes closed and with absorbent tissue wipe away any secretion.	
5 Tell patient not to rub his eyes.	5 The cornea is still anaesthetized; painful abrasions can result from the natural tendency to rub the eyes due to the unusual numb sensation.

Follow-up Phase

If the pressure is normal, advisable to have an eye pressure check at least every 2
years.

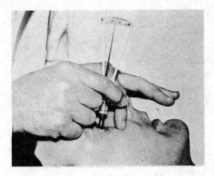

Figure 3.1. The Schøtz tonometer measures the ocular tension in mmHg. (Courtesy: F H Roy, MD.)

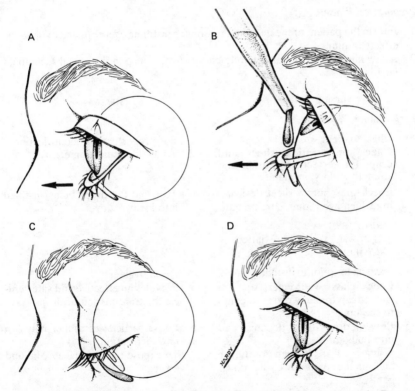

Figure 3.2. Administering eyedrops. a. Pull lower eyelid down—note arrow. b. Drop of medication is dropped into pouch. c. Ask the patient to look down as he gently closes his eye; keep eye closed for a minute or two. Medication is trapped next to eye. d. Normally the eye can retain only a fraction of the average eyedrop.

GUIDELINES: Instillation of Eyedrops (Fig. 3.2)

Purposes

1 To dilate or constrict the pupil.
2 To relieve pain and discomfort.
3 To act as an antiseptic in cleansing the eye.
4 To combat infection; to relieve inflammation.

Equipment

Prescribed drops.
2 × 2 gauze/lint squares or absorbent tissues.
Patient's prescription sheet.

Procedure

Preparatory Phase

1 Inform the patient of the need and reason for instilling eyedrops and explain the effects to him.
2 Allow him to sit with head slightly backwards or to lie in the dorsal recumbent position.

Nursing Action	Reasons
Performance Phase	
1 Check patient's name.	1 For proper patient identification.
2 Check prescription sheet and drops for correct medication and strength and expiry date.	2 To avoid medication error.
3 Check prescription sheet designating which eye requires treatment: RIGHT EYE ⎫ LEFT EYE ⎬ No abbreviations used. BOTH EYES ⎭	3 To avoid the drops being instilled into incorrect eye.
4 Wash hands prior to instilling drops.	4 Good hygiene.
5 Check glass eyedropper, squeeze rubber cap to allow drops to come to the tip.	5 Provides an effective and safe vehicle for transmission of drops.
6 Prevent drops from flowing back into bulb end.	6 Loose particles of rubber may slip into medication.
7 Using a swab between forefinger and thumb, pull lower lid down gently.	7 To expose inner surface of lid and fornix.
8 Instruct patient to look up (Fig. 3.2).	8 To prevent medication from going on to the sensitive cornea.
9 Instil one drop only into the centre of lower lid (lower fornix).	9 More than one drop at a time will overflow down patient's cheek.

Nursing Action	Reason
10 Ask patient to close both eyes gently—not to squeeze them.	10 Squeezing would express medication; closing allows medication to be distributed evenly over eye.
11 Wipe excess solution with swab.	11 Instruct patient not to rub eye.
12 Wash hands after instilling drop.	12 To prevent transferring microorganisms to self and other patients.

NOTE: Eye ointments are frequently used—procedure is similar to instillation of drops. Ointment from tube is gently squeezed as a ribbon of medication along lower eyelid, with care taken not to touch eye with end of tube. A separate applicator may be used to reduce contamination in multidose used tubes.

Follow-up Phase

Record on patient's prescription sheet—medication, strength, which eye, time.

GUIDELINES: Irrigating the Eye (Conjunctival Irrigation)

Reasons for Irrigating

1 To irrigate chemicals or foreign bodies from the eye.
2 To remove secretions from the conjunctival sac.
3 To provide moisture on the surface of the eyes of an unconscious patient.

Equipment

1 For small amounts of solution—an eyedropper.
2 For larger amount of solution—undine or plastic bottle with prescribed solution.
3 For copious use (chemical burns)—intravenous set with sterile normal saline.

Procedure

Preparatory Phase

1 Verify that you have the correct patient; check chart, address patient by name.
2 The patient may sit or lie in the dorsal recumbent (supine) position.
3 Have patient tilt head towards the side of the affected eye.

Nursing Action	Reason

Performance Phase

1 Bathe eyelashes and eyelids before irrigating the conjunctiva with prescribed solution at room temperature.	1 Any material on the lids and lashes can be removed before exposing the conjunctiva.
2 Place a receiver on the affected side of the face to catch outflow. If possible ask the patient to hold in position.	2 This involves the patient and gives him a sense of control.

Nursing Action	Reason
3 Evert the lower and upper eyelids.	3 The inner parts of the eyelids are less sensitive than the cornea.
4 Instruct patient to look up, down and from side to side when irrigating; avoid touching any part of eye with appliance.	4 To prevent injury—never touch the cornea.
5 Allow irrigating fluid to flow from inner to outer canthus along conjunctival sac.	5 This prevents the solution from flowing towards the lacrimal sac, duct and nose which would aid in transmitting infection.
6 Use only enough force to flush secretions from conjunctiva (allow patient to hold cotton wool near the eye to catch fluid).	6 Too much force may be injurious to the eye tissues. (Involve patient in his treatment).
7 Occasionally have patient close his eyes.	7 This allows upper lid to meet lower lid with the possibility of dislodging additional particles.

Follow-up Phase

1 Swab patient's eye (closed) and dry face with gauze or cotton wool.	1 Make patient comfortable.
2 Record type and amount of fluid used as well as its effects on the patient.	

EYE INJURIES (TRAUMA TO THE EYE)

Health Teaching and Preventive Measures

1 Appropriate glasses should be used for protection against very bright light, sun shining on snow, fumes of sprays or chemicals, etc.
2 Goggles should be worn if there is danger of flying gravel (power-mower lawn cutting), flying wood chips (while chopping wood), flying metal or glass particles (in machine factory).
3 Children should be reminded of dangers of sling shots, gun pellets, fireworks ('sparklers'), darts, arrows, etc.
4 Eyeglasses and sunglasses should have impact-resistant lenses.
5 Many schools and colleges have laws which require all students to use industrial-quality safety eye wear in workshops/laboratories.
6 Anhydrous ammonia used as agricultural fertilizer is a very destructive agent. Goggles must be worn when handling this chemical. Sufficient water should always be present.
7 Ideally, protective lenses or goggles ought to be worn when using a hammer, mowing the lawn, etc. They are also highly recommended in various sports—hockey, tennis, hunting, etc.
8 The Health and Safety at Work Act requires people in certain occupations to wear suitable eye protection.

Treatment and Nursing Management

1   Irrigate eye with saline solution, or universal buffer solution if chemical burns.
2   Have sterile fluorescein strips available for staining the cornea; the greenish dye facilitates detection of abrasion of ulcer.
3   Irrigate eye again with saline or prescribed solution.
4   Assist doctor in determining extent of injury; treat accordingly.
5   Encourage follow-up care.

Types of Eye Injuries

Acid or Alkali Burns

1   Prevalence of hair sprays and other spray products have caused an increase in the incidence of chemical eye burns (chemical conjunctivitis and keratitis).
2   Acid or alkali on lids or in eye creates an emergency.
3   Action
   a. Copiously flush the lids, conjunctivae and cornea.
      (1) Immerse patient's head in a bowl or sink filled with water.
      (2) Flush the eye with syringe if available, or
      (3) Hold patient's head with eye open under running water.
   b. Flush continuously for at least 15 min.
4   As soon as possible have a doctor see patient for further treatment.

Actinic Trauma

1   Excessive sunlight (or other strong light such as a sun lamp, bright sun on snow) can cause ultraviolet-ray damage to the cornea. Welder's flash or arc eye occurs when electric arc welders or welder's mate are exposed to the ultraviolet light.
2   Damage may be superficial and resolve in 48 hours; however, punctate keratitis may develop.
3   An ophthalmologist should be consulted immediately.
4   Treatment.
   a. Reassure patient.
   b. Instil anaesthetic drops (e.g., amethocaine 1%) as prescribed.
   c. Cover both eyes with eyepads.
   d. Report to ophthalmologist.

Contusions and Haematoma

Injury caused by blow with blunt object.

1   Haemorrhage into orbit from trauma (black eye).
2   Bleeding into tissues of orbit produces discoloration of lids and surrounding skin, resulting in swelling.
3   The eyeball itself may have sustained injury.
4   Treatment.
   a. It is best to refer all cases to an ophthalmologist for full examination.
   b. Apply cold compresses for first 24 hours.
   c. Then heat may be applied (at 15-min intervals during the day).
   d. Admission to hospital if serious injury to the eyeball.

Corneal Abrasion

1   Can be detected through staining with fluorescein strips.
2   Pain can be relieved with local anaesthetic drops or by eyepad over eye for 24–36 hours. Local anaesthetic drops, though very useful in relieving discomfort, can mask symptoms that may otherwise be noted. In some instances they also delay the healing process of the corneal epithelium.
3   Infection prevented by application of antibiotic drops and/or ointment.
4   A firm pad and bandage are placed over the closed eye for 24 hours to promote healing.
5   Complication to be guarded against—corneal ulcer (see p 000).

Foreign Bodies

Dust particles, tiny insects, etc., frequently cause considerable discomfort to the sensitive conjunctiva and cornea.

NOTE: All eye emergency patients should have visual activity checked in each eye both with and without glasses, as part of history taking and preliminary examination *prior to any* form of treatment.

GUIDELINES: Removing a Particle From the Eye (when it is lodged underneath the upper eyelid (Fig. 3.3))

Equipment

Local anaesthetic drops—e.g., amethocaine 1%   Saline
Corneal loupe (lens) and Binocular loupe (lens)
Fluorescein strips
Cotton wool applicator sticks
Antibiotic preparation—drops/ointment

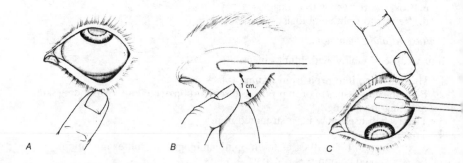

Figure. 3.3. Removing a particle from the eye when it is lodged underneath the upper eyelid.

Procedure

Nursing Action	Reason
1 As patient looks upwards evert lower lid to expose the conjunctival sac (see Fig. 3.3a).	1 Dust particles are often washed downwards by the upper lid.
2 With cotton applicator dipped in saline, gently attempt to remove particle.	2 Wipe gently across inner lid—from inside-out. Use binocular loupe if necessary.
3 If offending particle cannot be seen, proceed to examine upper lid.	
4 Ask patient to look downwards while you evert the upper lid, standing behind the patient.	4 Serves as a safety measure since cornea is away from area of activity. Looking downwards relaxes the levator muscle which is attached to the upper border of the tarsal plate.
5 Encourage patient to relax, move slowly and reassure him that it will not hurt.	5 This will prevent squeezing the eyelids shut, a manoeuvre which contracts the orbicularis muscle, making eversion of lid impossible.
6 Evert by grasping upper eyelashes with fingers and place index finger of other hand on outer surface of the lid; pull lid outwards and upwards and remove finger.	6 Particles may be washed under the lid; visual exposure assists in detection. Eyelid will remain everted by itself.
7 With cotton applicator moistened in saline, gently remove particle (see Fig. 3.3c).	

Nursing Alert: It is very important to take a history and record visual activity. Determine what the nature of the particle is—wood? (fungus infection may result); metal? what kind—magnetic? copper? was it a projectile?
If particle cannot be seen underneath eyelids, it may have become embedded on the cornea—examine cornea using corneal loupe. If seen refer to ophthalmologist.

NOTE: Always stain eye with fluorescein in case the particle has caused a corneal abrasion.

GUIDELINES: Removing Contact Lenses

Purpose

Since contact lenses are designed to be worn while awake, if a person is injured and incapacitated due to accident, sickness or other cause, the lenses should be removed.

Nursing Alert:
1 If the injured person is unconscious or unable to remove his lenses a (technician) optician or ophthalmologist should be called.
2 If expert professional help is not available and the lenses must be removed:
   a. Determine the type of lens.

(1) Small *corneal lenses* are most widely used. The diameter is less than the coloured part of the eye.

(2) Larger *scleral lenses* are worn by a few. These cover the front part of the eye.

b. *When not to remove lenses:* If coloured part of the eye is not visible when opening the eyelids, await the arrival of an optician or ophthalmologist.

Procedure

Preparatory Phase

1   Since the patient will undoubtedly be in the recumbent position, it is acceptable to remove the lens while he is in this position.

2   Wash your hands thoroughly.

Nursing Action

Corneal Lens

1   For right eye, stand on right side of patient so hands will have easier access to eye.

2   Lightly place left thumb on upper eyelid; right thumb on lower eyelid close to the edge and parallel with lids (Fig. 3.4a). Thumbs are placed in a leverage position on the eyelids.

3   Gently pull lids apart and observe if contact lens is visible (Fig. 3.4b). If contact lens is not visible wait for an experienced practitioner.

4   If lens is visible, it should slide with the movement of the eyelids while thumbs are still kept at the edges of the eyelids.

5   Gently open the lids wider beyond the edge of the lens and maintain this position.

6   Press gently downwards with right thumb on eyeball (Fig. 3.4c). This should cause the contact lens to tip up on one edge.

7   Then slide the eyelids and thumbs together gently (Fig. 3.4d). The lens should slide out between the lids where it can be taken off.

8   FORCE SHOULD NOT BE USED! Cornea may be irreparably damaged.

9   If lens can be seen but cannot be removed, gently slide it to the white sclera.

10   For left eye, move to left side of patient and repeat.

Scleral Lens

1   For right eye, stand on right side of patient.

2   Place left index finger parallel with and at the edge of the lower eyelid (Fig. 3.5a).

3   Press the lid downwards and backwards until the edge of the scleral lens becomes visible (Fig. 3.5b).

4   Maintain pressure but pull finger with lower lid towards the patient's right ear (Fig. 3.5c). This should cause the lid to slide under the lens. Avoid force.

5   Grasp scleral lens with right finger and thumb.

Soft Contact Lenses

May be removed by gently grasping them between the fingers. This is rarely necessary, since soft contact lens may remain on the eye for many hours without harm. An ophthalmologist can be called to remove lenses if the patient is unable to do so. Also

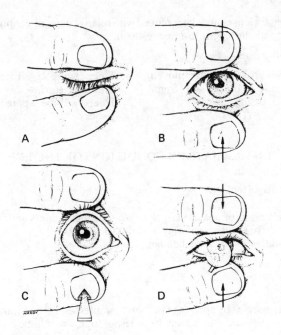

Figure 3.4. Removing corneal contact lens.

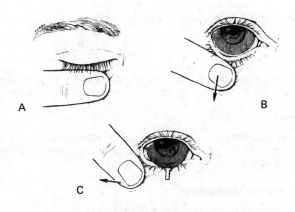

Figure 3.5. Removing scleral contact lens.

note: if the contact lens cannot be removed with relative ease, discontinue efforts and wait for the ophthalmologist to remove them.

Disposition of Lenses

1   When lenses are found and removed, place in a case or bottle; label 'right' and 'left'.

1   Since right and left lenses are often different, storing them with proper labels will be appreciated by the patient.

INFLAMMATORY CONDITIONS OF THE EYE

Superficial Lid Infections

Blepharitis—infection of eyelid margins, with crusting, redness and irritation.
   Hordeolum (stye)—infection of eyelash follicle.
   Chalazion—infection of a meibomian gland.

Treatment

Blepharitis

1   Cleanse lid margins by applying hot moist compresses three to four times daily.
2   Carefully wipe loose crusts away from lashes; apply antibiotic ointment and/or drops.

Stye

Apply heat, antibiotic ointment. Continue treatment for several days until infection clears. Keep patient's hands away from eyes and wash hands after eye care.

Chalazion

Chronic chalazion may require incision and curettage.

Conjunctivitis

Conjunctivitis is an inflammation of the conjunctiva resulting from an allergy, from bacterial, viral or rickettsial infection, or from physical or chemical trauma.

Clinical Features

1   Redness, pain/discomfort, swelling, lacrimation, photophobia.
2   Discharge, according to offending organism—abundant purulence indicates infection caused by pneumococcus or gonococcus.

Treatment and Nursing Management

1   Conjunctival swab to determine causative organism.
2   Bathe eye with saline. If profuse discharge, irrigation may be performed.
3   Instil drops, apply ointment as prescribed—to clear infection in 1–3 days.

4   Prevent dissemination of infection to other eye or other persons.
   a. Wash hands before and after treatment.
   b. Restrict washcloth and towels to infected eye and change frequently.
5   Give patient dark glasses to wear (*never cover with eyepad or plastic shade*).

Uveitis

Uveitis is inflammation of the uveal tract (iris, ciliary body, choroid).

Classification

1   Location:
   a. Anterior uveitis—iritis, iridocyclitis.
   b. Posterior uveitis—choroiditis, chorioretinitis.
   c. Panuveitis—entire uveal tract.
2   Granulomatous or nongranulomatous

	a. Granulomatous	b. Nongranulomatous
Location:	Any part, mostly posterior	Anterior
Onset:	Insidious	Acute
Pain:	None or minimal	Marked
Circumcorneal flush:	Minimal	Present
Course:	Chronic	Acute
Prognosis:	Poor	Good

Complications

1   Anterior uveitis—adhesions which impede aqueous flow, leading to secondary glaucoma. May cause cataracts.
2   Posterior uveitis—adhesions impede aqueous flow from posterior to anterior uvea, causing metabolic disturbances of the lens and leading to cataracts.
3   Retinal detachment may result from traction exerted on retina by vitreous strands.

Treatment

1   Directed to specific type of uveitis.
2   Atropine drops—to reduce likelihood of adhesions forming between iris and lens.
3   Steroids, locally—for anti-inflammatory and antiallergic action. Steroids, systemically, occasionally.
4   Analgesic—for pain.

Sympathetic Ophthalmia

Sympathetic ophthalmia is a severe granulomataus bilateral uveitis that may occur after any surgical or traumatic perforation involving the uveal tract. Rare, but *severe*.

Clinical Features

Photophobia, blurring vision and injection ('bloodshot') in sympathizing eye.

Treatment

1 Administer corticosteroids, locally and systemically, to reduce the amount of intraocular scarring.
2 Instil atropine drops to prevent adhesions between iris and lens.
3 Possibility of preventive enucleation of originally injured eye before sympathetic ophthalmia occurs.

Nursing Management

1 Understand the patient's condition and the objectives desired for him by the ophthalmologist.
2 Recognize the difficult decision facing the patient if enucleation approach is suggested.
3 Assess the psychosocial implications of the individual situation, offer sustaining support and collaborate in planning immediate and long term aims.

CORNEAL ULCER

Keratitis is an inflammation of the cornea, which when combined with a loss of substance results in *corneal ulcer*.

Clinical Features

1 Pain, marked photophobia, increased lacrimation.
2 Injected ('bloodshot') eye.
3 When a corneal ulcer progresses deeper to involve iris, iritis develops; pus forms in the anterior chamber and collects as a white or yellow deposit (hypopyon) behind the cornea.
4 If cornea perforates, iris may prolapse through cornea.

Treatment and Nursing Management

1 Prevention is much easier than treatment.
   a. Foreign bodies must be removed quickly.
   b. Corneal abrasions must be treated promptly.
2 Suggest the wearing of dark glasses to relieve photophobia.
3 Explain to patient that doctor may administer mydriatics preparatory to examining the eye, may instil topical anaesthetic to relieve pain and will instil fluorescein to outline ulcer.
4 Administer antibiotic or chemotherapeutic agent as prescribed for specific type of infection.
5 Apply heat to the eye.
6 Administer systemic antibiotics when prescribed.

Nursing Alert: Always question patient about allergies to medications, prior to treatment, whether topical or systemic drugs prescribed.

EYE CONDITIONS POSSIBLY REQUIRING SURGERY

Caring for the Patient Having Eye Surgery

Nursing Objectives and Management

To Understand the Psychological Effect of an Eye Problem on a Patient

1 Recognize that dependence on sight is exaggerated when faced with possible diminution or loss of sight.
2 Observe that the concern of the patient may be manifested as fear, depression, tension, resentment, anger and even rejection.
3 Encourage the patient to express his feelings in order to determine the underlying problems.
4 Provide diversional and occupational therapy to keep patient occupied mentally within the limits of his decreased vision so as not to accentuate his feelings of depression or despair over loss of vision.
5 Demonstrate interest, empathy and understanding, but try not to be oversolicitous.
6 Recognize individual differences which affect the method of dealing with patient anxiety.
7 Assure patient that rehabilitative programmes and personnel are available if his condition requires them.

To Assess the Physical Needs Which Have to be Met While Maintaining the Highest Level of Self-sufficiency

1 Always orientate the new patient who has diminished vision to his surroundings, his room and the people in his immediate environment.
2 Encourage patient to care for himself so that he will be self-sufficient and not feel that he is a burden.
3 Supervise him as he attempts to feed himself so that he does not become discouraged.
4 Promote proper elimination by adequate diet, laxatives or suppositories as required.
5 Provide a rest period daily.
6 For safety reasons, discourage his smoking, also reading and shaving—this is done by member of the health team.
7 Caution him against rubbing his eyes or wiping them with a soiled tissue or handkerchief.
8 Instruct him to wear dark glasses if he has had mydriatic eye drops instilled (e.g., atropine, cyclopentolate).
9 Maintain a safe environment that is free of obstacles such as footstools or loose rugs.
10 Doors should be completely open or closed.

To Assist in the Immediate Preoperative Preparation of Patient

1 In preparation for general anaesthesia evacuation of lower bowel may be ordered by glycerine suppositories administered night before operation.
2 Arrange long hair of female patient so that it may be conveniently out of the way.

3 Cut eyelashes of affected eye if ordered by doctor, using small, curved, blunt-ended scissors, blades covered with petroleum jelly so that lashes will adhere to them and not drop into the patient's eye.

4 Check local hospital policy regarding preoperative skin preparation; in many hospitals, this is done in the operating theatre.

5 Remove dentures, artificial eyes and any other prostheses before patient goes to the theatre.

6 The doctor may prescribe preoperative antibiotic eyedrops to reduce the risk of infection. An eye swab might also be ordered for culture and sensitivity.

7 Instruct patient regarding postoperative restrictions—no reading, no showers, baths or shampoos, no bending from waist or lifting heavy objects, no sleeping on operated side. Tell him he will have an eyepad, shield or both when he returns from the operating theatre.

8 Make sure the eye specified on the consent form and eye to be operated upon are the same, and marked by doctor—(skin).

9 Instil prescribed preoperative drops in the correct eye.

To Provide Optimum Care for the Patient Immediately Following Eye Surgery

1 Place patient in the dorsal recumbent position with a pillow under his head, or permit him to lie on unoperated side.

2 Position bed rails (cot sides) if policy of hospital—this offers the patient a sense of security.

3 Place a call bell within easy reach of the patient; have him call the nurse rather than risk stress or strain in an attempt to be self-sufficient.

4 Direct anyone who enters his room to announce himself; also, let patient know when you are leaving the room. Otherwise he may be left talking to himself.

5 Avoid disturbing the head with such activities as combing the hair; delay combing the hair until patient is allowed out of bed.

To Provide a Relaxing Convalescence

1 Consult ophthalmologist before recommending diversional or recreational therapy that is not fatiguing to the eyes—no reading; television in moderation; radio.

2 Recognize the soothing and relaxing effect of soft pastels for the wall and ceiling colours.

3 Regulate lights so that they are not too bright and do not produce a glare.

4 Inform patient before he leaves hospital regarding eye glasses, follow-up visits, type of work he can do and when he can do it.

5 Instruct the patient or family as follows on instillation of drops/application of ointment, and proper cleansing of eyes:
   a. Wash hands before and after treating eyes.
   b. To clean around the eye, use sterile wet gauze and wipe gently across lid from inner corner to outer corner.
   c. To apply medications, pull down lower lid, have patient look up and place eye drop in middle of inside of lower lid, place ribbon of ointment along the entire length of the inside of lid (from inside → out).
   d. Tape protective covering (eyepad or shield) over the operated eye at bed time.

6   Inform patient of large print books, talking book tapes, records, machines and where available.
7   Initiate follow-up visits with ophthalmologist. The nurse makes the first appointment for the patient.

Health Teaching and Discharge Planning

1   Measures listed above are pertinent for transfer teaching and learning for the patient, so that he may practise these at home.
2   Upon discharge from the hospital, check the following:
    a. Does the patient have a return appointment date with doctor confirmed?
    b. Does he have his medications properly identified and labelled? Does he (or a responsible member of family) know how to use his prescribed medications?
    c. Does the patient understand the restrictions placed upon him and the reason for them?

Corneal Transplantation (Keratoplasty)

Kertoplasty is the transplantation of a donor cornea to repair corneal scarring, or deformed cornea, as in keratoconus.

Types of Grafts

1   Full thickness—most common.
2   Partial thickness—lamellar.

Donor Corneal

Preferably cornea of donor eyes should be used within 48–72 hours after donation. A procedure—cryopreservation—is sometimes used. However, great care and handling is required when freezing to retain transparency of cornea.

1   Because an intact endothelium is required for ultimate transparency of corneal grafting, it is necessary in the preservation process to properly freeze, defrost and quickly use the graft to reduce the likelihood of damage to the graft.
2   Eye bank laboratories cut the cornea from the enucleated eye and place it in several solutions before freezing.
3   During defrosting, the cornea is gently rotated in a glass tube at a certain temperature for a certain period of time. When only a small ice ball adheres to the cornea, it is allowed to melt without shaking the vial.
4   Fluid from the vial is decanted and is replaced with fresh, diluted human albumin for several minutes before using immediately.
5   The technique described above requires trained skills.

Objectives of Treatment and Nursing Management

To Recognize and Alleviate the Concerns of the Patient Preoperatively

1   Psychological preparation for surgery is simplified because the patient is usually optimistic about the immediate transplant.

2   If cultural or spiritual concerns need to be voiced by the patient, the nurse, and possibly the hospital chaplain should be available so that the patient faces surgery in the best frame of mind possible.

To Keep Intraocular and External Pressure on the Operated Eye at a Safe Level

This is to protect the eye from loss of aqueous fluid or from injury because of the possibility of dislocating the newly transplanted cornea.

1   Prevent sudden turning of the head.
2   Minimize those activities or sources of irritants which may cause sneezing (dusting or sweeping, heavily scented flowers, sprays) (no pepper on meal trays).
3   Avoid conversation which annoys or disturbs the patient; caution visitors not to upset the patient, since emotional disturbances may increase his intraocular pressure.
4   Instruct patient not to sleep on operated side.

To Provide Rest for the Operated Eye in Order to Enhance the Healing Process

1   Apply eye coverings as ordered by doctor. Sometimes (rare these days) both eyes may be covered.
2   Recognize that healing is slow, due to the avascularity of the cornea.

To Utilize Measures that Will Prevent Infection of the Eye

1   Assist doctor on 'first dressing', and subsequent dressings by nurse in practising meticulous aseptic technique during eye treatment to reduce the possibility of infection.
2   Discourage patient from touching the dressings.

To Recognize the Differences Between Care Requirements of the Patient Having a Full Thickness Corneal Transplant and Those of the Patient Having a Lamellar Transplant

1   Full thickness type.
    a. May need longer bed rest.
    b. Restrict the patient's activities according to doctor's specifications: the patient may be fed, bathed and provided with bedpan/commode.
    c. Allow patient to raise his head slightly towards unoperated side.
    d. Initiate passive range of motion activities and deep breathing exercises to prevent circulatory and pulmonary complications.
2   Lamellar type.
    a. With doctor's sanction, help the patient out of bed and into chair.
    b. Keep the patient's eye covered according to doctor's orders.

To Implement Care that Will Prevent Complications

1   Avoid urinary retention by providing adequate fluids.
2   Prevent constipation or straining during defecation by avoiding constipating foods and maintaining adequate hydration.
3   Administer analgesics as necessary to relieve pain.
4   Report unrelieved pain since it may indicate that graft has slipped, that haemorrhage is occurring (hyphaema), or possible early infection, inflammation or postoperative (secondary) glaucoma.

5 Introduce additional activities gradually each day, but continue to avoid those which require straining.
6 Emphasize the importance of follow-up visits to ophthalmologist.

Nursing Alert: For eye patients requiring bed rest, e.g., following keratoplasty, injury, retinal detachment surgery, measures should be taken to prevent pulmonary and/or circulatory complications. This may include passive range of motion activities, antiembolic stockings, special positioning.

Detached Retina

Retinal detachment is the detachment of the sensory retina from the pigment epithelium of the retina.

Altered Physiology

1 The retina perceives light and transmits impulses from its nerve cells to the optic nerve.
2 Tears or holes in the retina may result rapidly from trauma, highly myopic subjects, systemic and metabolic conditions, degenerative process (e.g., macular degeneration).
3 A tear in the retina allows vitreous and transudate from choroid vessels to seep behind the retina and separate it from the pigment epithelium.

Clinical Manifestations

1 Patient complains of flashes of light or blurred vision due to stimulation of the retina by vitreous pull.
2 He notes sensation of particles moving in his line of vision (normally most individuals can see floating filaments when looking at a light background).
3 Delineated areas of vision may be blank (a relative scotoma); there is no perception of pain.
4 A sensation of a veil-like coating coming down, coming up, or sideways in front of the eye may be present.
    a. This veil-like coating or shadow, is often misinterpreted as a drooping eyelid or elevated cheek.
    b. Straight ahead vision (central vision) may remain good in early stages.
5 Unless the retinal holes are sealed, the retina will progressively detach and ultimately there is a loss of central vision as well as peripheral vision.
6 Retinal detachments do not cure themselves; they must be corrected surgically.

Treatment and Nursing Management

Preoperative Nursing Management

1 Instruct the patient to remain in bed as ordered by doctor; both eyes may be covered (according to doctor's request).
2 Ophthalmologist will determine proper position to be maintained according to the area of detachment; such an area must be in a dependent position if adherence is to take place.

3   Administer sedation and tranquillizing drug for comfort and relief of anxiety; explain what to expect preoperatively and postoperatively.

Surgical Intervention

Objective

To seal the retinal hole, thereby ensuring that the retina will adhere to the retinal pigment epithelium.

1   Possible types of surgery.
   a. Electrodiathermy—the passing of an electrode needle through the sclera to allow subretinal fluid to escape. An exudate forms from the pigment epithelium, adhering it to the retina.
   b. Cryosurgery or retinal cryopexy—a supercoated probe is touched to the sclera, causing minimal damage; as a result of scarring, the pigment epithelium adheres to the retina.
   c. Photocoagulation—a light beam (either laser or xenon arc) is passed through the dilated pupil, causing a small burn and producing an exudate between the pigment epithelium and retina.
   d. Scleral buckling—a technique whereby the sclera is shortened to allow a buckling to occur which forces the pigment epithelium closer to the retina by implanting a silicon plombe or encircling band.

Postoperative Nursing Management

1   Period of bed rest, covering of eye(s) with eye pad, shield, dark glasses and position maintained as according to prognosis or daily examination by the doctor.
2   Take precautions to avoid bumping the patient's head and causing the retina to detach further.
3   Allow additional activity according to progress following treatment.
4   Provide for diversional therapy, since this patient often becomes depressed.
5   Hospitalization ranges from 5 to 10 days.

Prognosis

1   Untreated retinal detachment progresses to complete retinal detachment and legal blindness in that eye.
2   Surgical reattachment by surgical intervention is completely successful in approximately 50% of cases. Secondary operations are usually required.
3   Return of visual acuity with a reattached retina depends upon:
   a. Amount of retina detached prior to surgery.
   b. Whether the macula was detached.
   c. Length of time the retina was detached.
   d. Amount of external distortion caused by scleral buckling.
   e. Possible macular damage as a result of diathermy or cryocoagulation.
4   Retinal tears that may lead to retinal detachment may be present in the other eye. These will also require surgical treatment.

Health Teaching and Discharge Planning

1   When he goes home, the patient is able to care for himself; he may not care for all bodily needs in an hurried manner, being careful to avoid falls, jerks and bumps.

2   It is advisable to stay home for the first several weeks to avoid accidental injury.
3   Watching television, looking at friends, and using eyes in straight line vision is harmless, but rapid eye movements, as in reading should be avoided for a few weeks.
4   For comfort of the eyes and eyelids, the use of a soft *clean* cloth, wrung out of hot water is most relaxing and soothing when applied several times during the day for 10 min.
5   The first follow-up visit to the ophthalmologist should take place in 2 weeks and other visits at longer intervals thereafter.
6   Within 3 weeks, light activities may be pursued; in 6 weeks, athletic and heavier activities are usually possible.
7   Acquaint the patient with the symptoms that indicate a recurrence of the detachment: floating spots, flashing light, progressive shadow; if they occur, recommend that he contact his doctor immediately.

Cataracts

A *cataract* is an opacity of the crystalline lens or its capsule; it is one of the leading cause of temporary blindness, particularly in the elderly.

Predisposing Factors

1   A cataract may be present at birth (congenital cataract).
2   May be due as a result of disease such as diabetes mellitus or trauma in young subjects.
3   Can be the result of poison (toxic cataract).
4   Most commonly, cataract occurs in adults past middle age (senile cataract) as a result of the ageing process.

Altered Physiology

1   Normally the lens is a semisolid body of clear, gelatinous protein encased in a capsule lying behind the iris, in front of the vitreous; the lens processes refractive powers (approximately one-fifth of the total).
2   Chemical changes in the lens protein may cause coagulation; as a result, the lens loses its pristine transparency and gradually become opaque.
3   Physical changes result in a swelling of the fibres, which in turn causes a distortion of the image.
4   Metabolic changes that reduce vitamin C and B_{12} in the lens may be instrumental in forming opacities.
5   Although a cataract may be readily diagnosed, the basic cause of a senile cataract is unknown.

Clinical Manifestations

1   Alterations in vision are noted.
   a. Objects seem distorted and blurred.
   b. Glare annoys the patient when there are bright lights.
   c. Visual loss is gradual, but eventually the opacity becomes complete.
2   The pupil, usually black, becomes grey and later milky-white.

Treatment

1 Surgical removal of the lens is indicated.
2 Proper time for cataract removal is determined by patient's eyesight, occupation, general health and convenience.
3 Usually a patient with one cataract can manage without surgery.
4 If cataract occurs in both eyes, he need not suffer blindness before he can be helped by surgery.
5 Following surgery and the healing process, the patient is fitted with appropriate spectacle lenses or contact lenses.
6 Intraocular lens implants may be implanted at the time of cataract extraction or as an independent procedure.

Traditional Surgical Procedures

Extracapsular Extraction

1 This surgery is conservative; it is simple to perform and may be done under local or general anaesthetic.
2 The lens capsule is incised and the lens matter is withdrawn.
3 Usually performed for traumatic cataract.
4 The posterior capsule is left in place. This may interfere with vision, and a second operation (a capsulotomy) may be required to produce a clear pupil.
5 A standard size incision (18–20 mm) is used.

Intracapsular Extraction (currently universally accepted method)

1 In this surgery, the lens as well as the capsule is removed through an 18 mm incision.
2 Cryosurgery may be used as the technique for this operation; a pencil-like instrument with a metal probe is cooled to about $-35°C$; when the lens capsule is available after dissection, the cryosurgical instrument touches the lens and freezes to it so that the lens is easily pulled out.
3 Approximately 5–7 days of hospitalization are required, although this figure is being reduced considerably and varies depending on the surgeon's preference, on the number and size of sutures used and on the patient's occupation and reliability.

Objectives of Treatment and Nursing Management

Preoperative Care

1 To make the patient comfortable in his new surroundings.
   a. Explain the plan of care.
   b. Escort the patient as he walks around the unit.
2 To allay his concerns, if he has any, regarding surgery.
   a. Determine how he feels about his operation.
   b. Assess his knowledge level regarding the purpose of surgery and his expectations afterwards.
   c. Encourage his questions and provide the answers.

3 To reduce the conjunctival bacterial count to minimize the chance of postoperative infection.
  a. Obtain conjunctival culture if ordered.
  b. Administer local antibiotics as prescribed.
  c. Employ aseptic technique in any eye treatment or procedure.
  d. Instruct patient not to touch his eyes.
4 To introduce rehabilitative measures that the patient will practise postoperatively.
  a. Following general anaesthesia, instruct patient to take deep breaths, move extremities without jerking his head.
  b. Point out the hazard of squeezing the eyelids shut. Teach him how to close his eyes slowly.
5 To prepare the eye to be operated upon in the immediate preoperative period.
  a. Instil mydriatic if prescribed.
  b. Note whether pupil dilates after instillation of mydriatic.
6 Determine whether a properly identified and executed consent for operation and anaesthesia has been obtained. There should be no discrepancies between the patient's understanding of the surgery and the informed consent for surgery and anaesthesia.
7 Administration of preoperative medications.
  a. Sedatives.
  b. Antiemetics.
  c. Narcotics.
  d. Ocular hypotensive agents (if intraocular pressure raised).
    (1) Cholinesterase inhibitors—acetazolamide (Diamox).
    (2) Osmotic hypotensives.
      (a) Oral–glycerine.
      (b) Intravenous—mannitol.

Postoperative Care

1 To prevent pressure build-up within the eye (intraocular) which may exert stress on the sutures.
  a. Admonish patient to refrain from coughing or sneezing.
  b. Advise patient to avoid rapid movement, but allow him to turn to the unoperated side.
  c. Admonish patient not to bend from the waist.
2 To promote comfort of the patient and reorientate him to surroundings.
  a. Allow patient to turn on unoperated side to relieve back strain.
  b. Offer analgesics as prescribed to control pain; report severe pain to doctor.
  c. Instruct those who enter room to announce themselves and to inform patient when leaving room.
  d. Provide a quiet environment to promote patient's relaxation.
  e. Allow patient to be ambulatory as permitted by doctor.
3 To control symptoms that may lead to serious complications.
  a. Sudden pain in the eye may be due to a ruptured vessel or suture and may lead to haemorrhage, iris prolapse or infection—inform doctor immediately.
  b. Nausea may lead to vomiting and increase intraocular pressure—administer antiemetic drugs as prescribed.

New Surgical Procedures

Phacoemulsification (Fig. 3.6)

1   Overview of this type of surgery.
   Phacoemulsification is the mechanical breaking up (emulsifying) of the lens by a hollow needle vibrating at 40 000 cycles per second.
   a. The needle tip moves forwards and backwards.
   b. It is powered by an ultrasound generator to produce the frequency necessary to emulsify the cataract.
   c. This action is coupled with simultaneous irrigation and aspiration of the emulsified particles from the anterior chamber through the needle tip.
   d. Only a 2–3 mm incision is required and the actual procedure takes 20–30 min (performed by a specially trained ophthalmic surgeon).
   e. Hospitalization of about 2 days is usually required.
   f. Normal activities may be resumed the day after surgery.
   g. Contact lenses can be used in about 3–6 weeks.
2   Criteria to be met for this operation.
   a. Pupil must be able to dilate fully.
   b. Anterior chamber must be deep enough to accommodate the manipulation of the probe-aspirator.
   c. Cornea should be healthy.
   d. The highly sophisticated phacoemulsifier utilizes expensive materials which are resupplied for each use.
3   Preoperative nursing management.
   a. Take advantage of the opportunity to discuss fears, concerns and any questions patient may have regarding his surgery, patient is usually admitted the day before surgery.
   b. Acquaint the patient with his surroundings and his plan of care; provide him with information regarding postoperative care, since this is more flexible and liberal than for other kinds of cataract surgery.
   c. Prepare the patient to receive oral glycerine and intravenous mannitol on the day of surgery, this is to decrease intraocular pressure.
      (1) Monitor vital signs and cardiovascular status.
      (2) Stop the intravenous infusion if untoward signs develop (shortness of breath, chest pain, etc.).
   d. Administer prescribed eye drops to dilate the pupil and to paralyse the muscle of accommodation (ciliary muscle).
   e. Administer sedation, antiemetics and/or narcotics as in intracapsular cataract extraction.
4   Postoperative nursing management.
   a. Remove the eye pad and patient is allowed out of bed when fully recovered from anaesthesia.
   b. Administer eye medications as prescribed; these may be to prevent infection and to keep posterior capsule in place.
   c. Offer analgesic if he is in any discomfort.
   d. Remind the patient to use his eye drops upon discharge from hospital, usually the first or second postoperatively.

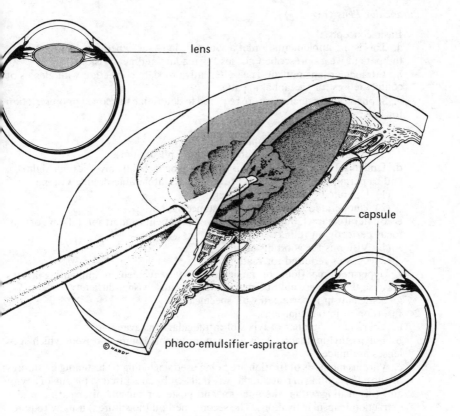

lens

capsule

phaco-emulsifier-aspirator

Figure 3.6. Cataract is shown in orb at upper left. Kelman ultrasonic needle (Cavitron Corps.) is inserted through 2–3 mm incision at corneal–scleral junction to emulsify lens cortex and nucleus and aspirate them. Drawing at right shows cataract removed and posterior capsule intact. Cataract surgery requires a 19–20 mm incision. (Copyright June 1975, the Amer. J. Nurs. Co. Reproduced with permission from Amer. J. Nurs., 75: No. 6).

    e. Explain the time plan for his permanent lenses and describe the need for and use of temporary lenses.

5   Considerations and possible disadvantages.
    a. The posterior lens capsule may later opacify; a percentage of these patients (25–30%) may require additional surgery—capsulotomy—perforation of capsule.
    b. The cornea may be affected by high frequency vibrations during operation, which may later cause degeneration of the cornea.
    c. Possible complications include infection, haemorrhage and fluid (aqueous) leakage from the eye.

Intraocular Lens (Fig. 3.7)

1   Basic concepts.
   a. This is the implementation of a synthetic lens—designed for distance vision, the patient wears prescribed glasses for reading and near vision.
   b. Intraocular lens implant is an alternative to sight correction with glasses or contact lenses for the aphakic patient.
   c. Sophisticated calculations are required to determine the power or prescription for lens:
      (1) Corneal curvature.
      (2) Depth of anterior chamber.
      (3) Axial length of eyeball (by diagnostic ultrasound).
   d. Unilateral cataract: objective is to leave patient slightly myopic (nearsighted), and to permit binocular vision, preventing an intolerable double vision.
      (1) Operated eye used for reading.
      (2) Unoperated eye is used for distance vision.
   e. Bilateral cataract: objective is to leave the patient emmetropic (all rays of light focus perfectly on retina).
      (1) Vision is for good distance.
      (2) Glasses required for reading.
   f. Hypermetropia (long or farsightedness) is avoided in implanting a lens because the image would be magnified and cause visual difficulty.
   g. Astigmatism is corrected with spectacles.
2   Insertion of intraocular lens.
   a. There are a number of types of intraocular lens available.
   b. Polymethyl methacrylate is a common durable compound from which such lenses are made.
   c. Various methods of fixation are being used, including (i) fastening by sutures or clips; (ii) holding in place in the way that a hub cap is fitted to the rim of a tyre; and (iii) sealing within the anterior and posterior capsule after extracapsular extraction (capsular fixation). The second method (no sutures) usually requires miotic eye drops (pilocarpine) to keep the iris from dilating too widely—thereby causing displacement of the implant.
3   Advantages of intraocular lens.
   a. Provides an alternative to individuals who cannot wear contact lenses or cataract glasses.
   b. Cannot be lost or misplaced like conventional glasses; does not need to be replaced.
   c. Provides a permanent form of near normal vision.
4   Complications (specific to implantation).
   a. Iritis or vitritis—can be controlled with steroids.
   b. Rosy vision, due to keeping pupil from full constriction; excessive light enters pupil, causing a dazzling of macula.
   c. Degeneration of cornea, chronic uveitis (see p. 115).
   d. Malposition or dislocation of lens.

Health Teaching

During rehabilitative phase of cataract extraction.

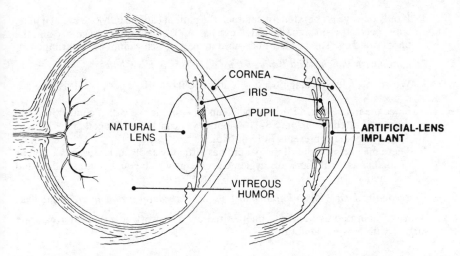

Figure 3.7. Illustration at left indicates position of natural lens; drawing on right shows artificial-lens implant following removal of cataract. (Newsweek—1b Ohlsson.)

To Encourage the Patient to be Independent

1 Assist patient in getting around his room, locating needed personal items, utilizing bathroom facilities.
2 Gradually increase his activities each day.

To Demonstrate to the Patient and a Responsible Member of His Family How to Administer Eye Medications

To Promote Patients Interest in Diversional Activities as He Recuperates Try to prevent him becoming bored

To Acquaint Patient With the Step-by-step Requirements of a Healthy Convalescence

1 The use of dark glasses after the eye dressings are removed.
2 Hospitalization—usually 5–7 days following intracapsular extraction.
3 Fitting for temporary corrective lenses for the first 6 weeks if prescribed.
4 Application of eye shield or pad over the eye at night to avoid accidental injury during sleep.
5 Prescription for permanent lenses 6–8 weeks after surgery for intracapsular extraction.
6 Prescription for contact lenses about 3–6 weeks after phacoemulsification.

To Assist the Patient in Adjusting to the Spectacles

1 If spectacles are to be worn they will be quite thick, causing the perceived image to be about one-third larger than that seen by the patient before cataract formation; peripheral vision is markedly distorted.
2 It is necessary to relearn space judgement—walking, using stairs, reaching for articles on the table, such as a cup of tea or coffee.

3 If only one eye is operated for cataract, the patient can use only one eye at a time, with spectacles, since the operated eye has a 30% increase in image size and the unoperated eye still has 'normal'-sized images, which cannot be superimposed.

To Familiarize Patient With Contact Lenses, if This is His Choice

1 With contact lenses, magnification is only about 8%–10%; peripheral vision is not distorted.
2 Since the image size difference between an aphakic eye with a contact lens and the unoperated eye is only 8–10%, both eyes can be used together.
3 Space judgement presents little difficulty.
4 There may be problems if the patient has difficulty applying lenses, has a tremor of the hands, or if there are hygienic problems which could cause swelling and infection.

To Recognize That With an Intraocular Lens Magnification Problems are Negligible

Both the operated eye and the unoperated eye can work together after cataract surgery with lens implantation.

Glaucoma

Glaucoma is a condition in which the pressure within the eyeball is higher than average; it is associated with progressive visual field loss. If allowed to proceed untreated, will lead to atrophy of the optic nerve and eventual blindness.

Incidence

1 Glaucoma is the cause of blindness in 1 of 7 persons who become blind.
2 The incidence of glaucoma is increasing as the number of elderly people in our population rises.
3 It is estimated that about 2% of persons over the age of 40 years in Britain have glaucoma.
4 Persons with family history of glaucoma are more susceptible than others.

Altered Physiology

1 Pressure within the eye is determined by the rate of aqueous production by the ciliary processes of the ciliary body, and the resistance to outflow of aqueous from the eye.
2 Inflow of aqueous is through the posterior chamber and pupil; outflow is at the meshwork located at the juncture of iris and cornea. Clogging at the meshwork by blood fibrin, or inflammatory cells account for the build up of pressure which produces secondary glaucoma.
3 Thickening of the meshwork appears spontaneously in those older individuals who appear to have hereditary predisposition; chronic simple glaucoma results and is the most common type.
4 When the iris is abnormally anterior and its root blocks the angle, cutting off aqueous outflow, pressure is increased—acute glaucoma results; this is the least frequent type.

Classifications

1 Primary glaucoma.
   a. Angle closure (narrow angle, closed angle, acute congestive glaucoma) —acute, subacute or chronic.
   b. Open angle (wide angle, chronic simple glaucoma)—chronic.
2 Primary congenital or infantile (buphthalmos, hydrophthalmos).
3 Secondary—due to other ocular disease, injury, neoplasms or following surgery.

Diagnosis

1 Because of relative ease of developing glaucoma, unless a person past 40 years has a complete medical (physical) examination periodically, including measurement of eye pressure (tonometry), the condition may not be discovered until it is considerably advanced (chronic simple type).
2 Tonometry (Fig. 3.1).
   A reading of 24–32 mmHg suggests glaucoma.
3 Gonioscopy—an examination of angle of eye, differentiates angle closure from open angle type glaucoma.
4 Tonography—application of electronic tonometer with a special device that records intraocular tension over a period of 4 min. Also gives indication of aqueous flow.
5 Water provocative test—breakfast is withheld, initial tonometer reading recorded. The patient then drinks one litre of water, and intraocular pressure recorded after 30, 45 and 60 min. A rise of more than 8 mmHg indicates poor outflow mechanism.
6 Examination of optic disc and blood vessels by means of ophthalmoscopy.
7 Visual field examination—perimeter or tangent screen.

Acute (Angle-closure) Glaucoma

Clinical Manifestations

1 With intraocular pressure increasing rapidly, severe pain occurs in and around eye.
2 Artificial lights appear to have rainbow colours around them (halos).
3 Vision becomes cloudy blurred.
4 Pupils semidilated and fixed; nausea and vomiting may occur.
5 Although onset may be insidious, severity of symptoms may develop within hours to include disturbances suggestive of gastrointestinal, sinus, neurological and dental problems as well as eye pain.
6 If untreated, irreversible blindness may result.

Medical Treatment

Miotic Drops (Parasympathomimetics)

Action—pupil contracts, iris is drawn away from cornea; aqueous may drain through lymph spaces (meshworks) into canal of Schlemm. Drops usually used:

Drops	Action	Effect and Precautions
Philocarpine hydrochloride	Acts directly on myoneural junction	Action lasts 6–8 hours
Carbachol (Doryl)	Acts directly on myoneural junction	Used if pilocarpine is ineffective
Physostigmine saliaylate (Eserine)	Cholinesterase inhibitor	Action lasts 6–8 hours. Allergenic, unstable, short in action

Carbonic Anhydrase Inhibitors

Action—restricts action of enzyme which is necessary to produce aqueous. Tablets that may be used:

Drug	Action	Effect and Precaution
Acetazolamide (Diamox)	Carbonic anhydrase inhibitor	Decreases production of aqueous
Methazolamide (USA only) (Neptazane) Ethoxzolamide (Cardrase) Dichlorphenamide (Daramide)		CAUTION: Side-effects— gastric disorders, shortness of breath, dermatitis, tingling of extremities, acidosis, ureteral stones

Hyperosmotic Agents

Medication	Action	Effect and Precautions
Intravenous mannitol urea	Reduces intraocular pressure, by increasing blood osmolality	Useful in treatment of acute attacks and preoperatively
Oral glycerol		Safer than intravenous method

Surgical Treatment

Peripheral iridectomy (sector or keyhole)—usually the operation of choice—an incision through corneal scleral junction so that portion of iris may be drawn out and excised.

Result: iris is prevented from bulging forwards and causing the angle at cornea and iris to be crowded. Consequently, drainage is facilitated and intraocular pressure is reduced and there is relief of pupillary block.

Others that may be performed: iridencleisis and trabeculectomy.

Chronic (Open-angle) Glaucoma

Clinical Manifestations

1 Insidious—mild discomfort (tired feeling in eye).
2 Slowly developing impairment of peripheral vision.
3 Possible halos around lights.
4 Progressive loss of visual field.

Treatment

Medical

1 Often treated with a combination of miotic drops and carbonic anhydrase inhibitors.
2 Remission may occur; however patient should continue to see ophthalmologist at 3–6-month intervals.
3 If medical treatment is not successful, surgery may be required, but delayed as long as possible.

Surgical

Surgery that may be performed.

Objective

To provide filtering of fluid in order to decrease intraocular pressure.

1 Iridencleisis.
2 Trephine.
3 Sclerectomy.
4 Cyclocryosurgery.
5 Trabeculectomy.

Nursing Management

Operative procedures are mainly performed under general anaesthesia.

1 Patient remains in recovery room until vital signs are stable and until he has orientated to time and place.
2 Administer analgesic or narcotics if required as prescribed.
3 Assist the patient in getting out of bed the first time: usually the patient is ambulatory the day after operation.
4 Provide adequate suitable diet to eliminate straining on defecation.
5 Remind patient of periodic eye check-up since pressure changes may occur.

Health Education

1   Even though glaucoma cannot be cured, it can be controlled.
2   Circumstances that may increase intraocular pressure are to be avoided, if possible.
   a. Emotional upsets—worry, fear, excitement, anger.
   b. Constricting clothing such as tight collar, belt, girdle.
   c. Exertion such as snow shovelling, pushing, heavy lifting.
   d. Upper respiratory tract infections.
3   Recommended activities.
   a. Exercise in moderation to maintain general well being.
   b. Moderate use of eyes for reading and watching television.
   c. Maintenance of regular bowel habits (straining on defecation causes increased intraocular pressure.
   d. Continuous daily use of eye medications as prescribed.
   e. Normal intake of fluids is not restricted even for alcohol or coffee unless these are known to increase eye pressure in the particular patient.
   f. Check-ups with ophthalmologist in order to keep condition under control.
   g. Wearing a medical identification tag indicating patient has glaucoma or glaucoma identification and treatment card, similar to steroid cards.

Nursing Care of the Nonseeing Patient

1   Upon entering the room of a nonseeing patient, address him by his name; use a clear, natural voice.
   a. Tell him your name and that you are a nurse.
   b. Indicate why you are there; do not touch him before he knows you are there.
   c. Inform his family and other visitors of this procedure when entering the room of the patient (or approaching bed side) so that he is not startled.
2   Acquaint the patient with his surroundings if he is in an environment new to him.
   a. If he is in bed:
      (1) Take his hand and show him how to find the call bell and how to use it.
      (2) Help him in using wash basin, soap and towel; tell him you have drawn the bed curtains when he should need privacy.
   b. If he is out of bed:
      Assist him to acquaint himself with his surroundings, chairs, bed, doors, bedside table and where his personal things are kept.
3   Guide him when walking.
   a. First, remember not to direct the visually handicapped person by steering him from behind—he may bump into things.
   b. Walk *slightly* ahead of him and have him place his hand in the space at the bend of your elbow, walk normally, at an *unhurried* pace.
   c. Describe where you are walking and inform him when you are going through a narrow passage or are approaching a curb, steps or an incline.
   d. Inform him that you are leading him to the bed, chair or toilet and permit him to feel the front of the object with his knees or hands.

Nursing Alert: Never permit a nonseeing patient to smoke in bed unattended. If he insists on smoking, have some responsible person remain with him until the cigar, cigarette or pipe is extinguished.

4   If for any reason a patient has both eyes bandaged (very rare these days) postoperatively, bed rails *may be used*, if so:

   a. Hold the patient's hand as you direct him to feel the side rails.

   b. Tell him the side rails are there to remind him not to attempt to get out of bed unassisted.

   c. Place the bell cord within easy reach and inform the patient that someone will answer his bell when he signals. If call light is multipurpose, place a piece of tape over the nurse signal area so that the patient can feel the proper switch.

5   Assist the patient in enjoying his meals.

   a. Read the proposed menu and have him make his own selection within his dietary prescription.

   b. Help him to assume a comfortable position when the tray arrives.

   c. Guide his hand to show him where the utensils, plate, cup, etc., are located. Describe food placement on the tray in terms of the face of a clock. If feeding patient, describe food; hot, cold, colour, flavour.

   d. Plan to have the various items of food always arranged in the same pattern on the tray, so that he will know for example where the salad, beverage, bread, etc., are. On his plate the servings should be placed in a specific arrangement so that he knows the meat, vegetables, etc., are in a certain place.

   e. Assist him by cutting the meat into bite size pieces, buttering the bread, adding sugar, milk/cream to tea or coffee. Permit him to do as much for himself as he can without embarrassing himself by spilling or knocking food onto the floor.

   f. Provide pleasant conversation or radio background music to make mealtime a satisfying time.

6   Gain his co-operation when he is taking medications.

   a. Tell him you have his medication ready for him; indicate how many tablets there are and that they are in a tiny medication container.

   b. Offer him half a glass of water or fruit juice to assist in swallowing the tablets.

   c. Tell him what the medication is for, if he asks.

7   Attend to the psychological and sociological needs of the person with no vision.

   a. Recognize that time does not pass as rapidly when one is inactive.

   b. When giving care, mention day of week, date, time and always involve patient in the conversation.

   c. Plan for him to have diversions that interest him—radio, talking books, braille books, visitors, television.

   d. Take time to stop and converse with him.

FURTHER READING

Chawla, H B (1981) Essential Ophthalmology, Churchill Livingstone

Chapman, E K (1978) Visually Handicapped Children and Young People, Routledge & Kegan Paul

Darling, V H and Thorpe, M R (1981) Ophthalmic Nursing, 2nd edition, Baillière Tindall

Dorrell, E (1978) Surgery of the Eye, Blackwell

Havener, W H and Gloeckner, S L (1972) Atlas of Cataract Surgery, C V Mosby

Jackson C R S (1975) The Eye in General Practice, 7th edition, E & S Livingstone

Klemz, A (1977) Blindness and Partial Sight, Woodhead-Faulkner

Last, R J (1968) Eugene Wolff's Anatomy of the Eye and Orbit, 6th edition, Lewis
Leydbecker, W and Crick, R R (1981) All About Glaucoma, Faber
Lim, A S M and Constable, I J (1979) Colour Atlas of Ophthalmology, Kimpton
Martin-Doyle, J L C and Kemp, M H (1975) A Synopsis of Ophthalmology, Wright
Miller, S J H (1978) Parson's Diseases of the Eye, 16th edition, Churchill Livingstone
Parr, J (1978) Introduction to Ophthalmology, Oxford University Press
Rooke, F C E et al. (1980) Ophthalmic Nursing, Its Practice and Management,
   Churchill Livingstone
Roy, F H (1975) Ocular Differential Diagnosis, 2nd edition, Lea & Febiger
Ruben, M (1975) Understanding Contact Lenses, Heinemann
Ryan, S J and Smith, R E (1974) The Eye in Systematic Disease, Grune & Stratton
Sachsenwerger, R (1980) Illustrated book of Ophthalmology, Wright
Saunders, W H et al. (1974) Nursing Care in Eye, Ear, Nose and Throat Disorders,
   C V Mosby
Stephenson, R W (1973) Anatomy, Physiology and Optics of the Eye, Kimpton
Thomas, P (1978) Pharmacology of the Eye, Lloyd-Luke
Trevor-Roper, P D (1980) Lecture Notes in Ophthalmology, 6th edition, Blackwell
   Scientific Publications
Vaughan, D et al. (1974) General Ophthalmology, 7th edition, Lang Medical

Articles

Bissett, P (1978) The six senses—1. Sight, Nursing Mirror, Supplement i-iv, 146, No. 1
Brown, N (1979) The A-Z of cataract treatment, Geriatric Nursing, 9: 55–59
Brown, N P (1978) Changes in the ageing eye: which are inevitable? Modern
   Geriatrics, 8: 49–54
Fitzpatrick, P J and Thompson, G A (1978) Diagnosing tumours of the orbit, Modern
   Medicine, 23, No. 4
Fletcher, D (1981) Intra-ocular foreign bodies—an eye for treatment, Nursing
   Mirror, 152: 34–35
French, E (1977) Glaucoma awareness prevents blindness, The Canadian Nurse, 73:
   21–25
Garston, J B (1976) Retinal detachment—3, Nursing Times, 72: 413–415
Hughs-Lamb, B (1981) Caring for the visually handicapped, Nursing, 28: 1221–1224
Kennedy, J and Heywood, M (1980) I see what I feel, New Scientist, 91: 386–389
Marsh, R J (1979) Ophthalmic herpes zoster, Nursing Times 75: 240–243
McAllister, J (1978) Displaced crystalline lens, Nursing Mirror, 147: 24–26
McMillan, G H G (1977) Occupational eye injuries—treatment in a nurse based
   service, Occupational Health, 29: 235–240
Mitchell, D R (1978) Treatment of eye injuries, Nursing Mirror, 146: 17–18
Murray, A (1979) The problem of glaucoma, Medical News
Ratcliff, G (1981) Perceptual disorder—there is more to vision than meets the eye,
   Nursing, 28: 1217–1220
Rowell, M (1981) Let me see the future, Nursing, 28: 1212–1216
Ruben, M A (1978) Nurses guide to contact lenses, Nursing Mirror, 147: 13–16
Short, J M (1978) Enucleation of the eye, Nursing Times, 74: 184–185
Smith, R (1979) The management of cataract, Medical News, March

Travers, J P (1978) Primary open angle glaucoma, Nursing Times, 74: 103–104
Traynar, (1981) Daycare cataract surgery, Nursing Times, 77: 1024–1025
Treplin, M C W and Arnott, E J (1978) Use of the microscope in ophthalmics, Nursing Mirror, 147: 30–33
Voke, J (1979) A case of spots before the eyes, Nursing Mirror, 148: 30–31
Voke, J (1980) Acting on impulse (colour vision), Nursing Mirror, 151: 35–37

Organizations

British Contact Lens Association, 51 Strathyre Avenue, Norbury, London SW16 4RF
British Talking Book Service for the Blind, Nuffield Library, Mount Pleasant, Alperton, Wembley, Middlesex, HA0 1RR
British Wireless for the Blind Fund, 226 Great Portland Street, London W1N 6AA
Catholic Blind Institute, Christopher Grange Centre, Youens Way, East Prestcott Road, Liverpool, L14 2EW
Greater London Fund for the Blind, 2 Wyndham Place, London W1H 2AQ
Guide Dogs for Blind Association, 9–11 Park Street, Windsor, Berks
Jewish Blind Society, 1 Craven Hill, Lancaster Gate, London W2 3EW
London Association for the Blind, 14–16 Verney Road, London SE16 2DZ
National Association of Deaf, Blind and Rubella Handicapped, 164 Cromwell Lane, Coventry CV4 8AP
National Library for the Blind, 35 Great Smith Street, London SW1 3BU
Royal Commonwealth Society for the Blind, Commonwealth House, Heath Road, Haywards Heath, Sussex
Royal National Institute for the Blind, 294 Great Portland Street, London W1N 6AA
The Royal London Society for the Blind, 105–109 Salisbury Road, London NW6 6RH

Chapter 4

MUSCULOSKELETAL CONDITIONS

Special Problems Associated with Orthopaedic Conditions	140
Pain	140
Deformity	141
Psychosocial Problems	141
Diagnosis of Musculoskeletal Disorders	142
Musculoskeletal Trauma	143
Contusions	143
Sprains	143
Joint Dislocation	143
Fractures	144
Casts	150
Guidelines: Application of a Plaster Cast	156
Guidelines: Removal of a Cast	158
Traction	160
Guidelines: Application of Buck's Extension Traction	163
Fractures of Specific Sites	166
Fractures of the Upper Limb	166
Fractures of the Lower Limb	171
Cast-Bracing	174
Fractures of the Lumbar and Dorsal Spine	175
Fractures of the Pelvis	176
Hip Fractures (Treated by an Internal Fixation Device)	177
Special Nursing Considerations	180
Nursing Management of the Patient Undergoing Orthopaedic Surgery	180
Lower Limb Amputation	182
Upper Limb Amputation	186
Hip Arthroplasty (Total Hip Replacement)	189
Total Knee Arthroplasty	193
Low Back Pain	194
Rheumatoid Arthritis	197
Guidelines: Paraffin Hand Bath for Rheumatoid Arthritis	204
Osteoarthritis (Degenerative Joint Disease; Arthrosis)	205

Malignant Bone Tumour   207
Osteoporosis   209
Osteitis Deformans (Paget's Disease of the Bone)   210
Further Reading   212

SPECIFIC PROBLEMS ASSOCIATED WITH ORTHOPAEDIC CONDITIONS

Pain

Types of Pain

1 Sharp pain—may be from bone infection with muscle spasm or pressure on sensory nerve; fracture pain is sharp and piercing, relieved by rest and immobilization.
2 Soreness and aching—due to muscular pain.
3 Increasing pain—due to progression of an infectious process or malignant tumour or to vascular complication.
4 Pain increasing with activity—may indicate joint strain.
5 Pain that is worse in bad weather, felt in more than one part of body—may be secondary to arthritis.
6 Radiating pain—rupture of intervertebral disc and pressure on the nerve root.
7 Bone pain—deep and boring.

Nursing Assessment

1 What activities precipitated the pain?
2 Is the body in proper alignment?
3 Is there pressure from traction, splints, casts, other appliances?
4 How does the patient describe the pain? Can he localize it?
5 Does it radiate? Is it continuous?
6 What relieves the pain? makes it worse?

Nursing Management

1 Position the patient in correct alignment.
2 Support the painful parts under the joints.
   a. Move the patient slowly and steadily.
   b. Avoid bumping the bed.
   c. Elevate the affected limb.
3 Apply heat to relieve muscle spasm.
4 Apply cold to relieve pain in inflammatory conditions.
5 Give analgesic, analgesic with sedative or muscle relaxant as indicated.
6 Evaluate vascular status.
7 Help the patient to become involved in his rehabilitation programme—muscle and joint exercises; promote early function, utilization of proper posture and gait.

Deformity

Types of Deformity

1 Contracture deformities are caused by limitation of movement and disuse.
2 Pain and muscle spasm produce limitation of movement.
3 Inflammation limits joint movement and causes fibrous tissue to form, producing fibrous or bony ankylosis (abnormal rigidity of joint).

Nursing Assessment

1 When was the deformity noted?
2 Was the onset accompanied by injury?
3 Is the deformity increasing? Decreasing?
4 Is paralysis present?
   a. What were the time and mode of onset of paralysis?
   b. Are there sensory disturbances?
   c. Where is the paralysis located?
   d. Are there trophic changes?
   e. Is there any disturbance in control of bladder and bowel?

Nursing Management

1 Position the patient in accordance with principles of body mechanics.
2 Ensure that there is a firm base for the patient to lie on. Secure a monkey pole.
3 Avoid semirecumbent position for prolonged periods—promotes flexion deformities of the hip.
4 Encourage and assist patient to perform passive and active exercises—to maintain and improve muscle strength, maintain and restore optimal joint function, prevent deformities, stimulate circulation and build endurance.

Psychosocial Problems

Types of Psychosocial Problems (from prolonged periods of disability)

1 Immobility. (Patients tend to become depressed when mobility is restricted and tend to improve when the treatment programme is modified to permit some movement.)
2 Economic problems.
3 Depression.

Nursing Management

1 Encourage and reassure the patient.
2 Keep the patient busy—activity helps to prevent anxiety.
3 Develop a programme of activity to include both physiotherapy and occupational therapy to promote feelings of independence.
4 Encourage group activities.

DIAGNOSIS OF MUSCULOSKELETAL DISORDERS

Patient's History

How does the patient describe his problem and how it affects him.

Physical Examination

1   Observation for muscle atrophy or swelling.
2   Observation of gait and posture.
3   Examination of joints—shape, alignment, circumference, range of motion, stability, instability, presence of abnormal joint fluid.
4   Evaluation of bone—integrity, size, tenderness, masses.
5   Palpation for skin temperature, local swelling, tenderness.
6   Measurement of muscle strength, length of extremities, circumference of extremities.
7   Neurological evaluation—including cranial nerve testing, motor and sensory nerve testing, reflexes of extremities (frequently have orthopaedic significance).
8   Vascular assessment—peripheral pulses.

X-ray

1   Of bone—to determine bone density, texture, erosion, changes in bone relationships.
2   Of cortex—to detect any widening, narrowing, irregularity.
3   Of medullary cavity—to detect any alteration in density.
4   Of involved joint—to show fluid, irregularity, spur formation, narrowing, changes in joint contour.

Special X-ray Techniques

1   Tomography—shows in detail a specific plane of involved bone.
2   Myelography—injection of radiopaque dye into subarachnoid space at lumbar spine (to determine level of disc prolapse or site of tumour).
3   Arthrography—injection of radiopaque substance or air into joint cavity—outlines soft tissue structures and contour of joint.

Electromyography (EMG)

See p. 5.

Bone Scanning

Parenteral injection of bone-seeking radioactive isotope; increased concentration of isotope uptake revealed in primary skeletal disease (osteosarcoma), metastatic bone disease, inflammatory skeletal disease (osteomyelitis).

Arteriography

May localize disc disease where myelogram may be negative; useful in tumour surgery.

Computed tomography

Noninvasive x-ray that localizes pathology of bone and surrounding soft tissues.

MUSCULOSKELETAL TRAUMA

Contusions

A *contusion* is an injury to the soft tissue produced by a blunt force, blow, kick or fall.

Clinical Features

1   Haemorrhage into injured part (ecchymosis)—from rupture of small blood vessels; also associated with fractures.
2   Pain, swelling and discoloration.

Treatment

1   Elevate the affected part.
2   Apply cold compresses—to produce vasoconstriction and decrease oedema.
3   Apply pressure bandage (elastic or elastic adhesive)—to reduce swelling and oedema.
4   Apply heat to affected area after 6 hours—to promote absorption.

Sprains

A *sprain* is an injury to ligamentous structures surrounding a joint and is usually caused by a wrenching or twisting force.

Clinical Features

1   Rapid swelling—due to extravasation of blood within tissues.
2   Pain upon movement of joint.

Treatment

1   X-ray injured area—to ensure there is no bone injury.
2   Elevate and rest affected part.
3   Apply cold compresses (or ice bag) intermittently for 12–36 hours—vasoconstricting effects of cold retard extravasation of blood and lymph (oedema) and suppress pain.
4   After 24 hours apply mild heat and a compression bandage if indicated.
5   For more severe sprain (tearing of fibres and disruption of ligaments) patient may require surgical repair and/or cast immobilization so that joint will not lose its stability.

Joint Dislocation

A *dislocation of a joint* is a condition in which the articular surfaces of the bones forming the joint are no longer in contact (bones are 'out of joint').

Classification

1 Congenital (hip most often affected).
2 Pathological or spontaneous—from disease of articular or periarticular structures.
3 Traumatic—from injury.

Clinical Features

1 Pain.
2 Change in contour of the joint.
3 Shortening of limb.
4 Loss of normal movement.
5 Change in axis of dislocated bones.

Treatment

1 X-ray affected part—to rule out associated fracture.
2 Immobilize part while patient is transported to accident department.
3 Reduce dislocation (bring displaced parts to normal position—usually under anaesthesia).
4 Essentials of nursing management are the same as for reduction of fractures (see p. 145).

Fractures

A *fracture* is a break in the continuity of bone.

Classification of Fractures (Fig. 4.1)

General Classification

1 Complete—a fracture involving the entire cross section of the bone; usually displaced.
2 Incomplete—a fracture involving only a portion of the cross section of bone; usually undisplaced.
3 Open—there is communication between the fracture and the skin (formerly called compound fracture).
4 Closed—the fracture does not communicate with outside area (formerly called simple fracture).

Specific Types of Fractures (Fig. 4.1)

1 Greenstick—a fracture in which one side of a bone is broken and the other side is bent.
2 Transverse—the fracture is straight across the bone.
3 Oblique—a fracture occurring at an angle across the bone (less stable than transverse).
4 Spiral—a fracture twisting around the shaft of the bone.
5 Comminuted—a fracture in which bone has splintered into several fragements.
6 Complicated—where a nerve, tendon, blood vessel or organ may be damaged by the fracture.

7   Depressed—a fracture in which fragment(s) is (are) in-driven (seen frequently in fractures of skull and facial bones).
8   Impacted—a fracture in which the fractured bone has been compressed by another bone(s) (seen in vertebral fractures).
9   Pathological—a fracture that occurs through an area of diseased bone (bone cyst, Paget's disease, bony metastasis).
10 Avulsion—fragment of bone pulled off by ligament or tendon and its attachment.

Clinical Manifestations

1   Pain—continues with increasing severity until bone fragments are immobilized.
2   Loss of function; inability to use the part.
3   Localized swelling and discoloration of the skin—from trauma and from haemorrhage that follows.
4   Deformity (visible or palpable).
5   False motion; abnormal mobility.
6   Crepitation—grating sensation felt upon examination, due to rubbing together of the fragments (testing for crepitation can produce further tissue damage).
7   In open fracture bone may be visible through skin.

Emergency Management

See Volume 1, Chapter 5, Emergency Nursing.

Treatment

Reduction (setting the bone)

Objectives

To regain the function of the involved part.
To regain and maintain correct position and alignment.
To return patient to his usual activities in the shortest time and at the least expense.

1   Restore, as nearly as possible, the fracture fragments to anatomical alignment.
2   Methods.
  a. Closed reduction—bringing the bony fragments into apposition (ends in contact) by manipulation and traction (most commonly used to restore alignment).
    (1) Usually done under anaesthesia—to relieve pain and relax muscles.
    (2) Cast is usually applied—to immobilize limb and maintain reduction.
  b. *Traction*—applying force in two directions to obtain reduction and regain normal length and alignment.
    (1) May be used for fractures of long bones.
    (2) Traction applied to limb by:
      (a) Skin traction—by means of extension plaster.
      (b) Skeletal traction—by means of wires, pins or tongs placed through bone.
    (3) For nursing management see under Traction, pp. 161–163
  c. *Open reduction* (open operation)—operative intervention to achieve fracture reduction.
    (1) Bone fragments are replaced under direct vision.
    (2) Internal fixation devices (metal pins, wires, screws, plates, nails, rods) may

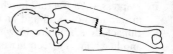

Simple (closed) fracture
— No open wound

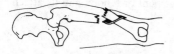

Compound (open) fracture—Wound in
skin communicates with fracture

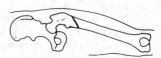

Extracapsular fracture—Bone broken
outside joint

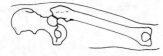

Intracapsular fracture—Bone broken
inside joint

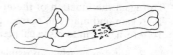

Comminuted fracture—Bone
splintered into fragments

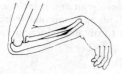

Greenstick fracture—Bone broken,
bent but still securely hinged at one
side

Longitudinal fracture—Break runs
parallel with bone

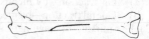

Figure 4.1. Types of fractures. (From: Nursing Care of the Patient in the O.R. Somerville, New Jersey, Ethicon, Inc.)

Transverse fracture—Break runs across bone

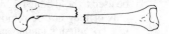

Oblique fracture—Break runs in slanting direction on bone

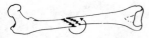

Spiral fracture—Break coils around bone

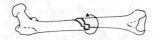

Pathologic fracture—Break is at site of bone disease

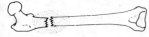

Impacted fracture—Bone broken and wedged into other break

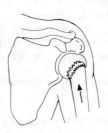

Fracture dislocation—Break complicated by bone out of joint

Depressed fracture—Broken skull bone driven inward

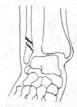

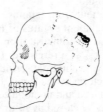

Figure 4.1. (continued).

be used to hold bone fragments in position until solid bone healing occurs (they may or may not be removed after bony union has taken place).
(3) For nursing management following open reduction, see Nursing Management of the Patient Undergoing Orthopaedic Surgery, pp. 180–182.
d. *Prosthetic replacement.*

Immobilization

1   Maintains reduction in place until healing occurs.
2   Methods:
   a. *External fixation.*
   (1) Plaster cast fixation.   (3) Continuous traction.
   (2) Splints.   (4) Pin and plaster technique.
   b. *Internal fixation.*
   Internal fixation devices (nails, plates, screws, wires, rods).
3   Nursing observation. Increasing pain following reduction of a fracture may indicate an ill-fitting cast or splint.

Rehabilitation

Regaining normal function of the affected part.

1   Instruct the patient to actively exercise joints above and below the cast at frequent intervals.
   a. Isometric exercises of muscles covered by cast—start exercise as soon as possible after cast application.
   b. Increase isometric exercises as fracture stabilizes.
2   After removal of cast, have patient start active exercises and continue with isometric exercises. See p. 156.
3   Instruct patient in methods of ambulation—frames, crutches, walking stick.

Treatment of Open Fractures

Objectives

To minimize chance of infection of wound, soft tissue injury and bone.
To promote soft tissue and bone healing.

1   Cleanse and debride the wound—to minimize chance of infection, debridement should be done as soon as possible.
   Take swabs for culture and sensitivity of wound, or organisms which may inhabit the wound.
2   Protect the patient from tetanus.
   a. Determine patient's status of immunization for tetanus.
   b. See schedule of administration Volume 1, Chapter 5.
3   Give antibiotics as prescribed (usually intravenous antibiotics are started quickly)—to avoid and treat serious infection; many open fractures are contaminated with bacteria at the time of admission.
4   Fracture is reduced and immobilized by cast, splint, traction or internal fixation.
   a. Wound may be closed by suture or by autogenous skin or flap graft; or it may be left open, especially when heavily contaminated.
   b. Soft tissue repairs (muscles, nerves, tendons) may be carried out.

5   Elevate injured extremity until initial swelling begins to subside.
   a. Examine and watch distal parts for evidence of ischaemia or neurovascular problems.
   b. Observe and record patient's temperature at regular intervals—for septic complications (gas gangrene, etc.).

Complications of Fractures

Immediate Complications

1   Shock—bone is very vascular; following trauma, large amounts of blood escape from circulating blood into soft tissues or through open wounds (especially in femoral and pelvic fractures).
   a. May be fatal within a few hours after injury.
   b. Treatment.
      (1) Maintain airway.
      (2) Maintain arterial blood pressure; replace depleted blood volume and correct electrolyte imbalance.
      (3) Control pain.
2   Haemorrhage.
3   Fat embolism.
   a. May occur after severe multiple fractures, particularly of the long bones (femur and tibia) and pelvis.
   b. After injury numerous fat globules appear in the bloodstream and act as emboli; abnormalities may develop in any part of the body, producing lethal changes in brain, lungs, heart.
   c. Assess patient for:
      (1) Tachycardia.
      (2) Fever.
      (3) Increasing respiratory rate, precordial chest pain, râles, wheezing, cough, dyspnoea, acute pulmonary oedema.
      (4) Cerebral symptoms—agitation, confusion, stupor, and coma—from fat emboli in the brain (may be first sign).
      (5) Petechiae (if systemic embolization has occurred)—in buccal membranes, conjunctival sacs, on the hard palate, on the fundus of the eyes and over the chest and anterior axillary folds.
      (6) Fat globules in urine.
   d. Treatment:

Nursing Alert: Personality changes, restlessness, irritability or confusion in a patient with fractures is an indication that immediate blood gas studies should be done.

Objectives

To correct homoeostatic disturbances.
To support the respiratory system.

   (1) Draw arterial blood for gas analysis—helps determine treatment and is a means for following the degree and progress of respiratory impairment.
   (2) Administer oxygen as indicated by results of blood gas analysis (respiratory failure is the most common cause of death).

(3) Assist with endotracheal intubation (for airway control); controlled volume ventilation and positive end-expiratory pressure (to decrease and inhibit formation of pulmonary oedema).

(4) Administer steroids—to control cerebral oedema; may be effective in management of pulmonary complications by decreasing inflammation in the alveolar membranes.

(5) Give low molecular weight dextran—improves pulmonary and systemic capillary flow by its desludging effect.

(6) Other modalities of treatment may (or may not) include:

(a) Diuretics (ethacrynic acid; frusemide)—for treatment of pulmonary oedema.

(b) Heparin—aids in prevention of platelet aggregation and blood coagulation; *may not be given*, since heparin increases lipase activity and therefore increases free fatty acid formation in lung parenchyma.

(7) Check immobilization devices (i.e., traction).

4 Thromboembolism (particularly of fractures of lower extremities).

5 Infection—all open fractures are considered contaminated. (See also gas gangrene and tetanus, Volume 1, Chapter 5.

6 Disseminated intravascular coagulation (DIC)—a group of bleeding states with diverse causes.

a. Many serious illnesses predispose to DIC, including massive tissue trauma.

b. Clinical manifestations: unexpected bleeding during or after surgery, ecchymosis, anaemia; patient may bleed from mucous membranes, venipuncture sites, gastrointestinal and urinary tracts.

c. Laboratory evaluation shows low fibrinogen, prolonged prothrombin and partial thromboplastin times, low factor VIII and thrombocytopaenia.

d. Treatment:

Objective

To control underlying disease. See Volume 2, Chapter 2 for treatment of DIC.

7 Peripheral nerve injury—bone ends may injure nerves.

Delayed Complications of Fractures

1 Delayed union—signifies that a specific fracture has not healed in the time considered average for this fracture.

2 Nonunion—failure of the ends of a fractured bone to unite (and union not expected to occur).

3 Avascular necrosis of bone—may occur when bone loses its blood supply following fracture or dislocation (notably in the hip) or in certain diseases.

CASTS

A *cast* is an immobilizing device consisting of layers of plaster bandages, fibreglass or resin impregnated bandages. Plaster of paris is manufactured from an inorganic material—anhydrous calcium sulphate (Gypsum). The new splinting materials require a slightly different technique in application.

Purposes

1   To immobilize and hold bone fragments in reduction.
2   To apply uniform compression of soft tissues.
3   To permit early weight-bearing activities.
4   To correct chronic deformities with wedging or special hinges or by serial cast changes.

Types of Casts (Fig. 4.2)

1   *Below elbow cast*—extends from below the elbow to the proximal palmar crease.
2   *Scaphoid cast*—extends from below the elbow to the proximal palmar crease, including the thumb (thumb spica).
3   *Above elbow cast*—extends from upper level of axillary fold to proximal palmar crease; elbow usually immobilized at right angle.
4   *Below knee cast*—extends from below knee to base of toes.
5   *Long leg (above knee) cast*—extends from junction of the upper and middle third of thigh to the base of toes; foot is at right angle in a neutral position.
6   *Spica or body cast*—incorporates the trunk and an extremity.
   a. *Shoulder spica cast*—a body jacket that encloses trunk and shoulder and elbow.
   b. *Hip spica cast*—encloses trunk and lower extremity.
   (1) Single hip spica—extends from nipple line to include pelvis and one thigh.
   (2) Double hip spica extends from nipple line or upper abdomen to include pelvis and extends to include both thighs and lower legs.
   (3) One-and-a-half hip spica—extends from upper abdomen, includes one entire leg, and extends to the knee of the other.

Application of Cast

See p. 156.

Complications

Constriction of Circulation
Trauma or surgery affecting a limb will produce swelling due to haemorrhage from bone and surrounding tissue and to tissue oedema. Vascular insufficiency due to unrelieved swelling can cause a reduction in or obliteration of blood supply to a limb.

1   *Symptoms and signs:*
   a. *Unrelieved pain or increasing pain.*
   b. Swelling.
   c. Blanching or discoloration.
   (1) Test nail beds and pulp of digits of injured limb for prompt capillary return. A rapid return of colour should appear on release of pressure.
   (2) The colour should be pink; blueness suggests venous obstruction.
   (3) Whiteness and cold fingers or toes suggest arterial obstruction.
   (4) Compare uninjured with injured limb.
   d. Tingling or numbness.
   e. No pulse or diminished pulse.
   Compare pulse on uninjured limb with that of injured limb.

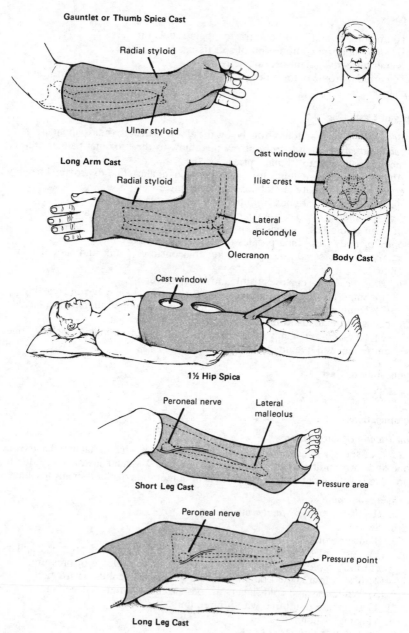

Figure 4.2. Pressure areas in different types of casts.

f. Inability to move fingers or toes; pain on extension of foot or hand may indicate ischaemia.

g. Temperature change of skin—cold extremity may indicate ischaemia.

2 *Nursing management:*

a. Bivalve the cast; split cast on each side over its full length into halves.

b. Cut the underlying padding—blood-soaked padding may shrink and cause constriction of circulation.

c. Spread cast sufficiently to relieve constriction.

Pressure of Cast on Tissues, Especially on Bony Parts

1 Causes necrosis, pressure sores, nerve palsies from prolonged pressure on nerve trunk.

2 *Symptoms:*

Severe initial pain over bony prominences; this is a warning symptom of an impending pressure sore. *Pain decreases when ulceration occurs.*

3 *Pressure sites:*

a. *Lower extremity*—heel, malleoli, dorsum of foot, head of fibula, anterior surface of patella.

b. *Upper extremity*—medial epicondyle of humerus, ulnar styloid.

c. When plaster jackets or body spica casts are used—sacrum, anterior and superior iliac spines, vertebral borders of scapulae.

4 *Nursing management:*

a. Examine the skin over the area by creating a 'window' in the plaster at the pain point (over bony prominence).

b. Or bivalve the cast but do not disturb the alignment; keep extremity in one portion of bivalved cast.

Nursing Alert: Do not ignore the complaint of pain of the patient in a cast. Suspect circulatory complications or a pressure sore.

Care of Patient While Cast Dries

Limb Cast

1 Explain to the patient that he will experience the feeling of heat under the plaster; however, plaster application is not painful.

2 Leave area enclosed in cast *uncovered* until the cast is dry—covers restrict escape of heat, especially in large casts.

3 Elevate limb on plastic covered pillow once the cast has set.

4 Avoid resting on hard surfaces or sharp edges that can cause denting of the cast and consequent pressure sores.

5 Avoid weight bearing or stress on cast for 48 hours.

Spica or Body Cast

1 Ensure that there is a firm base under the mattress—prevents sagging of bed from pressure of cast.

2 Support the curves of the cast with small plastic-covered flexible pillows—prevents cracking while cast is drying.

3   Avoid placing a pillow under head and shoulders while cast is drying—causes pressure on the chest.
4   Handle moist cast with palms of hands.

Observation of the Patient in a Cast

1   Listen to the patient's complaints (see complications).
2   Ask the patient to localize the exact site of pain.
3   Avoid giving analgesics for pain. Do not mask the pain until the cause has been determined.
4   Watch for signs of pressure and constriction of circulation such as colour, sensation swelling (see p. 150–152).
5   Inform doctor if symptoms persist. Cast may have to be removed.

Care of Patient After Cast Dries

Hip Spica Cast (Fig. 4.2)

1   Keep the cast level by elevating the lumbar sacral area with a small pillow when the patient is placed on the bedpan.
2   Protect the toes from the pressure of the bedding.
3   Encourage the patient to maintain physiological position by:
    a. Using the overhead 'Monkey Pole'.
    b. Placing good foot flat on bed and pushing down while lifting himself up on the trapeze.
    c. Avoiding twisting motions.
    d. Avoiding positions that produce pressure on groin, back, chest and abdomen.
4   Provide hygenic care of the patient.
    a. The perineal area of the cast may be protected by the application of waterproof plaster (sleek). This can be replaced if soiling occurs.
    b. With the newer splinting materials it is possible to clean the outside of the cast with a dry cleanser on an almost dry cloth.
    c. Pull stockinette taut, trim and fasten to cast edges with adhesive.
    d. Inspect skin for signs of irritation:
        (1) Around cast edge.
        (2) Under cast—pull skin taut and inspect under cast, using a torch for illumination.
    e. Massage accessible skin with an emollient lotion.
5   Turn the patient.
    a. Move the patient to the side of the bed, using a steady, even, pulling motion.
    b. Place pillows along the other side of the bed; one for the chest and two (lengthwise) for the legs.
    c. Instruct the patient to place his arms at his side.
    d. Turn the patient as a unit. Avoid twisting the patient in the cast.
    e. Turn the patient towards the leg not encased in plaster or towards the unoperated side if both legs are in plaster.
        (1) One nurse stands at other side of bed to receive patient's shoulders.
        (2) Second nurse supports leg in plaster while the third nurse supports the patient's back as he is turned.

(3) DO NOT GRASP CROSS BAR OF SPICA CAST TO MOVE PATIENT.

f. Turn patient to a prone position twice daily—provides postural drainage of bronchial tree; relieves pressure on back.

6 Encourage patient to drink liberal quantities of fluid—minimum 3 l a day—to avoid urinary calculi.

7 Have patient exercise the parts of the body that are not immobilized by the cast at regular and frequent intervals. Also encourage deep breathing exercises and coughing at regular intervals.

Nursing Alert: Watch for symptoms (*nausea*) of cast sydrome (acute obstruction of duodenum after spica or body cast is applied. See intestinal obstruction).

If symptoms occur

1 **Place patient prone to relieve pressure symptoms. Contact doctor.**
2 **Remove patient from cast if necessary.**
3 **Employ nasogastric suction.**
4 **Maintain normal electrolyte balance by intravenous replacement of fluid.**

Surgical intervention (duodenojejunostomy) may be necessary when conservative measures fail to relieve duodenal obstruction.

Leg Cast

1 Prevent or reduce swelling.
  a. Elevate the limb in the cast.
  b. After patient begins ambulation, encourage him to elevate the cast when he is seated.
2 Prevent irritation at cast edge—pad edges of cast with felt, avoid hard edges.
3 Examine toes and foot for:
  a. Blanching or cyanosis.
  b. Swelling.
  c. Inability to move toes.
4 Ascertain if patient is experiencing sensory disturbances to foot (numbness, tingling, burning, cold)—peroneal nerve injury from pressure at the head of the fibula is a common cause of footdrop; may be initial finding in vascular compromise.
5 *Be alert for evidences of thromboembolic complications.*
  High risk individuals (increased age, previous thromboembolism, obese, congestive heart failure, cancer of pancreas or lung, trauma) may require prophylaxis against thromboembolism.
6 Encourage the patient to move about as normally as possible.
  a. Do prescribed exercises faithfully.
  b. Do not cover a leg cast with plastic or rubber boots since this causes condensation and wetting of the cast. Avoid walking on wet floors or pavements.
  c. Report to the hospital accident unit if the cast cracks or breaks; instruct the patient not to try to fix it himself.
  d. Ensure that the patient understands the sheet of instructions given to him.

Arm Cast

1 Watch for symptoms of circulatory disturbance in hand (blueness or cyanosis, swelling, inability to move fingers, forearm pain on extension of fingers).

2   Reduce and control swelling.
    Elevate arm with each joint positioned higher than preceding joint (i.e., elbow higher than shoulder, hand higher than the elbow).

Nursing Alert: Guard against Volkmann's contracture–a severe fibrosis with resulting contracture of muscles which have become ischaemic by obstruction of the arterial flow to the forearm and hand. This complication is prevented by proper care; if allowed to develop the results are disastrous. Following supra condylar fracture of humerus the nurse should undertake half hourly check on radial pulse.

Exercising the Patient in the Cast: Health Teaching

1   Teach the patient to perform isometric exercises—contracting the muscles without moving the joint to maintain muscle strength and prevent atrophy (performed hourly when awake).
2   Leg cast—'Push down on the popliteal (knee) space, hold it, relax, repeat.'
3   Arm cast—'Make a fist, hold it, relax, repeat.'
4   Exercise every joint that is not immobilized.

GUIDELINES: Application of a Plaster Cast

Equipment

Prepare trolley with
Plaster bandages; 5, 7.5, 10, 15, 20 cm (2, 3, 4, 6, 8 in) widths
Cast padding (Velband Softex)
Stockinette (tubular knitted material)
Plaster slabs (for reinforcement)
Padding for bony prominences—usually orthopaedic felt or extra layer of Velband
Knives, scissors, indelible pencil
Polyethylene sheeting or newspaper—to protect floor
Disposable gloves—to protect hands of operator especially with new splinting materials
Large bucket of water at room temperature—21–24°C (70–75°F)

Underlying Considerations

1   The application of a cast requires two or three persons; one to apply the plaster (operator), one to dip and hand the plaster bandages to the operator, and a third person to hold the extremity in correct position. (Body spicas may require additional personnel.)
2   Plaster of paris bandages and splints set in 4–5 min. This time may be altered by varying the temperature and amount of water; nonplaster splinting material usually takes longer to achieve the initial set and the technique of application varies somewhat according to the manufacturer.
3   The operator should practise cast application on a model. Plaster sets rapidly and this is a skill that requires experience.
4   There should be no movement of the extremity while the cast is being applied.
5   In general, the joints above and below the involved bone are usually immobilized.

Procedure

Action	**Reason**

Preparation

1 Spread polyethylene sheeting to protect floor and patient.

2 Explain to the patient that there will be a feeling of warmth as the plaster is applied.

2 Heat is produced by crystallization as plaster sets. The reaction of water with plaster of paris liberates heat.

3 Apply stockinette and roll padding on the limb or part to be immobilized.

  a. Apply as smoothly and snugly as possible so that each turn overlaps the preceding turn by half the width of the roll.

  b. Extra pieces of padding may be placed over bony prominences; olecranon process, malleoli, patella.

3 Padding is used to pad the sharp cast margins for patient comfort and to prevent pressure areas, minimize circulatory problems and enhance cast removal.

4 Having unrolled the first 10–15 cm of the bandage submerge the plaster bandage vertically in water (room temperature) for a minute or so, or until bubbles cease to rise.

4 Water that is too warm will accelerate setting time, may cause a burn and may result in excessive plaster loss by loosening the adhesive agents which bond the plaster to the fabric.

5 Expel excess water by squeezing (not wringing) towards the centre of the bandage; hand bandage to operator with free end hanging loose.

5 The cast will dry more quickly (and thus will acquire maximum strength sooner) if a well-squeezed bandage is used.

Application

1 Commencing at the distal end, roll the bandage gently and evenly on the extremity, overlapping the preceding turn by half the width of the roll.

1 Roll inward towards the patient's body for ease of control.

2 Keep the bandage moving and in constant contact with the surface of the limb. Smooth and rub down successive layers or turns of each bandage into the layers below with the thumbs and thenar emineces (mound on the palm) in circumferential and longitudinal directions.

2 This keeps the cast uniformly thick. Rubbing the plaster as it is applied will form a smooth, solid and well-fused cast. Avoid indenting the cast with the fingertips since this will produce pressure sores on underlying skin.

3 Take tucks in the lower border of the bandage by lifting the bandage off the surface (without tension) and overlapping it in a V-shaped fashion.

3 Tucking the bandage helps to contour the cast to the changing circumference of the limb. Do not twist or reverse the bandage to change its direction since this produces sharp cutting edges.

Action	Reason
4 Trim the cast to size with a sharp knife by pulling the plaster edge against the cutting edge of the knife.	4 Do not pull too vigorously on the stockinette since this may cause pressure on bony pressure points.
5 Ask the patient if there is any discomfort or pain.	5 If a patient complains of pain, the cast and encircling dressings should be split to avoid constriction, circulatory problems and pressure sores.
6 Write the diagnosis and date of cast application with an indelible pencil on the cast.	6 This is often done when a cast is applied following surgery.
7 Support the cast with the palm of the hand while moving the patient. Avoid indentations from tips of fingers.	7 Finger indentation on a fresh cast can produce pressure sores.
8 Expose the cast to warm, circulating dry air.	8 Avoid covering the cast when it is drying as this delays drying time and causes a rise in temperature. Usually the cast will reach its maximum temperature 5–15 min after it is applied and will then cool rapidly. The ultimate cast strength is obtained after the cast is dry (up to 48 hours depending on outside temperature and humidity).
9 Clean plaster from equipment and store ready for use.	

GUIDELINES: Removal of a Cast

Equipment

Plaster cutter—an electric saw with circular blade that oscillates through the plaster
Plaster spreader
Plaster knife
Scissors
Plaster Shears

Procedure

Action	Reason
Preparation	
1 Describe to the patient how and where the cast cutter will be used and the expected sensations. Turn on the cutter and allow the patient to hear the motor.	1 Reassures the patient that the cutter produces vibrations but not pain.

Action	Reason
2 Determine whether or not the cast is padded.	2 An electric plaster cast cutter should not be used on unpadded casts.
3 Determine where the cut will be made. Mark, with a felt pen, the area to be cut.	3 The line should be in front of the lateral malleolus and behind the medial malleolus on a lower limb cast. An upper limb cast is usually split along the ulnar or flexor surface.
4 Dampen the cast along the portion to be cut.	4 Dampening diminishes the cloud of plaster dust.

Removal

1 Grasp the electric cutter as illustrated (Fig. 4.3a).	
2 Rest the thumb on the plaster.	2 The thumb serves as a depth gauge and acts as a guard in front of the blade.
3 Turn on the electric cutter. Push the blade firmly and gently through the cast while allowing the thumb to come in contact with the cast as the saw blade oscillates.	
4 As the blade cuts through the plaster, a sudden lack of resistance is felt; plaster will 'give' (or 'dip') when the cut is completed.	
5 Lift the cutting blade up a degree (but not out of the cutting groove) and advance the blade at a slightly higher or lower level. The cast is cut by a series of alternating pressure and linear movements along the line of the cut (Fig. 4.3b).	
6 Avoid drawing the cutting blade along the limb in a single motion.	6 This will cut the skin. If saw blade is in contact with padding too long

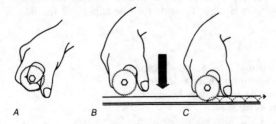

Figure 4.3. Operating a cast cutter. (Courtesy: Stryker Corporation.)

Action	Reason
	patient will feel burning sensation on skin from rapidly oscillating blade.
7 Cut the cast on both sides. Then rock the anterior portion of the cast over the posterior portion.	7 This manoeuvre allows the operator to determine if the cast is completely cut.
8 Insert the blades of the plaster spreader in the cut trough. Separate the two halves with the spreader at several sites along the cast split. Separate the cast with the hands.	8 Or spread the cast while cutting, to facilitate its removal.
9 Cut through the padding and stockinette with scissors, keeping the scissor blade that is closest to the skin parallel to the skin.	9 Use bandage scissors; place the flat blade closest to the skin.
10 Lift the limb carefully out of the posterior portion of the cast. Support the limb so that it is maintained in the same position as when in the cast.	10 When the support of the cast has been removed, stresses and strain are placed on parts that have been at rest.

After Removal of Cast

Action	Reason
1 Cleanse the skin gently with soap and water. Blot dry. Apply a skin cream.	1 Explain to the patient that the skin will be scaly and the limb will appear 'thin' from disuse. Reassure him that it will take a few weeks to regain normal appearance and function.
2 Emphasize the importance of continuing the prescribed exercises, reporting for physiotherapy, etc.	2 Exercises are necessary to redevelop and increase strength and function. Pain and stiffness may be expected after cast removal.

TRACTION

Traction is force applied in a specific direction. To apply the force needed to overcome the natural force or pull of muscle groups, a system of traction cords, pulleys, and weights is used. Traction may be applied to the skin or to the skeletal system.

Purposes

1   To regain normal length and alignment.
2   To reduce and immobilize fracture.
3   To lessen or eliminate muscle spasm.
4   To prevent deformity.
5   To give the patient freedom for 'in bed' activities.
6   To reduce pain.

Methods

Skin Traction

Accomplished by a weight that pulls on extension plaster or sponge rubber attached to the skin; traction on the skin transmits traction to the musculoskeletal structures.

1 Skin traction is used as a temporary measure in adults; used prior to surgery in treatment of intertrochanteric hip fracture (Buck's extension); Hamilton–Russell traction is used for applying traction to the femoral shaft with the knee flexed. Skin traction may be used definitively to treat fractures in children.
2 *Application and nursing assessment*—see p. 163–164.

Skeletal Traction

Traction applied to bone using wires, pins or tongs placed through bones; this is the most effective means of traction. It is applied by the orthopaedic surgeon under aseptic conditions.

1 Skeletal traction is used most frequently in treatment of fractures of the femur; dislocations of hips, and of fractures of the cervical spine.
2 *Nursing assessment and responsibilities:*
   a. Watch for signs of infection, especially around the pin tract.
   (1) The pin should be immobile in the bone and the skin wound should be dry.
   (2) If infection is suspected, percuss gently over the tibial tuberosity; this will elicit pain if infection is developing.
   (3) Assess for other signs of infection: heat, redness, fever.
   b. It may be necessary to clean the pin tracts using an aseptic technique to clear drainage around the skeletal pin, since plugging at this site can predispose to bacterial invasion of the tract and bone.
   c. Apply a cork or pin guards over the edges of the pin.
   d. Check traction apparatus at repeated intervals to see that the direction of pull is correct and the ropes are unobstructed; that weights are in proper position; and that patient is comfortable.
   e. See below for nursing management.

Cervical Traction

See p. 64.

Pelvic Traction

Used for treatment of back disorders or injuries.

Nursing Management

1 The patient is placed on a firm mattress with fracture boards underneath if necessary.
2 The traction cord and the pulleys should be in straight alignment.
3 The pull should be in line with the long axis of the bone.
4 Any factor that might reduce the pull or alter its direction must be eliminated.
   a. Weights should hang free.
   b. Traction cord should be unobstructed and not in contact with the bed or equipment.

c. Help the patient to pull himself up in bed at frequent intervals. Traction is *not* accomplished if the knot in the cord or the spreader bar is touching the pulley or the foot of the bed, or if the weights are resting on the floor.

5 The amount of weight applied in skin traction must not exceed the tolerance of the skin. The condition of the skin must be inspected frequently. Usually a maximum of 3 kg (7 lb).

6 There is always the possibility of bone infection when skeletal traction is used. Be alert for odours, signs of local inflammation or other evidence of osteomyelitis.

7 The patient's skin should be examined frequently for evidences of pressure or friction over bony prominences.

8 Provision should be made for supplying additional countertraction by increasing the pull in the opposite direction, i.e., by raising the bed in such a manner that the weight of the patient's body tends to oppose the pull of the traction.

9 Active motion of all unaffected joints should be encouraged.

10 *Every complaint of the patient in traction should be investigated immediately.*

Principles of Balanced (Suspension) Traction

Balanced (suspension) traction is produced by a counterforce other than the patient's body weight. The limb balances in the traction apparatus. The line of traction on the extremity remains fairly constant despite changes in the patient's position.

Nursing Management

1 The patient may sit, turn slightly, and move as desired.

2 The angle of hip flexion is approximately 20° (the angle between the thigh and the bed).

3 The cords and the pulleys should be freely movable; the traction should be applied securely to the leg.

4 Observe for skin irritation around the traction bandage.

5 Check the patient for odour and signs of infection.

6 Observe for pressure under the sling at the popliteal space.

7 Provide foot supports to prevent footdrop.

8 The traction must be continuous to be effective.

Principles of Weight and Pulley Traction

Weight and pulley traction is a form of traction in which the pull is exerted in one plane. It may utilize either skin or skeletal traction, and it may be either unilateral or bilateral. Example: Buck's extension.

Nursing Management

1 The foot should be inspected for circulatory difficulties within a few minutes and then periodically after the traction has been applied.

2 Special care must be given to the back at regular intervals, because the patient maintains a supine position.

3 Any complaint or burning sensation under the traction bandage should be reported immediately.

4 Observe for wrinkling or slipping of the traction bandage.

5 The patient should have foot supports to prevent footdrop.
6 Check peripheral pulses and the colour and temperature of the digits.
7 Check for calf tenderness and for possible Homan's sign for signs of deep vein thrombosis.

GUIDELINES: Application of Buck's Extension Traction

Buck's extension (unilateral or bilateral skin traction) is a form of skin traction used as a temporary measure to provide support and comfort to a fractured limb until definitive treatment is accomplished.

Equipment

Skin Extensions
Elastic bandages, 10 cm (4 in) ⎫
Felt or foam padding   ⎬   These are commercially available in ready made traction kits
Spreader block or metal spreader ⎭
Pulley, traction cords and weights (2.3–3.1 kg (5–7 lb) is usual—amount of weight is prescribed by doctor)
Tincture of benzoin (for adhesive traction)
Sheepskin pad
Elevator or blocks

Procedure

Nursing Action	Reason
Preparation	
1 Place bedboard under the mattress and elevator blocks under the wheels at the foot of the bed if indicated. This depends on the size of the patient and the weight applied.	1 ⁕Elevating the foot of the bed (countertraction) helps prevent the patient from sliding down towards the foot of the bed.
2 Question the patient to determine previous skin conditions (contact dermatitis). Inspect skin for evidences of atrophy, abrasions and circulatory disturbances. Ensure that the patient is not allergic to elastoplast.	2 The skin must be in healthy condition to tolerate skin traction.
3 Make sure that the skin of the limb is clean and dry.	3 A clean, dry skin helps adherence of extensions.
Application	
1 For nonadhesive traction bandage: **a.** Pad both malleoli and proximal fibula with padding.	**a.** Pressure sores and skin necrosis may result from pressure applied directly over malleoli. Pressure over

Nursing Action   **Reason**

the region of the fibular head
and common peroneal nerve may
produce peroneal palsy and 'drop-
foot'.

b. Apply Ventfoam (with the foam
surface against the skin) on each side
of the affected extremity, leaving a
loop projecting 10–15 cm (4–6 in)
beyond the sole of the foot.

2 For adhesive skin extensions.
a. Pad both malleoli and proximal   **a.** Tincture of benzoin may help pro-
fibula. Apply tincture of benzoin to   tect the skin, although the tape
the skin.   adheres satisfactorily without it and
                                         some manufacturers advise against
                                         using it with these products.

b. Gently stroke the tape onto the   **b.** Stroking the tape onto the skin
skin. Apply adhesive skin tape in the   promotes skin adherence and pre-
same manner as nonadhesive trac-   vents wrinkles and creases.
tion bandage.
c. Make 0.6–1.2 cm ($\frac{1}{4}$–$\frac{1}{2}$ in) oblique   **c.** Clipping the border of the tape
cuts along each border of the tape if   allows it to conform to the contour of
necessary.   the leg. Uneven tension contributes
                                         to skin breakdown.

3 Have a second person elevate and   3 The elastic bandage improves adher-
support the extremity under the   ence of tape to the skin and helps
ankle and knee while the elastic ban-   prevent slipping.
dage is applied (Fig. 4.4). Beginning
at the ankle, wrap the elastic bandage snugly over the tape up to the
tibial tubercle.

4 Attach a spreader block (or metal   4 The spreader block prevents pres-
spreader) to the distal end of the   sure along the side of the foot. The
tape. Attach a cord to the spreader   spreader should not be too narrow
block and pass it over a pulley fas-   (causes pressure sores on ankle) or
tened to the end of the bed (Fig. 4.5). too wide (pulls extension away from
                                         the heel).

5 Make sure knots are tied securely.   5 The cord should be unobstructed;
Gently attach the traction weight.   the weight should hang free of
Release gradually.   the bed and should not touch the
                                         floor.

6 Place a sheepskin pad under the leg 6 Sheepskin is used to reduce friction
(or use a commercial heel protector)   of the heel against the bed.
if desired.

7 Assess the patient to ensure he is in 7 The part of the body in traction
proper alignment.   should be in line with the pull of the
                                         weight.

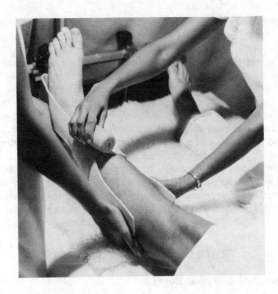

Figure 4.4. Apply elastic bandage for Buck's extension traction.

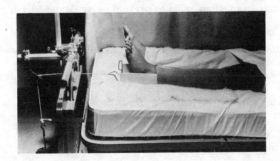

Figure 4.5. Lower limb in Buck's extension traction.

Nursing Assessment of the Patient Following Application of Buck's Extension

1   Palpate over area of extension daily. If area is tender to palpation, suspect skin irritation and report it immediately. The elastic bandage may have to be removed.
2   Inspect for skin irritation and pressure on:
   a. Achilles tendon.
   b. Peroneal nerve (as it passes around the neck of the fibula just below the knee).

3   Inspect dorsum of foot for loss of sensation, weakness of dorsiflexors of foot and toes, inversion of foot—may be caused by tight extensions and pressure on the common peroneal nerve.
4   Unwrap the elastic bandage and inspect leg if there is evidence of slipping of extensions.
5   Assess for complaints of persistent itching and burning.
6   Maintain the limb in a neutral position. Avoid external rotation.
7   The patient may not turn from side to side because the position of the leg on the bed will cause the bony fragments to move against each other.
8   Inspect and bathe back. To give back care instruct the patient to:
    a. Place hands on overhead trapeze (monkey pole).
    b. Bend the knee of unaffected extremity and place foot flat on bed.
    c. Push down on the uninvolved foot while at the same time pulling up on the trapeze (monkey pole)—allows the entire body and trunk to rise off the bed.
    The shoulders, back and buttocks must move as a single, straight unit.
9   See p. 159 for other aspects of nursing management.

FRACTURES OF SPECIFIC SITES*

Fracture of the Clavicle (Collar Bone)

1   The clavicle helps to hold the shoulder upwards, outwards and backwards from the thorax.
2   Aim of reduction: to hold the shoulder in the position described above.
3   Most fractures of the clavicle are treated by closed reduction and immobilization accomplished by one of the following methods:
    a. Clavicular strap. (Pad axilla to prevent nerve damage from pressure.)
    b. Sling.
    c. Figure 8 bandage.
    Watch for tingling in hands; too tight a clavicular strap or figure 8 bandage may cause circulatory impairment.
4   Open reduction and internal fixation may be done for marked displacement and angulation of bone ends.
    a. Following surgery the patient's arm is kept in a sling.
    b. Caution patient not to elevate his arm above shoulder level until the fracture has united; will impede healing of fracture.

Health Teaching

1   Exercise elbow, wrist and fingers as soon as possible.
2   Do shoulder exercises to obtain full shoulder motion as prescribed (Fig. 4.6).

Fractures of the Upper Limb

Fractures of the Surgical Neck of the Humerus (Fractures of the Proximal Humerus)

1   Most occur from falls in which the outstretched arm strikes the ground (impacted fracture). Osteoporosis is a predisposing factor.

* For fracture of the skull see p. 11.

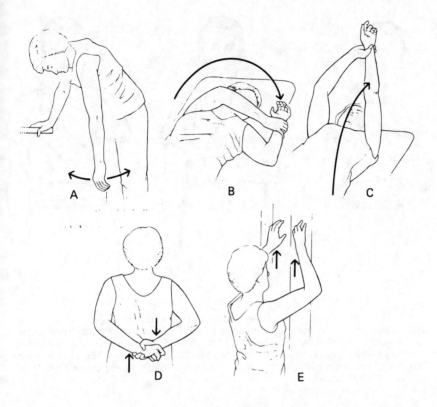

Figure 4.6. Exercises to develop range of motion of shoulder. a. Pendulum exercise. b. External rotation. c. Elevation. d. Internal rotation. In all of these the unaffected arm is used for power. e. Wall climbing.

2   The majority of impacted fractures of the surgical neck of the humerus do not require reduction. The weight of the arm helps to correct displacement.
   a. Place a soft pad under the axilla to prevent skin maceration.
   b. The arm is supported by a sling bandage for comfort (Fig. 4.7).
   c. Advise the patient that he will sleep more comfortably when supported in an upright position.
3   Displaced fractures are treated with reduction under x-ray control, open reduction or replacement of humeral head with prosthesis.
   a. A programme of exercises is usually started 4 days postoperatively with emphasis on range of motion of the shoulder (Fig. 4.6).
   b. Watch for postoperative infection, a common sequela of surgery on shoulder.

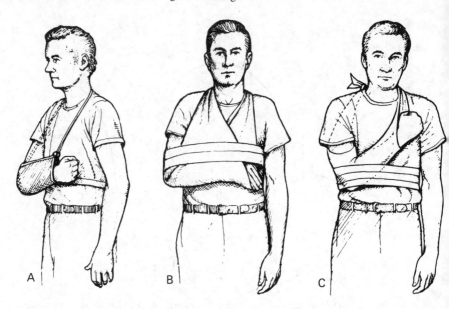

Figure 4.7. The types of immobilizing dressings used for upper humeral fractures. a. A commercial sling which permits easy removal of the arm for exercises and is comfortable on the neck. b. A conventional sling and bandage. c. A stockinette Velpeau and bandage used when there is an unstable surgical neck component, because this position relaxes the pectoralis major. This is not presently available in the UK. (From: Rockwood, C A and Green, D P (1975) Fractures. J B Lippincott

Health Teaching

Objective

To restore shoulder function and prevent adhesions.

1   Start active motion of shoulder joint early—to prevent limitation of motion and stiffness of shoulder.
2   Instruct patient to lean forward and allow affected arm to abduct and rotate (*termed pendulum exercise*) (Fig. 4.6a).

Fractures of the Shaft of the Humerus

1   Fractures of the shaft of the humerus are most frequently caused by direct violence—falls, blows to arm, road traffic injuries.
2   Most fractures at this site can be treated nonoperatively.
3   Hanging cast is frequently applied to oblique, spiral and displaced fractures with shortening of humeral shaft.

Nursing Alert: A hanging cast for treatment of fracture of the shaft of the humerus must be dependent (remain unsupported) to provide a traction force. Continuous

traction on long axis of arm is effected by the weight of the cast. The patient must avoid supporting the elbow in the lap while seated.

4   See that the patient sleeps in a fairly upright position to maintain uninterrupted 24-hour traction.
5   Exercise fingers immediately after the application of the cast.
6   Start pendulum exercises as directed—provides active exercise of shoulder to prevent adhesions of the shoulder joint capsule after cast removal (Fig. 4.6a).
7   Open reduction and internal fixation (usually by compression plate) are performed when satisfactory alignment cannot be obtained with closed treatment, when there is associated vascular injury, and when the fracture is the result of a pathologic (malignant) lesion. Internal fixation is often supplemented by methyl methacrylate (bone cement).
    Following a surgical procedure, the arm is placed in a sling and bandaged until bone union has taken place at the fracture site.

Supracondylar Fracture (above the elbow)

1   This fracture is close to the median nerve and brachial artery. An injury to the brachial artery, may produce ischaemia in the flexor forearm muscles and, consequently, Volkmann's ischaemia contracture.
2   Treatment of this type of fracture varies:
    a. Alignment corrected by manipulation under general or regional anaesthesia. Fragments are usually maintained by holding elbow in an acutely flexed position after reduction. (Degree of elbow flexion is determined by amplitude of pulse.)
    b. For more severe injuries Dunlop's traction is used. The forearm is held in suspension. These methods maintain traction, keep the fracture reduced, decrease oedema and aid circulation (reduces risk of Volkmann's contracture).
    c. Open reducion and pin and screw fixation in adults may be required.
3   Watch for signs of impaired circulation in forearm and hand.
    a. Observe hand for swelling or blueness of fingernails; compare with unaffected hand.
    b. Evaluate radial pulse; if it weakens or disappears, call orthopaedic surgeon *immediately* since irreversible ischaemia may develop.
4   Assess for paresthesia (tingling and burning sensations) in the hand—indicate nerve injury or impending ischaemia.
5   Encourage patient to move his fingers frequently.

Fractures and Dislocations about the Elbow

1   Usually occur from direct fall on elbow or on outstretched hand with elbow in flexion. May be undisplaced or displaced (avulsion; oblique and transverse fractures; comminuted fracture; or fracture-dislocation).
2   *Undisplaced fracture*—treated by short period of immobilization in a cast with elbow in 45–90° flexion or supported with a sling and pressure dressing to the elbow.
3   *Displaced fracture*—usually treated by open reduction and internal fixation or primary excision of the proximal fragment(s).
4   Watch for signs of impaired circulation in forearm and hand. Assess for local nerve damage from injury to the median, radial or ulnar nerves.

5   Range of motion exercises started upon order; flexion past 90° is avoided until bone healing is demonstrated by x-ray.

Fractures of the Head of the Radius

1   Usually produced by indirect trauma (fall on outstretched hand) or by direct trauma (blow).
2   *Undisplaced fracture.*
   a. Aspiration of haemarthrosis (blood in joint) at the elbow may be done to relieve pain and allow earlier range of motion.
   b. Immobilization by plaster slab or sling.
3   *Displaced fracture*—open operation with excision of radial head when indicated.
   a. Postoperatively the arm is immobilized in a posterior plaster splint and sling.
   b. Early active motion of elbow and forearm is encouraged when plaster splint is removed.

Health Teaching

1   Encourage patient to continue *daily* programme of repetitive, progressive exercises (as prescribed). The exercise programme is designed to restore full extension and supination.
2   Instruct the patient to avoid lifting heavy objects for 6 weeks after sling has been discontinued.

Fractures of the Shafts of the Radius and Ulna

1   Objective of treatment is to preserve function of forearm.
2   *Undisplaced fractures*—treated by immobilizing arm in an above elbow cast with elbow flexed 90°.
   a. Watch circulation and function of hand.
   b. Encourage active flexion and extension of fingers at frequent intervals to reduce oedema. Encourage shoulder motion.
3   *Displaced fractures*—internal fixation accomplished by compression plate or some other fixation device.
   a. Postoperatively, a closed drainage system may be used to decrease haematoma and resultant swelling.
   b. The arm is usually immobilized in plaster splints or cast until there is evidence that fracture is healing.

Health Teaching

Encourage patient to move his fingers and the shoulder of the involved limb.

Fracture of the Wrist

1   Colles' fracture is a fracture of the radius 1.2–2.5 cm ($\frac{1}{2}$–1 in) above the wrist with dorsal displacement of the lower fragment.
2   Treatment usually consists of closed reduction and plaster of paris splint or cast support.
   a. Elevate arm above level of heart for 48 hours after reduction.
   b. Watch for swelling of fingers—indicates decreased venous and lymphatic return. Check for constricting bandages or cast.

c. Instruct patient to do finger exercises to reduce swelling and prevent stiffness.
(1) Hold hand above level of heart.
(2) Move fingers from full extension to flexion (claw position). Hold to a count of 2 or more.
(3) Repeat at least 10 times every half hour while awake—as long as hand has a tendency to swell.

Fractures of the Hand

1 Numerous injuries to the hand require extensive reconstructive surgery which is beyond the scope of this book. The reader is referred to specialized texts on the hand.
2 Objective of treatment is to regain maximum function of the hand.
3 *Undisplaced fracture of the distal phalanx.*
a. Drainage of the haematoma under the fingernail may be necessary.
b. Finger is splinted (to adjoining finger or by a dorsal or volar splint)—to relieve pain and to protect finger tip from further trauma.
4 *Open fractures* may be handled by Kirschner wire fixation following debridement and irrigation.

Fractures of the Lower Limb

Objectives

To obtain adequate bony union with full length and normal alignment and without rotational or angular deformity.
To restore muscle power and joint motion.

Fracture of the Shaft of the Femur

Nursing Alert: Fracture of the shaft of the femur may be accompanied by marked concealed blood loss.

1 Closed reduction.
a. Fracture reduced and stabilized by means of balanced skeletal traction, using a Thomas splint with a Pearson knee flexion piece attachment (Fig. 4.8).
b. Thomas splint suspends the thigh; Pearson knee flexion piece attachment allows knee flexion and supports the leg below the knee.
c. Examine skin under the ring on Thomas splint.
d. Passive and active motion of knee joint may be ordered.
e. May be replaced with cast-brace (for fractures of shaft of the femur)—after 2–4 weeks of traction.
2 Open reduction with intramedullary (within the bone) fixation.
a. See nursing management following orthopaedic surgery.
b. Observe for complications: postoperative infection, osteomyelitis.
c. Or a cast-brace may be used in conjunction with internal fixation of fractured femur.

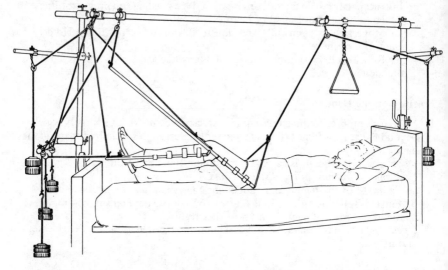

Figure 4.8. Balanced traction with Thomas leg splint with Pearson attachment.

Fractures of the Tibia and Fibula

1   Treatment of tibial fractures represents a challenge; there is a high incidence of open infected fractures since the tibia lies superficially beneath the skin.
2   These fractures may require prolonged immobilization—union is slow because there is often poor blood supply to the distal part of the tibia.
3   Tibial fractures generally heal in 12–16 weeks; compound and comminuted fractures take longer.
4   *Treatment* (broad range of opinion on treatment of these fractures):
    a. May be managed by simple manipulation and the reduction maintained by application of plaster cast (toe to groin; see Fig. 4.2).
        (1) In time this long-leg cast may be replaced with a below-the-knee functional cast which permits weight-bearing and knee joint motion.
        (2) As an alternative, a functional cast-brace (fabricated with orthoplast-like material and special hinges) may be used (Fig. 4.9).
    b. Or fracture may be treated by open reduction and early fixation (plate, compression plate, intramedullary nails or other devices) as indicated by aetiology, type of trauma and type of fracture.

Knee Surgery

Nursing Management

1   Elevate affected limb on pillow; keep knee straight.
2   Evaluate for effusion of the knee—a common complication following knee surgery.
    a. Remove pressure bandage and reapply if pain is severe.

b. Support patient undergoing aspiration of fluid from knee joint.

3 Encourage quadriceps exercise to prevent atrophy of the thigh muscles.

Rehabilitation After Fracture of Lower Extremity

1 Apply elastic stocking to uninvolved leg—maintains pressure on deeper leg veins, helps prevent stasis of blood, oedema and thrombophlebitis (deep vein thrombosis).

2 Elevate unaffected leg at intervals throughout day—to promote venous return.

3 Elevate affected limb to promote venous return and relieve pain.
   a. The early re-establishment of venous return helps absorb blood and tissue fluid (oedema from bleeding is a common cause of disability following fractures).
   b. Chronic oedema predisposes limb to fibrosis and ulceration.

4 Exercise as much as possible—promotes bone healing.

5 Avoid placing limb in dependent positions for prolonged periods.

6 Mobilize the patient as soon as possible. Instruct in methods of ambulation—frame, crutches, and stick.

7 Physiotherapy procedures may be utilized after cast removal (heat, cold, massage, exercise)—to restore joint mobility, increase muscle strength and endurance.

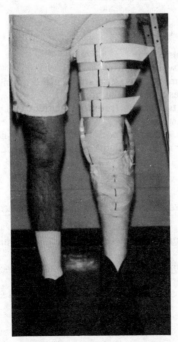

Figure 4.9. Cast-brace provides circumferential support to a segment of a fractured limb while allowing mobility of nearby joints.

8   Instruct patient to wear elastic bandage after cast is removed to support venous circulation.
9   Advise patient to move feet up and down in pedalling motion to exercise calf muscles.
10 Recommend that patient start moving affected limb under water if necessary, since water supports the limb and provides warmth, which helps promote muscle relaxation.

Cast-Bracing

A *cast-brace* (fracture-orthosis) consists of two separate weight-bearing casts (patellar weight-bearing cast on lower leg and ischial weight-bearing cast on thigh) which are joined at the knee by a pair of gliding-action hinges (Fig. 4.9). The foot and ankle joint may be included in the cast and a walking heel or boot applied; or the foot and ankle joint may be freed by a removable shoe attached to the cast by a brace joint.

The cast may be of plaster of paris or the newer splintage materials, e.g., bay cast.

Rationale

Cast-bracing is based on the concept that weight-bearing will promote osteogenesis (bone formation).

Purposes and Advantages

1   Allows motion of joints.
2   Permits progressive weight bearing.
3   Allows gradually increasing skeletal stresses and promotes fracture healing by transmission of forces through the bone.
4   Allows early return to walking (promotes patient independence).
5   Allows earlier hospital discharge.
6   Lessens detrimental effect on body physiology by shortening the period of recumbency—earlier return of bladder and bowel function, less chance of renal calculi, etc.

Clinical Indications

Fractures of tibia and of femoral shaft; supracondylar fractures of the femur (open or closed).

1   Tibial fracture—functional below-knee walking brace may be applied 2–3 weeks after fracture.
2   Femoral fracture—long leg cast-brace may be applied 3–5 weeks after patient has been in traction.
3   Cast-brace—applied after initial oedema has subsided and there is evidence of fracture stability.

Nursing Management

1   The patient may be permitted to get up 24–48 hours after cast is applied.
    a. As much weight is borne on affected extremity as can be tolerated.

b. Be sure patient uses proper crutch gait (three-point gait) so that normal gait and rhythm are established.
2 Advise patient that he should be closely monitored.
   a. Angular deformity may occur during first weeks of weight bearing.
   b. Standing weight-bearing anteroposterior and lateral x-rays are taken at intervals.
3 Watch for skin breakdown and circulatory problems.
   a. Watch for excessive swelling of exposed area of knee.
   b. Report signs of skin discoloration, numbness, breakdown.
4 Protect cast from soiling (urine and faeces)—cast may extend to groin.
5 Elevate cast when not walking—to promote venous return.
6 The cast is changed at intervals until clinical union is achieved.

Fractures of the Lumbar and Dorsal Spine

Fractures of the vertebrae of the dorsal and lumbar spine may involve the vertebral body, lamina articulating processes and spinous processes or transverse processes. (Fractures of the cervical spine are discussed on p. 63.)

Clinical Manifestations

Severe pain in back—may radiate.

Clinical Problems

1 Fractures of the vertebral bodies are compression fractures; they are frequently multiple and comprise the most common types of fractures of the spine.
2 The majority of vertebral fractures seem to be related to osteoporosis.
3 A spinal cord injury may occur with fracture or dislocation of a vertebra.

Treatment and Nursing Management

Objective

To determine if there is injury to the spinal cord.

1 Assess and treat the patient for spinal cord injury.
2 Evaluate for paralytic ileus and difficulty in micturition—may occur the first few days after compression fracture of the lower dorsal or lumbar spine—may be from retroperitoneal haemorrhage.
3 Use measures to prevent risk of deep vein thrombosis complications—elevate foot of bed, apply elastic stockings, encourage active ankle motion, high risk patients may be given anticoagulant therapy.

Treatment

For Stable Injuries to Vertebrae

1 Treat symptomatically for pain and encourage patient to mobilize—or
2 Place patient on a firm mattress and keep on bed rest until pain subsides.

a. Encourage patient to roll from side to side; patient should not sit up during acute stage.

b. Give analgesics and muscle relaxants as required since pain may be severe.

c. Patient is permitted to walk with assistance (wearing shoes) when discomfort subsides.

d. Encourage patient to do the prescribed back exercises—to increase or maintain the strength of back muscles (2–3 weeks after fracture).

(1) Exercises are prescribed that strengthen spinal extensor muscles.

(2) Exercises that encourage spinal flexion are contraindicated.

e. Patient may feel better with a corset-type brace or back support when he is mobilizing; remove appliance while in bed.

f. Patient with a more severe injury may require a more substantial back brace or cast.

For Unstable Fractures/Displacement

1   The patient is placed on a turning frame when there is neurological involvement.
2   In the absence of paraplegia the patient may be placed in a body cast for immobilization.
3   Mobilize the patient when physical examinations and x-ray evaluations determine there is no displacement or neurological deficit.

Fractures of the Pelvis

Clinical Manifestations

1   Inability to bear weight without discomfort.
2   Local swelling and tenderness at site of fracture.
3   Symptoms of haemorrhage and shock.

Treatment and Nursing Management

Objective

To carry out ongoing nursing assessment for injuries to the bladder, rectum, intestine and intra-abdominal organs.

1   Determine the extent of internal injuries.

a. Request patient to micturate. Urine is examined for blood.

b. Assess and evaluate for intra-abdominal haemorrhage—pelvic fractures may cause death from extraperitoneal and retroperitoneal haemorrhage.

c. Palpate peripheral pulses—absence of peripheral pulses may indicate possibility of torn iliac artery.

d. Monitor stools and urine for blood.

e. Look for other injuries—direct force to pelvic girdle may involve intra-abdominal organs.

f. Observe for impending shock.

g. Evaluate for other complications that are likely to develop as a result of shock, massive soft tissue injury and multiple fractures—intravascular coagulation, thromboembolic complications, fat emboli, pulmonary complications.

2 *Nonoperative treatment.*
   a. Consists of bed rest, skeletal traction, pelvic sling, plaster spica—to immobilize and stabilize fracture—or
   b. Pelvic sling—serves to exert a compression force against the iliac bone which helps mould the fracture back in place.
   c. Pelvic sling lifts the weight of the pelvis very slightly off the mattress.
      (1) Adjust pressure by moving the cords of the sling closer together or farther apart by direction of the surgeon.
      (2) Fold sling back over buttocks to enable patient to use the bedpan.
      (3) Reach under sling to give skin care—sheepskin may be used to line sling to prevent pressure sores.
      (4) Loosen the sling only upon order.
3 Operative treatment—for ruptured abdominal or pelvic viscera and occasionally for haemorrhage.
4 Mobilization and weight bearing are determined by x-ray and patient's reaction to mobility.

Hip Fractures (Treated by an Internal Fixation Device)

Clinical Manifestations

1 Shortening, adduction and external rotation of affected leg.
2 Pain.

Types of Hip Fractures

1 Intracapsular—femur is fractured inside the joint (femoral neck fracture).
2 Extracapsular—femur is fractured outside the joint (intertrochanteric fracture).

Treatment and Nursing Management

Objectives

To prolong the patient's life.
To prevent physical, psychological and social dependence.
To restore the mobility of the hip joint (if the patient was mobile before the fracture).

Preoperative Nursing Management

1 Alleviate the pain.
   a. Assist with whatever means of preoperative immobilization is ordered. This will commonly be either Hamilton–Russell traction, below knee skin traction (Buck's traction) or Ventfoam traction. This will relieve pain and allow the patient to be mobile in bed until surgery a few days later.
   b. Handle the affected limb gently.
   c. Give analgesics as patient's condition indicates.
   d. Keep the skin dry and relieve pressure areas—pressure sores develop rapidly in the preoperative period.
      (1) Inspect the heel *daily*—a patient with painful hip tends to let weight of leg press the heel against the bed; area loses sensation when blood/nerve supply diminishes and the skin becomes necrosed.

(2) Support leg with pillow if permitted—distributes pressure more evenly.

(3) Massage area around heel at intervals.

(4) Check traction frequently, especially elastic bandages.

2   Ensure that the patient is in as favourable a condition as possible preoperatively.

a. Co-ordinate ECG, blood chemistry studies (urea and electrolyte levels) and x-rays.

b. Prepare for arterial blood gas analysis—to evaluate patient's pulmonary state.

c. Determine if patient is oriented to time, place and person—mental confusion may be due to underlying systemic illness, particularly to cardiopulmonary disease with inadequate cerebral oxygen transport.

d. Carry out an ongoing nursing assessment—mental alertness, bright facial expression and good skin colour are considered favourable prognositc indications.

e. Give intravenous infusions *slowly*—patients with limited cardiac reserve cannot stand additional circulatory loading.

3   Use anticipatory nursing assessment and techniques to avoid complications.

Nursing Alert: Thromboembolism is the most common complication following hip fractures, and it frequently occurs without clinical signs.

a. Prevent thromboembolism with leg exercises, elastic stockings, early ambulation or antiembolic stockings.

b. Warfarin, low-molecular weight dextran, aspirin or low doses of heparin given subcutaneously may be effective in reducing the incidence of venous thrombi.

c. Elevate foot of bed 25°—to promote venous drainage.

Intraoperative Considerations

1   Surgical procedure is usually carried out as soon as possible after full medical assessment since these patients are usually elderly.

2   Stable fractures are usually reduced and fixed with a nail, nail-plate combination, multiple pins, screw, sliding nails, etc.

Postoperative Nursing Management

1   Encourage the patient to move by himself as much as possible to decrease the likelihood of complications (thromboembolism, diminished cerebral perfusion, aspiration of secretions and pneumonia, gastrointestinal stasis, urinary problems, increase in bone mineral loss, pressure sores).

a. Teach the patient to assist with turning by having him grasp the monkey pole for support.

b. When turning on unoperated side, keep the affected limb in a position of abduction. Place pillows between legs while patient is in side-lying position.

c. Start on exercise programme (see below).

2   Get the patient out of bed as soon as possible.

a. Bandage the lower limbs with elastic bandages, or apply tubigrip. This assists in minimizing dependent oedema.

b. With the use of the tilt-table the patient becomes accustomed to the upright position, and circulation and respiratory functioning improve.

c. Assist the patient into a chair during the day—helps avoid arterial hypotension, helps maintain strength, aids pulmonary function and is beneficial psychologically.

(1) With the aid of the overhead monkey pole encourage the patient to move into a sitting position. (Use a Hi-low bed.)

(2) Assist patient to stand on the *unaffected limb* and to transfer to the chair.

(3) If weight bearing is permitted, patient may be encouraged to walk with aid of a frame, applying as much weight to limb as is comfortable.

(4) Certain types of fractures must be supported and protected until bone union is secure and displacement of fractures unlikely. If this is the case the patient may have to be lifted into the chair.

(5) Allow the patient to get up at his own pace; avoid hurrying.

d. Encourage the patient to participate in activities of daily living (eating, bathing, hair care)—to condition the patient for future activities and to help maintain a degree of independence.

3 Start active exercises as soon as pain and soreness subside to prepare the patient to walk.

a. Encourage quadriceps setting exercises hourly—the quadriceps femoris muscle extends the leg and is one of the major muscles necessary for walking.

b. Do heel-cord stretching of both legs and abdominal and gluteal contractions (isometric contractions). Isometric muscle contractions strengthen the muscle but do not move the joint.

c. Assist the patient to perform arm strengthening exercises (flexion and extension of the arms). The muscles in the shoulder girdle and upper extremities must be strong enough to bear the patient's weight while he is using the walking frame.

d. Assist the patient to learn to use the walking frame with a nonweight-bearing (or partial weight-bearing depending on the fracture and its fixation) technique.

e. Remind the patient *not* to bear weight on the affected limb until the surgeon gives permission and the x-rays reveal sufficient healing. Early weight bearing before bony union occurs exerts too much stress and may cause bending or breaking of the pin, crushing of the bone or loss of fixation due to the device's cutting through the bone.

4 Watch for and prevent complications.

a. Thromboembolism—most common complication.

(1) Prophylactic anticoagulation medication may be given preoperatively and postoperatively; the following regimens have been advocated:

(a) Dicumarol, heparin (intravenous or low dose subcutaneously), low-molecular weight dextran, high molecular weight dextran. These methods require laboratory control and continuing medical surveillance.

(b) Aspirin, preoperatively and postoperatively, appears to reduce incidence of thrombotic complications.

(2) Examine for evidences of thrombophlebitis.

(3) Patient may require additional therapy if clinical evaluation, venograms or radioactive scanning studies demonstrate problems in lower limb veins or in pulmonary vascular system.

b. Pneumonia—have the patient breathe deeply and cough at intervals to clear tracheobronchial tree of secretions. Use IPPB or incentive spirometer.

c. Fat embolism—characterized by fever, tachycardia, dyspnoea and cough. (Fat embolism sometimes occurs after fractures of the long bones, particularly in elderly patients).

d. Knee contractures.

(1) Maintain the knee in a position of extension while patient is in bed.
(2) Flex the knee in a 90° angle while the patient is in the chair—avoid extending the knee for long periods when the patient is in a sitting position because extension produces undue strain on the fractured hip.
(3) Move the knee through assisted range-of-motion exercises.
e. Urinary tract infection.
(1) Avoid the routine use of an indwelling catheter—infection almost always follows the use of an indwelling catheter. (A urinary tract infection can cause a prolonged period of morbidity and incontinence in the elderly.)
(2) Watch the colour, odour and volume of urinary output.
(3) Maintain a liberal fluid intake (within limits of cardiorenal function).
f. Pressure sores.
(1) Encourage the patient to move about freely using the overhead monkey pole as an assistive device—peripheral arterial insufficiency, poor nutrition and lack of movement contribute to skin breakdown.
(2) Inspect the heels daily. Use protective heel padding (but inspect under it several times daily); massage reddened areas.
(3) Use ripple mattresses when necessary.
g. Infection—usually related to intercurrent medical problems, debility and infection elsewhere in the body.
h. Nonunion and avascular necrosis.

SPECIAL NURSING CONSIDERATIONS

Nursing Management of the Patient Undergoing Orthopaedic Surgery

Underlying Consideration

Orthopaedic operations usually require a longer period of convalescence and rehabilitation than other surgical procedures.

Nursing Management

Preoperative Care

1   Question patient to determine if he has had previous therapy with corticosteroids (especially patients with arthritis).
    a. Steroid therapy (current or past) may adversely affect patient's response to anaesthesia.
    b. Steroids (hydrocortisone, prednisolone) should be administered to cover the stress of surgery.
2   Have patient practise micturating in bedpan or urinal in recumbent position before surgery. This helps reduce necessity of postoperative catheterization.
3   Acquaint patient with traction apparatus, necessity for splints and cast—to familiarize him with his postoperative environment.
4   Prepare skin according to the local policy.

Postoperative Care

1   Check the blood pressure, pulse and respiratory rates frequently—rising pulse

rate or slowly falling blood pressure indicates persistent bleeding or development of a state of shock.

2 Assess changes in respiratory rate or in patient's colour—may indicate obstruction of respiratory exchange or pulmonary or cardiac complications.

3 Watch circulation distal to the portion of the extremity where cast, bandage or splint has been applied.

a. Prevent constriction leading to interference with blood or nerve supply.

b. Watch toes and fingers for normal temperature and healthy colour and swelling.

Nursing Alert: Abnormal coolness of skin, cyanosis, redness, or pallor indicates interference with circulation.

c. Notify surgeon and loosen cast or dressing at once.

4 Watch for excessive bleeding—orthopaedic wounds have a tendency to ooze more than other surgical wounds. Measure suction drainage if used.

5 Maintain sufficient pulmonary ventilation.

a. Avoid or give respiratory depressant drugs in minimal doses.

b. Change position every 2 hours—mobilizes secretions and helps prevent bronchial obstruction.

6 Maintain urinary output.

a. Maintain adequate fluid intake.

b. Watch for urinary retention—elderly men with some degree of prostatism may have difficulty in micturating.

Long-term Management

Orthopaedic operations frequently require prolonged periods in bed; movement may be limited by pain, casts or splints.

1 Watch for development of pressure sores.

a. Turn patient.

b. Wash, dry and massage skin frequently, every 2–4 hours.

c. Expose skin to air.

d. Maintain nutrition—administer plasma and vitamins as indicated to prevent hypoproteinaemia and avitaminosis, conditions which make pressure sores resistant to treatment.

2 Watch for complications due to prolonged disability.

a. Venous thrombosis.

(1) Mild swelling of limb.

(2) Pain, tenderness and distension of veins.

(3) Positive Homan's sign (pain upon dorsiflexion of foot).

(4) Tenderness—calf or anterior thigh.

b. Prevent venous complications.

(1) Encourage the patient to exercise by himself with a planned programme of exercise as soon as possible after surgery.

(2) Have patient flex his knee, extend the knee with hip still flexed, and then lower the limb to the bed.

(3) Encourage patient to move fingers and toes periodically.

(4) Advise patient to move joints which are not fixed by traction or appliance through their range of motion as fully as possible.

(5) Suggest muscle-setting exercises (quadriceps setting) if active motion is contraindicated.

(6) Bandage with elastic bandages, apply elastic hose or use antithrombolitic stockings.

(7) Treatment for venous thrombosis is discussed on p. 000.

   c. Give prophylactic anticoagulants as directed (heparin, warfarin, aspirin, etc.).

3 Give a normal balanced diet.

   a. Give supplemental vitamins (B and C) to elderly patients or those with chronic disease.

   b. Avoid giving large amounts of milk to orthopaedic patients on bed rest—adds to calcium pool in the body and demands more calcium excretion by the kidneys, predisposing to the formation of urinary calculi.

4 Watch for signs and symptoms of anaemia—especially after fracture of long bones.

   a. Haemoglobin determination usually done on third postoperative day or sooner.

   b. Give iron supplements as directed.

   c. Blood transfusion may be given to raise level of haemoglobin.

Lower Limb Amputation

Indications

1 Peripheral vascular disease (ischaemia of limb).
2 Trauma.
3 Uncontrolled infection (usually in bone).
4 Tumour.
5 Congenital deformities.

Treatment and Nursing Management (conventional approach)

Preoperative Care

Objective

To have the patient attain his highest physical and emotional level in preparation for wearing a prosthesis (artifical limb) and/or attaining mobility by other means.

1 Assist the patient undergoing circulatory patency tests (surface temperature, colour changes, oscillometric readings, arteriography).

   a. Amputation usually not performed until control of gangrene or advancing infection is achieved.

   b. Modern trend is towards selecting most distal amputation level (below knee) consistent with wound healing.

   c. The status of the sound limb is evaluated.

   d. Cardiac studies are carried out. Cardiac decompensation in older patients may contraindicate a prosthesis after surgery (rare).

   e. Culture and sensitivity tests of draining wounds (secondary to gangrene) often carried out.

2   Support the patient psychologically. Knowing what to expect helps reduce anxiety.

a. Explain various phases of rehabilitation involved—active participation in rehabilitation is essential for a successful outcome.

b. The surgeon will discuss the possibilities of obtaining and using a prosthesis—not all amputees can benefit from a prosthesis.

(1) Diabetes mellitus, heart disease, infection, cerebrovascular accident, arteriosclerosis obliterans and increasing age are factors limiting full rehabilitation.

(2) Wound breakdown, infection and delay in healing of amputation stump are significant limiting factors.

c. Amputation may be viewed as a surgical reconstructive procedure and as the first step in rehabilitation for the patient who has had prolonged periods of disability from peripheral vascular disease.

3   Build up the patient's nutritional status.

4   Preoperative physiotherapy. Have the patient strengthen the muscles of the upper limb, trunk and abdomen as a preparation for crutch walking. (Develop arm extensors and shoulder depressors, which are the muscle groups needed for crutch walking.) Instruct the patient as follows:

a. Flex and extend arms while holding weights.

b. Do push-ups from a prone position.

c. Do sit-ups from a seated position.

5   Teach the patient to crutch walk preoperatively—prepares for postoperative mobility, maintains mobility and arm function.

Postoperative Care

Objectives

To achieve optimal physical and emotional status in order to minimize problems in fitting and use of prosthesis.
To avoid complications.
To prevent prolonged disability.

1   Watch for signs and symptoms of haemorrhage.

a. Apply direct pressure and obtain assistance if haemorrhage occurs.

b. Raise foot of bed slightly to elevate stump. Do not flex patient's hips by elevating stump on pillow since this will produce a hip flexion contracture.

c. Reinforce dressing as required using aseptic technique.

d. Monitor suction drainage.

2   Prevent deformities in the immediate postoperative period. Contracture of the next joint above an amputation is a frequent complication.

a. Deformities include:

(1) Flexion deformities.

(2) Nonshrinkage of stump.

(3) Abduction deformities.

b. Encourage patient to turn from side to side.

c. Place patient in prone position twice daily—to stretch the flexor muscles and prevent flexion contracture of the hip.

(1) Keep patient's legs close together—to prevent abduction deformity.

(2) Place pillow under abdomen and stump while patient is prone.

d. Encourage patient to move stump—to avoid contractures.

e. Start range of motion exercises—contracture deformities develop rapidly and cause serious problems in management of prosthesis.

3   Observe and protect the remaining foot from injury.

a. Examine remaining foot and malleoli daily.

b. Keep pressure (bedclothes) off foot.

4   Assist physiotherapist with muscle strengthening and balancing exercises—to strengthen muscles, mobilize joints and increase balance sense.

Instruct patient as follows (stand behind patient and stabilize him at the waist, if necessary):

a. Arise from chair and stand.

b. Stand on toes while holding on to a chair.

c. Bend the knees while holding on to a chair.

d. Balance on one leg without support.

e. Hop on one foot while holding on to a chair.

5   Condition the stump—so that prosthesis can be fitted properly in future.

a. Shrink and shape the stump—to permit accurate measurement of prosthesis and maximum fit.

(1) Apply elastic stump shrinker or

(2) Use elastic bandages—to prevent oedema and shrink stump.

(a) Apply bandage smoothly with no folds—creases will produce skin abrasion (Fig. 4.10).

(b) Apply bandages snugly to adductor area to prevent formation of adductor roll.

(c) Bandages are worn constantly; rewrap when necessary.

(d) Prosthesis is measured and fitted when maximum shrinkage occurs.

b. Or—air splint may be applied to amputation stump to control oedema.

c. Have the patient do stump-conditioning exercises—to harden the stump.

(1) The patient pushes the stump against a soft pillow.

(2) Gradually he pushes stump against harder surfaces.

d. Teach the patient to massage the stump—to soften the scar, decrease tenderness and improve vascularity.

(1) Massage is usually started 1 week postoperatively.

(2) Initially massage is usually done by physiotherapist.

e. Protect the stump from infection.

(1) Protect dressing if patient is incontinent.

(2) Wash stump with mild soap and water.

(3) Expose stump to air and sun.

6   Watch for deterioration of remaining leg—from disuse, poor vascular supply, foot trauma. (Obliterative arteriosclerotic vascular disease may necessitate *bilateral* lower limb amputation.)

7   Keep the patient active—decreases occurrence of phantom-limb pain.

a. If patient is not a candidate for prosthesis/ambulation, teach him to participate in self-care activities in a special wheelchair designed for amputees.

b. Reassure patient that phantom-limb sensation (painful sensation that amputated foot is still there) will soon pass.

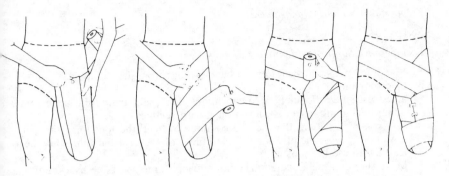

Figure 4.10. Shrinking and shaping the stump in a conical form helps ensure comfort and fit of the prosthetic device. Bandaging supports the soft tissue and minimizes the formation of oedema fluid while the stump is in a dependent position.

8　Accept the frustrations and behaviour of the patient.
　　a. The self-image has to be adjusted after amputation.
　　b. It will take time for the patient to make this modification.

Immediate or Early Postoperative Fitting of Prosthesis

Immediate postoperative fitting is a procedure in which a prosthesis is applied and used 24–48 hours after amputation. Immediately following surgery, a rigid plaster of paris dressing is applied with provision for the attachment of a pylon and artificial foot. The patient is brought into an upright position soon after surgery and allowed to bear a small amount of weight on the prosthesis. He progresses to walking as soon as tolerance permits.

Early postoperative prosthetic fitting is a procedure in which the rigid dressing is applied immediately and used 10–30 days after amputation. The difference between the two procedures lies in the time when weight bearing and walking take place.

Rationale of Rigid Dressing

This allows optimum pressure gradients to be exerted on the stump—to control oedema, support circulation, minimize pain on movement, help shape the stump and promote healing. It allows earlier fitting of the prosthesis, shortens the interval between amputation and walking, and is of tremendous psychological value to the patient.

Modifications of Immediate Prosthetic Technique

1　Simple plaster socket without prosthetic equipment—constitutes rigid dressing that splints and compresses amputation stump, but does not have prosthesis necessary for ambulation.
2　Air splint (pneumatic prosthesis)—applied upon completion of amputation and inflated. It provides uniform compression of the stump, controls stump oedema by adjustment of external pressure, gives easy access to stump for inspection.

Preoperative Nursing Management

See p. 182.

Postoperative Surgical and Nursing Management

1   Watch for signs and symptoms of haemorrhage from the stump.
2   Control pain.
   a. Assess for development of complications; increasing stump pain, haematoma, odour emanating from cast, infection, stump necrosis.
   b. Explain to patient that he will continue to 'feel' the foot for a time; this sensation may be helpful for the placement of the artificial foot while he is learning to use the prosthesis.
3   Make sure that the amputation stump remains in the plaster cast socket during the patient's hospitalization; if the socket inadvertently comes off, excessive oedema will form very rapidly, causing a delay in rehabilitation.
   a. Rebandage the stump immediately with elastic compression bandage (Fig. 4.10).
   b. Prepare for immediate reapplication of cast socket.
4   Observe and protect the remaining foot from injury.
5   Start patient on standing and ambulation activities.
   a. The timing depends on age, general physical status, condition of remaining foot, etc.
   b. Although the rigid dressing is vital to care, early weight bearing is not always desirable in patients with severe peripheral vascular disease.
   c. The patient may stand by his bed (or on tilt-table) within 48 hours postoperatively with the prosthetic foot touching down (no weight bearing)—helps minimize fear of pain and promotes confidence of patient in his ability to handle himself; allows prosthetist to check length of pylon.
   d. Weight bearing to tolerance of pain is carried out progressively.
   e. Progressively longer periods of standing and walking in parallel bars or frame are initiated (with protected weight bearing while prosthesis is in place).
   f. Progressive ambulation following first change of dressing is carried out under the supervision of physiotherapist or nurse. Gait training is continued under the direction of physiotherapist.
   g. A going-home prosthesis is fitted approximately 3 weeks following surgery. The permanent prosthesis is fitted when the stump is fully conditioned.

Rehabilitation

The patient will require rehabilitation services to learn mobility skills, transfers, wheelchair or automobile locomotion, etc.

Upper Limb Amputation

Indications

1   Trauma (acute injury, electrical burns, frostbite).
2   Congenital malformations.
3   Malignant tumours.

Surgical Management and Nursing Care

Preoperative Care (when time permits)

Objective

To optimize the rehabilitation of the patient.

1   Give the patient psychological support to help him adapt to changes in his life style.
   a. Listen to his fears and concerns.
   b. Discuss with him the available prosthetic replacement (by orthotist).
   c. Demonstrate aids to independence (one-handed knife for cutting, elastic shoelaces, one-handed methods of functioning)—usually done in co-operation with occupational therapist.
2   Instruct the patient in postoperative exercises (by physiotherapist).

Postoperative Care

1   When the patient returns from the operating theatre he will have either a rigid plaster of paris socket with provision for the application of a temporary prosthesis or a conventional compression bandage in place.
2   Monitor the amount and character of the suction drainage—used to eliminate haematoma and approximate the tissues.
3   Encourage active motion of stump aftr mobility restrictions have been removed.
   a. Muscle setting, joint mobilizing, range of motion are performed as soon as tolerated—to strengthen muscles and joints (under direction of physiotherapist).
   b. Exercise muscles of both shoulders—an upper limb amputee uses both shoulders to operate prosthesis.
   c. Carry out postural exercises—loss of weight of amputated limb may produce postural abnormality.
4   Assist with dressing change and suture removal; wound is inspected and sutures removed in 7–10 days.
   a. Rigid dressing.
   A new plaster socket with temporary prosthetic device is applied—increases patient's endurance—allows early prosthetic training and fitting of permanent prosthetic device.
   b. Compression dressing.
   (1) Rewrap the stump three to four times daily—to maintain proper tension in the bandage and to reduce the fluid and shape the stump so that a prosthesis may be fitted.
   (2) See Figs. 4.11 and 4.12 for technique of stump bandaging. Make sure that the patient and his family know the correct technique of application since stump bandaging will be continued until the permanent prosthesis is fitted (6 weeks to a year).
   (3) Keep stump snugly wrapped with elastic bandage for 24-hour period except for periods of bathing and exercise.
5   Start patient on one-handed self care activities as soon as possible—to promote independence. Occupational therapist teaches self-feeding, bathing, grooming, etc.

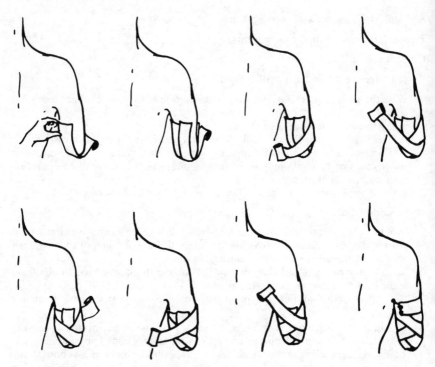

Figure 4.11. Steps in the application of an elastic bandage to a standard or long above-elbow stump. (From: Bender, L F (1974) Prostheses and Rehabilitation after Arm Amputation. Courtesy: Charles C. Thomas, Springfield, Illinois.)

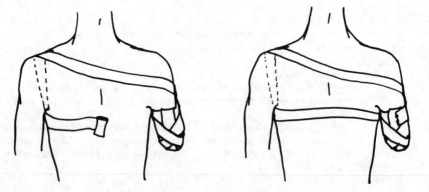

Figure 4.12. An elastic bandage applied to a short above-elbow stump usually must be wrapped one or more times through the normal axilla to hold the stump wrapping in place. (From: Bender, L F (1974) Prostheses and Rehabilitation after Arm Amputation. Courtesy: Charles C. Thomas, Springfield, Illinois.)

6 Assess for complications:
   a. Neuroma—sensitive tumour of nerve cells growing at end of severed nerve.
   b. Skin problems—from irritants in prosthetic components, lack of ventilation.
   c. Stump contraction or stump contour problems.
   d. Phantom sensation (feeling that limb is still present).
   e. Psychological problems (denial, withdrawal)—responses influenced by support and encouragement of rehabilitation team, by early introduction of one-handed activities, and by discussion of prosthetic options and capabilities.
7 The fitting of the prosthesis depends on the level of amputation, age of patient and whether or not weakness or limitation of range of motion of joints proximal to amputation site is present.
   a. Patient will require instruction in putting on and removing prosthesis, control of prosthesis, etc.
   b. Ultimate patient rehabilitation requires the services and supervision of rehabilitation team at the limb fitting centre.

Health Teaching

Instruct the patient to maintain careful stump hygiene to prevent skin irritation and infection.

1 Wash and dry stump thoroughly at least twice daily.
2 Wear stump sock. Change daily (and wash immediately)—to absorb perspiration and avoid direct contact between prosthetic socket and skin.
3 Avoid wrinkles in stump sock—may irritate skin.
4 Wipe the socket of prosthesis with damp cloth upon removal in evening.
5 Wear cotton tee shirt—to prevent contact between skin and shoulder harness and to absorb perspiration. Change daily.
6 Launder the washable portions of the harness as often as necessary; have two harnesses so that one can be laundered while the other is worn.
7 Have prosthesis checked periodically.

Hip Arthroplasty (Total Hip Replacement)

Arthroplasty is an operation to restore motion to a joint and function to the structures (muscles, ligaments, soft tissues) that control it. An inert substance is interposed between the reshaped ends of the bone to mould or maintain joint function, or the joint is replaced. The procedure depends on the anatomy and function of the joint (Fig. 4.13).

Total hip replacement (total joint arthroplasty) is the implantation of a metal femoral head (Vitallium or stainless steel) fitted into an acetabular plastic socket (high-molecular weight polyethylene) and affixed to surrounding bone with methyl methacrylate (bone cement). There are many types of implants available. Total joint arthroplasty is an exacting and meticulous procedure.

Clinical Indications

1 For patients (over 50) with unremitting pain, irreversibly damaged hip joints.
   a. Rheumatoid arthritis.
   b. Primary degenerative arthritis (osteoarthritis).

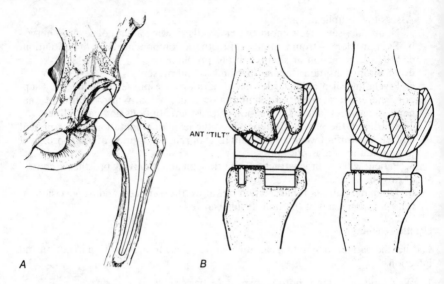

Figure 4.13. Examples of total joint arthroplasty. a. Total hip replacement. b. Total knee replacement. (Courtesy: Zimmer, USA.)

2   Complications of femoral neck fractures.
3   Failure of previous reconstructive surgery (osteotomy, cup arthroplasty, femoral head replacement for complications of nonunion and avascular necrosis).
4   Problems resulting from congenital hip disease.

Treatment and Nursing Management

Objectives

To decrease pain.
To restore, improve or maintain joint function.
To provide greater stability of arthritic hip.
To avoid complications.

Preoperative Care

1   Educate and prepare the patient for the procedure.
    a. Have the patient practise in-bed activities:
    (1) Learn to use bedpan or urinal for micturating in the recumbent position—acquaints patient with procedure of micturition while lying down; reduces probability of postoperative catheterization.
    (2) With the aid of the physiotherapist teach isometric exercises (muscle setting) of quadriceps and gluteal muscles; active ankle motion.
    (3) Fit with crutches and instruct patient to walk without weight bearing (if prescribed)—to develop crutch walking ability and facilitate patient's postoperative walking.

(4) Teach bed-to-wheelchair transfer without going beyond the hip flexion limits.

(5) Demonstrate deep breathing exercises—to assist in complete expansion of the lungs.

Urge patient to stop smoking in preoperative period.

(6) Demonstrate use of equipment that the patient may be required to use following surgery.

(7) Educate patient concerning his postoperative regimen; e.g., extended exercise programme will be carried out after surgery—atrophied muscles must be re-educated and strengthened.

2 Utilize all precautions to avoid infection.

a. Antibiotics usually given preoperatively, intraoperatively and postoperatively to reduce incidence of infection.

b. Give preoperative medication into uninvolved limb.

c. During the operative procedure in operating room:

(1) Theatre traffic reduced to a minimum.

(2) Theatre personnel wear special gowns with waterproof front and sleeves, double gloves and masks and hoods.

(3) Theatre may be ventilated by rapidly changing air delivered by filtering system (unidirectional or laminar)—reduces particulate matter and bacterial count of air such as the Charnley–Howarth tent.

(4) Instruments protected from airborne contamination.

(5) Wound may be irrigated with antibiotic solution during surgery.

Postoperative Care

Objectives

To maintain the affected limb in the desired position.
To prevent and treat complications.

1 Following arthroplasty traction may be applied to the limb if the surgeon wishes. The limb is usually kept in abduction (sometimes by a wedge of foam rubber) to prevent dislocation of prothesis until soft tissue is healed.

NOTE: There are numerous modifications with differing requirements in the postoperative positioning of these patients.

2 **a.** Two nurses lift the patient clear of the bed while a third nurse washes and massages the back.

b. Use pillows to keep the leg abducted.

c. The patient is nursed in a semirecumbent position. However, he will require to lie flat for short periods to help prevent hip flexion contractures.

(1) A suitable schedule may be semirecumbent for meals and evening, supine for 1 hour postmeals.

(2) Support the low back with a small pillow or towel when patient is supine—to relieve strain placed on muscles by the flat position.

d. As the patient becomes familiar with the turning routine, assist him to change position by using overhead monkey pole.

Patient must not adduct or flex operated hip—may produce dislocation.

3   Monitor blood loss—portable suction is used to decrease incidence of wound haematoma, which is a possible focus of infection.
4   Give narcotics as required the first 24 hours postoperatively and then taper to non-narcotic analgesia thereafter.
5   Encourage patient to carry out prescribed exercise programme, usually under direction of physiotherapist.
   a. Instruct him to think about the motion required to contract the appropriate muscles.
   b. Encourage him to breathe deeply while exercising.
   c. Exercise activities depend on procedure and on condition of patient.
      (1) Active motion of affected foot and ankle started first postoperative day.
      (2) Isometric exercise of quadriceps, gluteals, abductors started upon direction of orthopaedic surgeon.
      (3) Flexion, extension, abduction and rotation exercises started upon direction of surgeon; patient ambulates upon order.
6   Use anticipatory nursing measures to prevent complications.
   a. Thromboembolism (major threat following reconstructive hip operations).
      (1) Continue to exercise ankles and legs—accelerates blood flow and prevents venous stasis.
      (2) Antiembolic stockings for uninvolved extremity—to increase venous velocity; elastic stocking applied to operated extremity when elastic compression dressing is removed.
      (3) Check for calf oedema, tenderness, positive Homan's sign.
      (4) Aspirin may be given in the hope of reducing thromboembolic problems; low dose heparin, etc., may be used.
   b. Infection.
      (1) Infection may not become apparent until months or years after surgery.
      (2) Deep infection almost always requires removal of implant.
      (3) Give antibiotics as directed.
      (4) Watch for elevation of temperature and inspect wound at intervals.
   c. Complicating medical conditions (cardiac, gastrointestinal, genitourinary).
   d. Dislocation of prosthesis, loosening of bond between methyl methacrylate and metal or bone, fatigue fracture of metal component, avascular necrosis or dead bone caused by loss of blood supply.

Health Teaching

Instruct the patient as follows:
1   Continue to wear elastic stockings after going home until full activities are resumed.
2   Limit sitting to 30 min at a time.
   a. Avoid sitting in low chair. Keep knees apart.
   b. Avoid prolonged travel unless frequent changes of position are possible.
3   Continue quadriceps exercises and range of motion as directed.
      Have a *daily* programme of stretching, exercise and rest throughout lifetime.
4   Use self-help and energy saving devices.
   a. Handrails by toilet.

    b. Raised toilet seat if there is some residual hip flexion problem.
    c. Bar type stool for shower and kitchen work.
5 Lie prone twice daily for 30 min.
6 Report for follow-up evaluation and testing; supportive equipment (crutches, stick) is modified as needed.
7 Walking stick may be discarded when sufficient muscle tone has returned to permit normal gait.

Total Knee Arthroplasty

A *total knee arthroplasty* is an implant procedure in which both tibial and femoral joint surfaces are replaced because of destroyed knee joint(s). Different types of implants are used, depending on degree of destruction and stability of joint. Most implants have metallic femoral and polyethylene tibial components.

Indications

Disabling pain and loss of function from degenerative or rheumatoid arthritis of knee.

Preoperative Nursing Management

1 Patient is advised of implant he will receive and what will be expected of him postoperatively.
2 See p. 190.

Postoperative Nursing Management

The postoperative nursing management is essentially the same as that for total hip arthroplasty.

1 The knee may be immobilized in full extension with either a plaster cast or a firm compression dressing with extension splint.
2 Static quadriceps setting exercises are started preoperatively and resumed on second postoperative day—quadriceps muscle is important in achieving full extension of the knee.
3 Suction drainage tubes removed when bloody drainage ceases (usually 48 hours).
4 Gentle knee motion usually started after first dressing is changed.
    a. Give pain medication before exercise period if necessary; cold applications may be beneficial.
    b. Patient assisted in straight leg raising until he is able to lift leg independently.
    c. Patient encouraged to perform active flexion and extension exercises.
    d. Exercises progress to active extension of knee through its fullest arc of motion within the limits of pain.
    e. A pulley and sling setup may be used for assisted hip and knee flexion.
5 Patient may transfer out of bed into wheelchair with extension splint in place; no weight bearing is permitted at this time.
6 Partial weight bearing (with crutches or parallel bars) may be achieved by end of 1 week; patient usually has 70–90° flexion.

If knee motion is less than 70° by 10–14th postoperative day, gentle manipulation is carried out under anaesthesia.

7   Use bilateral supportive walking equipment—proper supportive equipment enables patient to walk while bearing weight to tolerance.
   a. Protect wrist and finger joints from extreme stress, especially if patient has rheumatoid arthritis.
   b. Use forearm trough walker, forearm trough cane, axillary crutches, etc.
8   Complications:
   a. Early: wound dehiscence, infection, thromboembolic complications, peroneal nerve palsy.
   b. Late: deep infection, loosening of prosthetic components, implant wear and dislocation, fatigue fracture of tibial plateau.

Health Teaching

Instruct the patient as follows:

1   Use the resting splint at night for 3–4 weeks to maintain knee at full extention.
2   Use stationary bicycle to improve range of motion and strengthen muscles.
3   See p. 192

LOW BACK PAIN

Low back pain is characterized by acute pain in the low back associated with severe spasm of the paraspinal muscles, often with radiation.
Muscle spasm is a condition in which muscles are painfully contracted.

Aetiology (multiple causes)

1   Mechanical (joint, muscular or ligamentous strain).
2   Congenital malformations.
3   Degenerative disc disease; acute herniation of discs.
4   Poor posture; obesity.
5   Lack of physical activity and exercise.
6   Arthritic conditions.
7   Predisposing endocrine and systemic diseases.
8   Diseases of bone (Paget's disease, metastatic carcinoma).
9   Infections of disc spaces or vertebrae.
10   Spinal cord tumours.

Diagnosis

1   History—to determine when, where and how the pain occurs and its relationship to activity and rest; to rule out medical causes.
2   Neurologic evaluation—to spot localized weakness of extremities and reflex and sensory loss; to exclude neurogenic disease.
3   Evaluation of muscular system—for changes in strength, tone and flexibility of key posture muscles.

4   Electromyography—to record changes in electric potential of muscle and of nerve leading to it.
5   X-ray—of lumbar spine (anteroposterior, lateral and oblique).
6   Bone scan—to detect early malignant or infectious conditions.

Treatment and Nursing Management

Objectives

To relieve muscle spasm.
To gain normal elasticity of affected muscles.
To return normal joint motion.
To correct underlying conditions.

1   Advise the patient to rest in bed in a semirecumbent position (hips and knees flexed—to relax muscles, remove stress from lumbar sacral area, relieve tension on sciatic nerves and open the posterior part of the intervertebral spaces.
   a. Acute spasm should subside in 3–7 days if there is no nerve involvement or other serious underlying disease.
   b. Do prescribed isometric exercises hourly while on bed rest if possible.
2   Use heat to relax muscle spasm and relieve discomfort.
   a. Apply moist warm heat (moist towels, hydrocolator packs).
   b. Follow heat by massage.
3   Or utilize ice applications, which may be equally effective for secondary muscle spasm.
4   Use appropriate medications to relieve pain. (Rest in bed may eliminate the need for pain medications.)
   a. Give oral pain medication and muscle relaxants.
   b. Use parenteral pain medication in acute severe pain syndromes.
   c. Pelvic traction may be utilized.
5   Have patient start abdominal muscle strengthening exercises after acute symptoms subside—the abdominal muscles are the anterior supporting muscles of the spine.
6   Encourage patient to do prescribed back exercises (Fig. 4.14). Exercise keeps postural muscles strong, helps recondition the back and abdominal musculature and serves as an outlet for emotional tension.
   Pelvic tilt (small of back is pressed against a flat surface)—decreases lordosis.
7   Advise patient to start activity as soon as possible—activity speeds recovery and helps prevent loss of muscle function.
8   Psychiatric intervention may be needed for patient with both chronic depression and low back syndrome. Encourage patient to discuss problems which may be contributing to his backache.
9   Use lumbosacral support early—helps control pain and gives patient confidence.
10 Prepare patient for myelogram if he shows no improvement after 7–10 days of conservative treatment; operative intervention may be necessary. (See Treatment of Herniated Nucleus Pulposus p 67.)

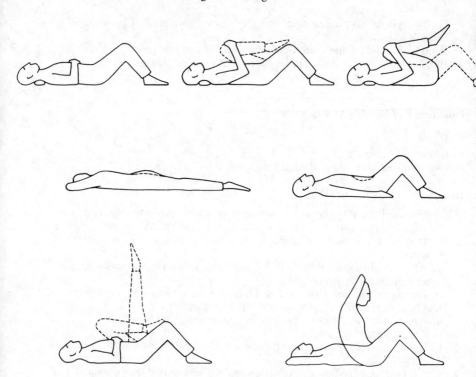

Figure 4.14. Back exercises are designed to strengthen abdominal muscles and stretch the contracted back muscles. They help keep posture muscles strong and flexible and aid in reducing nervous tension which increases low back pain.

Health Teaching

Instruct the patient as follows:

1   Tension can contribute to spasm in the back muscles.
2   Avoid prolonged standing, walking, sitting and driving.
3   Rest at intervals throughout the day.
4   Avoid assuming tense, cramped positions. Avoid forward flexion.
5   Use a hard plywood board under a firm mattress.
6   Pick up objects or loads correctly.
     a. Maintain a straight spine.
     b. Flex knees and hips while stooping—places stress on bony components rather than on soft tissues.
7   Stay with the exercise programme, which should be supervised and reviewed frequently. Continue with generalized conditioning of body (walking, swimming).
8   Reduce weight if indicated.

RHEUMATOID ARTHRITIS

Rheumatoid arthritis is a chronic systemic disease primarily affecting connective tissue in any or all of the body systems. It is characterized most prominently by recurrent inflammation involving the synovium, or lining of the joints, that leads to destructive changes in the joints. The cause is unknown and the course is variable.

Clinical Manifestations

1 Inflammation of the joints characterized by pain, swelling, heat, redness and limitation of function.
2 Subcutaneous nodules over bony prominences, bursae and tendon sheaths.
3 Enlarged lymph nodes; particularly nodes draining inflamed joints.
4 Constitutional symptoms (may accompany or precede arthropathy):
   a. Easy fatigability and malaise.
   b. Fever.
   c. Weight loss, general weakness.
   d. Anaemia.

Pathophysiology Underlying Joint Destruction

Inflammation of joint (synovitis) → synovial effusion → granulation tissue covering articular cartilage (pannus) → joint capsular and subcondral bone destruction → pain → loss of mobility of joint → muscular weakness about the joint → damage to tendons and ligaments → joint instability and deformity → joint malfunction and disuse → muscular atrophy and contracture deformity.

Diagnosis

1 History, physical examination.
2 Laboratory tests.
   a. Blood count (most patients are anaemic).
   b. Tests which reveal disease activity and provide guidelines for therapy include:
      (1) C-reactive protein test (CRP)—positive in rheumatoid arthritis.
      (2) Erythrocyte sedimentation rate—elevated during periods of active arthritis.
   c. Tests for rheumatoid factor in the serum: positive in 70–80% of patients with rheumatoid arthritis:
      (1) Latex fixation test.
      (2) Antinuclear antibody test.
   d. Serum protein electrophoresis—increased globulins (gamma and alpha globulins); decreased albumin.
3 Roentgenograms of involved joints—to determine extent, rate of progress and structural changes within bones; reveals swelling of soft tissue, erosion of bone at articular margins, narrowing of joint space.
4 Thermography—pinpoints areas of inflammation and increased metabolic activity in the body by pictorially recording (mapping) the heat emitted from the skin over the affected areas.
5 Synovial fluid analysis—to distinguish between inflammatory, traumatic or degenerative arthritis.

6   Arthroscopy—endoscopic examination of knee joint; allows observation of synovial lining, articular cartilage and minisci; permits examination of knee during passive movements and allows biopsy under direct vision; detects pathology earlier than other methods.

Objectives of Treatment and Nursing Management

Objective

To maintain independence and prevent crippling deformities by:

1   Controlling synovitis.
2   Maintaining joint mobility and muscle power.
3   Relieving pain and promoting comfort.
4   Decreasing the activity of the disease.
5   Educating and helping the patient and family to adjust to a chronic disability.

The treatment programme includes rest, exercise, drug therapy and education.

To Maintain Joint Mobility and Muscle Power

Inflammation, scarring and mechanical damage to joint structures produce pain and disability.

1   Regular rest at specified periods is needed to control fatigue—arthritis affects the whole body.
   a. Complete bed rest for patients with active widespread inflammatory disease.
   b. Have patient rest in a recumbent position (one pillow under head) on a firm mattress—to take the weight off the joints.
   c. Advise patient to establish one or more daytime rest periods of 30–60 min.
   d. Encourage patient to rest in bed 8–9 hours at night.
   e. Instruct patient to lie in prone position twice daily to prevent hip flexion and knee contractures.
   f. Pillows should not be placed under painful joints—promotes flexion contractures.
2   Painful joints should be rested with splints—to locally decrease synovitis; to reduce pain, stiffness and swelling (in wrists and fingers)—to combat deformity and enhance function (Fig. 4.15).
   a. Lightweight plastic splints are useful if they do not impede activity.
   b. The joint should be supported in a functional position (if splinting is indicated) with resting splints, bivalved casts, etc.
      (1) A resting splint is used at night to keep the knee in full extension.
      (2) The wrist is splinted with slight dorsiflexion—useful in patients with carpal tunnel syndrome (compression of median nerve within carpal canal).
   c. Splints may need modifications as joint structures change.
   d. Metatarsal bars or pads (for shoes) or Plastizote inserts may be used to decrease pressure on painful arthritic feet.
3   Have patient do exercises—to maintain function of all joints, to strengthen muscles that support the joints, to improve circulation and to promote endurance.
   a. Encourage the patient to follow a prescribed *daily* programme of exercise

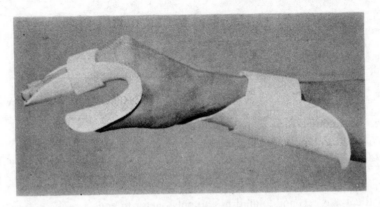

Figure 4.15. Rest splint for hand. Rest of the hand is important when soft tissues are acutely inflamed. Instruct the patient to maintain full range of motion of all joints and maintain tendon excursion while wearing a rest splint to prevent loss of important hand function. (Photo courtesy: Western Pennsylvania Hospital, Pittsburgh, Pennsylvania.)

composed of conditioning exercises and specific exercises for particular joint problems (after inflammatory process is controlled).

(1) Avoid excessive exercise—may lead to rapid joint destruction.

(2) Stop exercise before tiring.

(3) Pain lasting more than ½ hour after activity indicates exercise is too vigorous; decrease but do not stop activity.

(4) Exercise slowly and smoothly in short, frequent bouts.

b. See that patient performs isometric exercises—to help prevent muscle atrophy which contributes to joint instability.

c. Have patient move joints through full range of motion once to twice daily to prevent loss of joint motion.

(1) Assist patient in performing required joint motion if necessary.

(2) Avoid grasping painful joints; grasp belly of muscle.

d. Have patient do progressive resistive exercises—for muscle building, depending on activity of arthritis.

e. Self-help devices can be used to help with daily activities.

(1) Eating utensils with built-up handles.

(2) Raised chair seats, toilet seats.

(3) Special fastenings on clothing.

f. Crutches or cane held in hand opposite affected knee/hip can be used—to reduce the load on the affected knee/hip.

4   Control pain.

Instruct patient as follows:

a. Apply moist heat to reduce muscle spasm and postrest stiffness; provide as much relief from pain as possible so that exercise programme can be carried out.

(1) Take warm tub bath or shower upon arising—shortens period of morning stiffness.

(2) Use hot paraffin baths for fingers, hands.

b. Use cold packs or ice when indicated for hot, swollen joints; heat is sometimes contraindicated when a joint is acutely inflamed. Cold will relieve swelling and pain and help restore function.

c. Employ gentle massage to relax muscles.

d. Take joints through range of motion after heat treatments.

e. Advise rest to alleviate pain.

f. Take medication to relieve pain (although the primary function of salicylates in rheumatoid arthritis is anti-inflammatory).

g. Take non-narcotic analgesic if there is pain at night.

To Give Medications to Reduce Inflammation and Pain in Joint Tissues and Surrounding Structures and to Suppress the Disease Process as Much as Possible, as Well as to Allow More Effective Exercise

1   See Table 4.1 for drug therapy.

2   Patient may respond to all drugs, to only one or to none.

To Support the Patient Who is Depressed and Anxious Because of the Constant, Unremitting Nature of the Disease

1   Maintain a close patient–nurse–doctor relationship—successful management usually requires a long period of treatment.

2   Adopt a positive and optimistic attitude.

3   Emphasize that something can and will be done to relieve the patient's pain and mobilize his joints.

a. Encourage him to express his feelings—patient becomes hostile and angry because of chronic pain, stiffness and loss of mobility.

b. Let the patient know that you are aware of his fears and that his future is important to the health team.

4   Give tranquillizers and mood elevating drugs as prescribed.

5   Try to prevent patient from adopting a dependent role.

Health Teaching

Instruct the patient as follows:

1   *The primary goal is to maintain function of all joints.*

2   Maintain independence.

a. Rely on your own capabilities.

b. Conserve energy and simplify daily activities using self-help devices, work simplification methods and energy-saving methods.

c. Work at an even pace.

d. Alternate periods of work, exercise and rest. Avoid overdoing on good days.

e. Alternate sitting and standing tasks; do not remain seated too long.

3   Avoid dietary fads and 'quack' treatments.

4   Take the medication exactly as prescribed.

a. Aspirin is the primary drug (used for its anti-inflammatory effect). It must be taken over a long period and at high doses to achieve desired response.

b. Report ringing in the ears, since this is a guide to adequate dosage.

c. Take with food (a buffering agent).

Table 4.1. Drugs Used in Rheumatoid Arthritis

Drug	Action	Nursing Implication and Assessment for Drug Intolerance
Anti-inflammatory Agents *Salicylates*		
Acetylsalicylic Acid Aspirin (may be buffered or enteric coated)	An example of a prostoglandin inhibitor—drugs of this group form the cornerstone of treatment Exerts anti-inflammatory effect Optimum dosage will produce blood salicylate levels of 20–25 mg/100 ml Can be used in combination with other analgesics and anti-inflammatory agents	Take salicylates with antacid or milk to protect against gastric irritation Watch for complaints of tinnitus, gastric intolerance, or gastrointestinal bleeding and purpuric tendencies
Phenylbutazone (Butazolidin)	Nonsteroidal antirheumatic agents for adjunctive treatment of rheumatoid arthritis Exerts analgesic, anti-inflammatory action Sometimes remarkably effective in control of articular symptoms Patient should be under close medical supervision Can cause salt and water retention Usually used only for short peroids	Observe for untoward effects Gastrointestinal effects: Nausea, vomiting, epigastric distress, precipitation and reactivation of peptic ulcer Haematological effects: Bone marrow depression, anaemia, leucopenia, agranulocytosis, thrombocytopenia purpura *Irreversible blood element depression may occur rapidly despite careful supervision and frequent testing* May precipitate gout
Indomethicin (Indocid)	Additionally available as suppositories	Gastrointestinal effects, C.N.S. effects
Ibuprofen (Brufen)	Anti-inflammatory action	Headache Epigastric distress. Less so than other drugs of this group
Antimalarial Compounds		
Hydroxychloroquine Sulphate (Plaquenil)	Appears to be no rational basis for the comparative success of these drugs	Stress that patient should have regular ophthalmologic examination every 4–6 months; *drug has potential retinal effects* Toxic effects: Headache, dizziness, gastrointestinal complaints, occular toxicity and retinopathy

(continued)

Table 4.1 (*cont.*)

Drug	Action	Nursing Implication and Assessment for Drug Intolerance
Gold Salts		
Gold sodium thiomalate Myocrisin	Gold salts are useful when rheumatoid activity is uncontrolled by previous therapy Gold salt therapy is cumulative with slow onset of beneficial effects Mechanism of action unknown; exerts an inflammatory-suppressive effect Can produce a long-sustained remission when treatment continued indefinitely	Toxic effects: Dermatitis, stomatitis, nephritis, blood dyscrasias Before administering, shake the vial vigorously Administer deep intra-muscularly into the ventrogluteal area to avoid local irritation or necrosis of nerves, a potential lethal complication of injection
Corticosteroids		

Prednisolone Adrenocorticotrophic hormone (ACTH)	Corticosteroids used in treatment of incapacitating active rheumatoid arthritis when other conservative measures fail to control the disease
	Use of corticosteroids for long periods has wide range of adverse effects
	Steroids should be used with caution in small doses and for limited periods
		Toxic effects:
		  Osteoporosis and fractures
		  Gastric ulcers, organic psychosis, infection
		  Hirsutism, acne, moon facies, abnormal fat deposition, oedema, emotional dis-orders, menstrual disorders

Intra-articular Corticosteroid Injections		
	Given when rheumatoid arthritic reaction has been suppressed and one or two joints are not responding to treatment Given when only one or two joints affected Given to patient with extremely painful joints so he can undergo physiotherapy Relieves pain, benefit may last from weeks to months	An inflamed joint may respond to local injection when it has failed to come under control with other general systemic measures Joints most amenable to corticosteroid injections are ankles, knees, hips, shoulders and hands

(continued)

Table 4.1   (cont.)

Drug	Action	Nursing Implication and Assessment for Drug Intolerance
Immunosuppressive Drugs		
Cyclophosphamide Endoxane Azathioprin (Imuran)	Mechanism underlying action of these drugs not known; thought to affect the production of antibodies at the cellular level Suppress auto-immune mechanism Used only in advanced rheumatic arthritis that is unresponsive to conventional therapy These drugs have teratogenic potential	*Highly toxic:* Bone marrow depression, gastrointestinal ulceration Skin rashes, alopecia *Reduces patient's resistance to infections* Patient must be monitored with weekly blood evaluation and urinalysis Advise patient of contraceptive measures

5   Use prescribed heat or cold treatments for muscle relaxation and relief of pain.
6   Do the prescribed exercises to preserve joint motion and to gain muscular strength and co-ordination.
  a. Exercise also in water (pool; bathtub)—water provides buoyancy, support and relaxation.
  b. Review *Handbook for Patients* which has specific exercise instructions. Available from: Arthritic and Rheumatism Council, 8/10 Charing Cross Road, London WC2. (Other publications also available.)
7   Some doctors may wish patients to wear stretch nylon gloves at night to relieve numbness and tingling of fingers.
8   Protect musculoskeletal system from further damage.
  a. Lower yourself gently into a chair, using the sidearms. Collapsing into a chair produces knee and hip joint trauma.
  b. Use an elevated chair if knee and hip joints are affected.
  c. Straighten up before walking.
  d. Avoid carrying heavy objects, especially up stairs.
  e. Avoid tension and stress on fingers and thumb joints.
  f. Avoid obesity, which places greater strain on weight-bearing joints.
9   Seek sexual counselling (positions and techniques) if arthritic involvement of the hip is a barrier to sexual performance, e.g., Sexual Personal Relationships of the Disabled, 14 Peto Place, London NW1 4DT.
10   See your doctor on a regular basis. Function re-evaluation must be carried out periodically to determine if there is loss of joint function.
11   Surgical procedures are available for relief of pain and deformity (when recommended by doctor).

12 The therapeutic programme must be maintained for a lifetime; there is no cure at this time.

GUIDELINES: Paraffin Hand Bath for Rheumatoid Arthritis

Purposes

1 To relieve pain.
2 To decrease duration of morning stiffness of fingers, hand and wrist.

Equipment

Wax bath with thermostat control
Low melting point wax
Aluminium foil/Polythene sheet
Towel

Procedure

Nursing Action	Reason
Preparatory Phase	
1 Explain to the patient what he can expect.	
2 Have the patient wash his hands before inserting them into warm wax.	
Performance Phase	
3 Heat and melt wax to 53°C (120–130°F).	
4 Dip the hand and wrist in warm wax rapidly (Fig. 4.16) while keeping the fingers still.	4 The heat is transferred from the wax to the skin by conduction.
5 Immerse the hand in wax again; allow the wax to harden and reimmerse.	5 This builds up a glove of warm wax about 0.3 cm (1/8 in) thick which also acts as a splint.
6 Allow the wax to harden after each immersion.	
7 Wrap hand with protective aluminium foil and cover with a towel.	7 Wrapping with foil and a towel helps to retain the heat.
8 Allow wax to remain on hand 15–20 min.	
9 Peel off wax and place in salvage bucket.	9 When cleaned the wax can be reused.
10 Put fingers and wrist through range of motion exercises after wax has been removed.	10 Heat relieves the patient of pain and enables him to exercise his fingers and wrists with greater mobility.

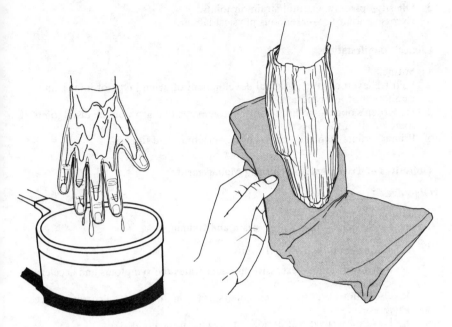

Figure 4.16. Paraffin hand bath.

OSTEOARTHRITIS (DEGENERATIVE JOINT DISEASE; ARTHROSIS)

Osteoarthritis, the most common of all joint diseases, is degeneration of the articular cartilage in the joints. It is characterized by bony spur formation at the edges of the joint surfaces and by thickening of the capsule and the synovial membrane.

Underlying Principles

1 Osteoarthritis is to be regarded essentially as a senescent process—the result of prolonged wear and tear of the joint surfaces which produce changes not only in the bony structures but also in the cartilaginous and soft tissue components of the joints.
2 The tests for rheumatoid factor are usually negative, the blood count and erythrocyte sedimentation rate are normal, and systemic manifestations are absent.
3 The nature of the disease should be explained to the patient and he should be reassured that the disease is usually not progressive or incapacitating unless there is severe involvement of weight-bearing joints.

Predisposing Factors

1 Ageing—occurs mainly in middle aged and elderly.

2   Trauma—mild or continuous irritation.
3   Obesity—places unnatural strain on joints.
4   Excessive joint use—strenuous physical labour.

Clinical Manifestations

1   Stiffness.
2   Pain (relieved by rest); gradual development of aching type of joint pain.
3   Limitation of joint motion.
4   Heberden's nodes—nodular bony enlargements that grow on the distal joints of some or all of the fingers.
5   Primary joints involved—hips, knees, vertebrae and fingers.

Objectives of Treatment and Nursing Management

Objectives

To relieve discomfort.
To protect the joints from undue strain and trauma.

To Relieve Strain on the Affected Joints

1   Rest involved joints—excessive use aggravates the symptoms and accelerates degeneration.
    a. Use splints, braces, cervical collars, traction, lumbosacral corsets as necessary.
    b. Have prescribed rest periods in recumbent position.
2   Advise the patient to avoid activities that precipitate pain.
3   Use heat—relieves pain, muscle spasm and stiffness and allows a more effective follow-up exercise programme.
4   Try cold applications if heat is not effective.
5   Give analgesics for pain control.
6   Give anti-inflammatory agents when synovial inflammation is present.
7   Support the patient undergoing intra-articular (into the joint) injections of long-acting steroids.
8   Teach the patient to use correct posture and body mechanics.
9   The patient may sleep with a rolled terry towel under the neck—for relief of cervical osteoarthritis.
10 Have patient use crutches, braces or walking stick when indicated—to reduce weight-bearing stress on hips and knees. Hold walking stick in hand opposite side of involved hip/knee.

To Avoid Trauma and Further Degeneration of the Weight-bearing Joints

Instruct the patient as follows:

1   Use postural exercises to correct poor posture.
2   Wear corrective shoes and metatarsal supports for foot disorders—also helps in the treatment of arthritis of the knee.
3   Carry out weight reduction programme under nursing and medical supervision—to decrease stress on weight-bearing joints.

4 Stop excessive weight-bearing activities such as standing for prolonged periods, undue stair climbing, lifting, carrying heavy loads, engaging in excessive vigorous overhead reaching.
5 Avoid engaging in excessive activity and unusual exercise or effort.

To Restore Function to the Maximal Extent

1 Use range of motion exercises to maintain joint mobility and muscle tone for joint support; to prevent capsular and tendon tightening; and to prevent deformities.
2 Avoid flexion and adduction deformities—if deformities are avoided, pain is more apt to disappear.
3 Use isometric exercises and progressive resistance exercises to improve muscle strength around the involved joint.
4 Support the patient undergoing orthopaedic surgery for unremitting pain and disabling arthritis of joints.

Health Teaching

See Objectives of Treatment and Nursing Management.

MALIGNANT BONE TUMOUR

Osteogenic sarcoma is a primary malignant bone tumour usually characterized by early haematogenous dissemination of cancer and the establishment of micrometastases in the lung.

Clinical Manifestations

1 Pain.
2 Limitation of motion and joint effusion.
3 Significant weight loss (an ominous finding).
4 *Physical findings:*
   a. Palpable, tender, fixed bony mass.
   b. Increase in skin temperature over mass.
   c. Venous distension.
5 *Sites of occurrence*—lower end of femur, upper ends of tibia and humerus.
5 *Sites of metastases*—lung, other bone, local recurrence, brain.

Diagnosis

1 X-ray will usually reveal bone tumour.
2 Bone scan—helpful in detecting initial extent of malignancy, planning therapy, defining level of amputation and following course of radiation/chemotherapy.
3 Serum alkaline phosphatase—usually increased.
4 Open biopsy of bone and permanent tissue section—to confirm suspected diagnosis.
5 Intravenous urogram and creatine clearance—to evaluate renal function.
6 Chest x-ray and lung scan—to determine if metastases are present.

Treatment and Nursing Management

Objective

To destroy or remove malignant tissue by the most effective method possible.

Assumption

The treatment of osteogenic sarcoma requires a multidisciplinary approach, preferably in a cancer treatment centre.

1   Surgical ablation of the tumour (requires amputation of extremity)—to achieve local control of primary lesion. Usually requires a radical approach, removing the affected bone and if possible the proximal joint. (See Nursing Management Following Amputation.)

2   Chemotherapy—to eradicate micrometastatic lesions.
    a. Chemotherapy used in combination to achieve a greater patient response at a lower toxicity rate and to minimize potential problems of drug resistance.
    b. Chemotherapy usually started 3 weeks after surgical treatment.
    c. Combinations of chemotherapeutic agents may be given in varying courses separated by rest periods.
        (1) Vincristine, high dose methotrexate with citrovorum factor, adriamycin and cyclophosphamide in various combinations.
            (a) Vincristine—given intravenously before methotrexate infusion—may promote methotrexate uptake by tumour cells.
            (b) High-dose methotrexate—given by infusion to destroy malignant cells.
            (c) Citrovorum factor—'rescue' of the patient from methotrexate by allowing larger doses of methotrexate; prevents excess toxicity.
        (2) Or adriamycin (antitumour antibiotic) given in high doses; may be given alone or in combination with other agents.
            (a) Nausea and vomiting may occur the day after drug administration.
            (b) Appears to have cardiotoxic effect—administration followed by ECG, serum SGOT, serum creatine phosphokinase (CPK) monitoring.
        (3) Chemotherapy may be used in combination with radiation therapy.
        (4) Or immunotherapeutic approach may be selected.

3   See Nursing Management of Patient Undergoing Chemotherapy.
    a. Encourage patient who has to cope with discomfort from disagreeable toxic effects, alopecia and uncertain outcome of disease.
    b. Oropharyngeal mucositis of oral membranes is a frequent severe manifestation of gastrointestinal toxicity of methotrexate.
        (1) Instruct patient to cleanse mouth regularly. Cleanse mouth after eating and at bedtime.
        (2) Stomatitis with superinfection of oral membranes with *Candida albicans*—may be controlled with oral nystatin.
        (3) Bone marrow depression (leucopaenia and thrombocytopaenia)—may require platelet transfusion.

4   Orthopaedic surgical procedures may be carried out to implant a prosthetic replacement of the area affected by the tumour. This work is still experimental but enables the patient to retain his normal body features.

OSTEOPOROSIS

Osteoporosis is a state in which there is a reduction in the amount of normal bony material in the skeleton. It is characterized by generalized loss of density and tensile strength throughout the skeleton.

Causes

1 Postmenopausal or 'senile' osteoporosis—there is a relationship between bone loss and reduction of oestrogen levels after menopause.
2 Immobilization from injury or inactivity.
3 Nutritional disorders; malabsorption syndrome (extensive diverticulitis).
4 Endocrine disorders; Cushing's syndrome, hyperparathyroidism, large doses of steroids (secondary osteoporosis).

Clinical Manifestations

Majority of patients have no symptoms.

1 Back pain.
   a. Sharp, severe pain aggravated by motion—usually due to vertebral fracture.
   b. Dull ache in lower thoracic/lumbar region.
2 Tendency to kyphosis; loss of stature—postmenopausal women may lose 2–15 cm (1–6 in) in height from vertebral compression.
3 Tendency to fractures—vertebral bodies, upper femur, humerus and distal portion of forearm.
4 Renal calculi—from hypercalcaemia.

Nursing Alert: Osteoporotic bone fragility leads to vertebral collapse and hip fractures. It is the principal cause of fractures in the aged (as a result of minimal or questionable trauma).

Diagnosis

1 X-rays—show increased radiolucency of bones.
2 Bone biopsy—may be necessary to rule out malignant disease.

Treatment and Nursing Management

Objectives

To keep the patient active.
To provide optimal nutrition.
To prevent fractures.

1 Administer short-term oestrogen therapy as directed—appears to slow progression of bone loss, relieve osteoporotic pain and provide positive calcium-phosphorus balance.
   a. Oestrogen may produce breast and endometrial hyperplasia.
   b. Oral oestrogen appears to increase risk for vascular accidents and thromboembolic disease.

c. Oestrogens may be contraindicated in high-risk patients (e.g., strong family history or previous malignancy of breast/endometrium).

2   See that the patient understands that the diet must supply adequate vitamin D and calcium (milk, milk products) and protein—to encourage bone mineralization. Vitamin D is necessary for calcium absorption.

Calcium supplementation (calcium carbonate and multivitamins (for vitamin D)) may be required if dietary measures are not successful.

3   Ensure daily exercise (walking) to prevent bone demineralization.

4   For vertebral compression fractures from osteoporosis.
   a. Give analgesics as required.
   b. Provide bracing and support when needed—to allow as much activity as possible as early as possible.

Health Teaching

Instruct the patient as follows:

1   Sleep with a bedboard under the mattress.
2   Make environment safe to prevent falls.
3   Increase muscle tone of trunk flexors and extensors by isometric exercises.
4   Keep physically active to strengthen muscles and prevent disuse atrophy and further bone demineralization.
5   Weigh periodically—indicates whether or not disease is stabilized.
6   Bend and lift correctly to avoid compression fractures of vertebral bodies.
7   Have daily outdoor activity—to provide vitamin D (sunlight) and stimulate osteoblastic cells.
8   Oestrogen replacement therapy should be considered for women with premature menopause (surgical or spontaneous)—to arrest or prevent bone loss.

OSTEITIS DEFORMANS (PAGET'S DISEASE OF THE BONE)

Osteitis deformans is a bone disease of unknown cause marked by excessive bone resorption (bone loss) and disordered formation of bone. Increased bone turnover and loss of normal bone architecture are characteristic. In time the involved bone becomes sclerotic and brittle.

General Factors

1   Bony overgrowth and deformities occur and sometimes cause pressure on soft tissue structures.
2   May develop in any part of the skeleton—usually the skull, vertebral column, pelvis or long bones.
3   Eventually produces marked hypertrophy and bowing of the long bones and irregular deformities of the flat bones.
4   Increased blood flow to affected bone(s) may lead to increased cardiac output and high-output cardiac failure.

Nursing Alert: Osteitis deformans predisposes to spontaneous fractures and malignant bone tumours.

Clinical Manifestations
1 Bone pain; tenderness on pressure.
2 Bone deformity:
   a. Bowing of femur and tibia.
   b. Kyphosis—producing a decrease in height.
3 Enlargement of the skull.
4 Deafness—from pronounced thickening of skull and bony overgrowth which impinges on vital structures.

Diagnosis
1 Skeletal x-rays—involved bones appear to be expanded and have greater than normal density.
2 Serum alkaline phosphatase (serves as index of bone resorption)—markedly elevated.
3 24 hour urinary hydroxyproline excretion—used to assess skeletal metabolic activity; reflects increased bone resorption.
4 Bone scan—to evaluate location and activity of disease.

Treatment and Nursing Management
1 No particular treatment is recommended in patient without symptoms.
2 Agents used to suppress clinical manifestations (particularly bone pain):
   a. Calcitonin—a polypeptide hormone comprising 32 amino acids—retards bone resorption by decreasing the number and activity of osteoclasts.
   b. Salmon calcitonin (Calsynar) and porcine (Calcitaire) is available for clinical use.
   (1) Improves or relieves bone pain and produces a fall in serum alkaline phosphatase and urinary hydroxyproline secretion (showing its effect on osteoclasts); halts progression of bone lesions.
   (2) Nausea may be a side-effect of drug.
   (3) Patient may be taught to give his own injection.
   c. Mithramycin (Mithracin)—cytotoxic antibiotic that appears to have a hypocalcaemic effect; reduces urinary calcium and hydroxyproline levels; gives symptomatic improvement (relief of bone pain and headaches).
   (1) Hepatic, renal and haemorrhagic toxicity associated with this drug.
   (2) Drug is given by intravenous injection and patient is monitored for signs of toxicity by measurement of platelet counts, etc.
   d. A diphosphonate, sodium etidronate (EHDP)—used in inhibiting excessive bone resorption; reduces levels of both total urinary hydroxyproline and serum alkaline phosphatase; produces remission of clinical symptoms.
3 Supportive and symptomatic treatment:
   a. Give salicylates—to combat pain; may reduce hypercalcaemia.
   b. Small fractional doses of x-ray irradiation—to relieve pain.
   c. Watch for occurrence of fractures—stress fractures occur with minimal trauma.
   (1) Fractures usually treated with internal fixation.
   (2) Avoid immobilization—increases hazard of hypercalcaemia and stone formation.

(3) For temporary immobilization due to fracture, limit calcium intake and provide high fluid intake—to avoid serious hypercalcaemia and the development of renal calculi.

d. Watch for evidences of bone sarcoma (see p. 207).

FURTHER READING

General Books

Apley, A G (1978) System of Orthopaedics and Fractures, Butterworths
Bradley, D (1980) Accident and Emergency Nursing, Baillière Tindall
Brunner, N (1975) Orthopaedic Nursing, C V Mosby
Crawford Adams, J (1978) Outline of Fractures, Churchill Livingstone
Crawford Adams, J (1978) Outline of Orthopaedics, Churchill Livingstone
Duthie, R B and Ferguson, A B (1973) Mercer's Orthopaedic Surgery, Williams & Wilkins
Farrell, J (1982) Illustrated Guide to Orthopaedic Nursing, 2nd edition, J B Lippincott
Huskisson, E C and Hart, F D (1973) Joint Disease, Williams & Wilkins
Kennedy, J M (1974) Orthopaedic Splints and Appliances, Baillière Tindall
Larson, C B and Gould, M (1974) Orthopaedic Nursing, C V Mosby
Little, J M (1975) Major Amputation for Vascular Disease, Churchill Livingstone
Mourad, A (1980) Nursing Care of Adults with Orthopaedic Conditions, Wiley
Pinney, E and Stone, E M (1978) Orthopaedics for Nurses, Baillière Tindall
Roafe, R and Hodkinson, L J (1980) Textbook of Orthopaedic Nursing, 3rd edition, Blackwell Scientific
Rowe, J and Dyer Stewart J D M (1977) Care of the Orthopaedic Patient, Blackwell
Smith & Nephew Medical (1979) Plaster of Paris Technique, Smith & Nephew
Stewart, J D M (1975) Traction and Orthopaedic Appliances, Churchill Livingstone
Swinson (1979) Rheumatology, Hoder & Stoughton
Wright, V and Haslock, I (1977) Rheumatism for Nurses, Heinemann Medical

Articles

Amputation

Annals of the Royal College of Surgeons of England (1980) Symposium—Limb Replacement and Limb Rehabilitation, 62: 87–105
Burkhalter, W E et al. (1976) The upper extremity amputee, Journal of Bone and Joint Surgery, 58A: 46–51
Clark-Williams, M J (1978) The problems of the lower limb amputee, The Practitioner, 220:
Humm, W (1974) Care of the lower limb amputee, Nursing Times, 70: 1935–1941
Kerstein, M D et al. (1975) What influence does age have on rehabilitation of amputees, Geriatrics, 30: 67–71
MacInnes, M S A (1977) Bilateral amputation of the legs, Nursing Times, 73: 1033–1035

Robinson, K (1976) Amputation of the lower limb, British Journal of Hospital Medicine, 60: 629–637

Arthritis

0Brandt, K D (1974) Medical management of patient with arthritis, Clinical Orthopaedic, 6: 13–27

Fox, J (1980) Revision arthoplasty of the hip, Nursing Times, 76: 1930–1933
Golding, D N (1978) Rheumatoid arthritis, Update Publications
Simpson, A (1982) A joint approach, Nursing Mirror, 153: 28–29
Wright, V (1977) Rheumatoid arthritis (series of articles), Nursing Times, 73: 1794–1797, 1832–1835, 1878–1881, 1915–1918, 1955–1958

Arthritis Surgery

Bridgewater, S E (1975) Charnley hip replacement, Nursing Times, 71: 1000–1002
Coventry, M B et al. (1974) 2012 total hip athroplasties: a study of postoperative course and early complications, Journal of Bone and Joint Surgery, 56A: 273–284
Harris, W H (1974) Comparison of warfarin, low molecular-weight dextran, aspirin and subcutaneous heparin in prevention of venous thromboembolism following total hip replacement, Journal of Bone and Joint Surgery, 56A: 1552–1562
Ring, P A (Ed) (1975) Risks and total hip replacement, British Medical Journal, 2: 296–297
Stinchfield, F E (1975) Symposium: Statistics on total hip replacement, Clinical Orthopaedic Journal, 95: 2–262

Back

Gambrill, E (1981) Acute back pain, Update Publications, 23: 1699–1798
Jackson, R K (1973) Lumbar disc lesions. Fact and fallacies, Update Publications, 15: 451–459

Fractures

Crout E, Cape, S, Thompson, C and Hurlow, A (1979) Boning up on a brace, Nursing Times, 75: 46–49
Hunt, D M (1980) New material for the immobilzation of fractures, British Journal of Hospital Medicine, 24: 273–275
Massie, S (1980) Cast bracing of femoral shaft fractures (series of articles), Nursing Times, 76: series of articles
Micheli, L J (1975) Thromboembolic complications of cast immobilization for injuries of the lower extremities, Clinical Orthopaedic Journal, 108: 191–195
Monahan, P R W et al. (1975) Dislocation and fracture-dislocation of the pelvis, Injury, 6: 325–333
Murray, D G et al. (1974) Fat embolism syndrome, Journal of Bone and Joint Surgery, 56A: 1338–1349
Pusey, R (1978) Potts fracture, Nursing Times, 74: 1293–1295
Sarmianto, A (1974) Fracture bracing, Clinical Orthopaedic Journal, 102: 152–158
Sarmianto, A (1974) Fractures of the tibia, Clinical Orthopaedic Journal, 105: 2–294

Musculoskeletal tumours

Campbell, C J et al (Eds) (1975) New therapies for osteogenic sarcoma, Journal of Bone and Joint Surgery, 57A: 143–144

Cortes, E P et al (1974) Amputation and adriamycin in primary osteosarcoma, New English Journal of Medicine, 291: 998–1000

Sweetman, R (1980) Tumours of bone and their treatment today, British Journal of Hospital Medicine, 24: 452–456

Turoff, N B, Booker, M and Lewis, M (1978) Ewing's sarcoma—unusual presentation, Journal of Bone and Joint Surgery, 60A: 1109–1110

Chapter 5

CONDITIONS OF THE KIDNEYS, URINARY TRACT AND REPRODUCTIVE SYSTEM

1. Renal and Genitourinary Conditions

Manifestations of Disorders of the Genitourinary Tract	217
Diagnostic Investigation for Urological Disease	219
Tests of Renal Function	226
Urine Examination	226
Guidelines: Technique for Obtaining Cleancatch Midstream Specimen of Urine	229
Catheterization	230
Guidelines: Catheterization of the Urinary Bladder	230
Guidelines: Management of the Patient with an Indwelling Catheter and Closed Drainage System	237
Management of Continuous Irrigating System	239
Guidelines: Assisting the Patient Undergoing Suprapubic Drainage (Cystostomy)	240
Urine Retention	242
Nursing Assessment for Fluid and Electrolyte Imbalance	245
Acute Renal Failure	246
Chronic Renal Failure	249
Guidelines: Assisting the Patient Undergoing Short-Term Peritoneal Dialysis	251
Haemodialysis	258
Kidney Transplantation	263
Nursing Management of the Patient Undergoing Renal/Urological Surgery	267
Infections of the Urinary Tract	271
Cystitis	272
Pyelonephritis	274
Tuberculosis of the Kidney	276
Acute Glomerulonephritis	277
Nephrotic Syndrome	279

Hydronephrosis　280
Nephroptosis　281
Urolithiasis　282
Tumours of the Kidney　286
Injuries to the Kidney　287
Neurogenic Bladder　289
　Guidelines: Intermittent Self-Catheterization; Clean (Nonsterile)
　　Technique　292
Injuries to the Bladder (and Urethra)　294
Cancer of the Bladder　295
Urinary Diversion　297
Problems Affecting the Urethra　303
　Urethral Stricture　303
　Urethritis　304
　Urethritis from Gonorrhoea　305
Conditions of the Prostate　306
　Benign Prostatic Hyperplasia (Hypertrophy)　306
　Prostatitis　307
　Cancer of the Prostate　309
　Management of the Patient Undergoing Prostatic Surgery　311
Hydrocele　316
Varicocele　317
Tumours of the Testicle　317
　Guidelines: Self-Examination for Testicular Tumour　318
Epididymitis　319
Orchitis　320
Vasectomy　321
Conditions Affecting the Penis　322
　Ulceration of the Glans Penis　322
　Carcinoma of the Penis　323
　Other Conditions　323
　Circumcision　323
Sexually Transmitted Diseases　324

2. Gynaecological Conditions

Menstruation　324
　Disturbances of Menstruation　324
Diagnostic Studies for Gynaecological Conditions　327
　Pelvic Examination　327
　Guidelines: Vaginal Examination by the Nurse/Doctor　330
　Other Diagnostic Tests　331
　Guidelines: Colposcopy　334
　Dilatation and Curettage (D&C)　335
Conditions of the External Genitalia and Vagina　336
　Contact Dermatitis of the Vulva　336
　Pruritus　337
　Condylomata　337
　Kraurosis Vulvae and Leucoplakia　337

Vulvitis and Abscess of Greater Vestibular Gland (Bartholin's Gland)   338
Cancer of the Vulva   338
Vaginal Fistula   340
Vaginal Infections   342
Guidelines: Vaginal Irrigation (Douche)   345
Guidelines: Perineal swabbing   347
Problems Resulting from Relaxed Pelvic Muscles   348
    Cystocele   348
    Rectocele   350
    Displacement of the Uterus   351
Tumours of the Uterus   352
    Cancer of the Cervix   353
    Cancer of the Corpus Uteri   354
    Myoma of the Uterus   355
    Nursing Care of the Patient Receiving Radiation Therapy of the Uterus   356
Hysterectomy   357
Endometriosis   360
Ovarian Cancer   361
Pelvic Infection   362
Fertility Control   364

3. Conditions of the Breast

Conditions of the Nipple   369
    Fissures and Bleeding   369
    Paget's Disease of the Breast   370
Inflammation of the Breast   372
Fibrocystic Disease   373
Tumours of the Breast   373
    Fibroadenomata   373
    Guidelines: Examination of the Breast by the Nurse   374
    Cancer of the Breast   375
Further Reading   387

1. Renal and Genitourinary Conditions

MANIFESTATIONS OF DISORDERS OF THE GENITOURINARY TRACT

Pain

1. Pain is only occasionally a symptom of some of the most severe forms of urinary tract lesions.
2. Urologic pain is generally seen in more *acute* conditions.
3. Pain in flank radiating to lower abdomen, upper thigh, testis or labium typically is due to renal colic (kidney stones).
   a. Often accompanied by nausea, vomiting, paralytic ileus.
   b. Pain is produced by distension of ureter and renal pelvis due to retained

urine above the point of obstruction or a blood clot; severity is related to the rapidity with which distension develops.

4 Pain over suprapubic area (bladder pain) due to infection and urinary retention.

5 Urethral pain from irritation of bladder neck, from foreign body in canal or from urethritis due to infection or trauma.

6 Pain in scrotal area from inflammatory swelling of epididymis or testis, torsion of testis.

7 Testicular pain due to injury, mumps orchitis, torsion of spermatic cord.

8 Perineal or rectal discomfort from acute prostatitis, prostatic abscess.

9 Back and leg pain from cancer of prostate with metastases to pelvic bones.

10 Pain in glans penis is usually from prostatitis; penile shaft pain is from urethra.

Changes in Micturition (Voiding)

1 Haematuria (red blood cells in urine).
   a. Haematuria is considered a serious sign and requires investigation.
   b. Colour of bloody urine dependent upon pH of urine and amount of blood present.
      (1) Acid urine is dark, smoky colour.
      (2) Alkaline urine is red.
   c. Haematuria may be due to systemic cause such as blood dyscrasias, anticoagulant therapy, neoplasms, trauma, extreme exercise.
   d. Painless haematuria may indicate neoplasm in the urinary tract.
   e. Haematuria from renal colic (stones in kidney).
   f. Bloody spotting reveals bleeding from urethra, bladder neoplasms.
   g. Haematuria also seen in renal tuberculosis, polycystic disease of kidneys, septic pyelonephritis, thrombosis and embolism involving renal artery or vein.

2 Proteinuria (albuminuria).
   a. Normal urine does not contain persistent protein in significant quantities.
   b. Proteinuria characteristically seen in all forms of acute and chronic renal disease (more characteristic of glomerulonephritis than pyelonephritis).
      (1) The protein is mainly albumin, but globulin is also present.
      (2) Albumin and globulin escape through damaged glomerular capillaries in a greater amount than can be reabsorbed by the tubules, or damaged tubules fail to reabsorb normal amount filtered.
   c. Proteinuria occurs in systemic diseases when there are varying degrees of renal anoxia, as in cardiac decompensation, diabetic glomerulosclerosis.
   d. Mild proteinuria may occur from other sources—urethritis, prostatitis, cystitis.

3 Dysuria (painful or difficult micturition)—seen in wide variety of pathological conditions, usually at bladder level or beyond.

4 Frequency—micturition occurs more often than usual, compared to patient's usual pattern (or to a generally accepted norm of once every 3–6 hours).
   a. Determine if habits regarding fluid intake have been altered; it is essential to know normal micturition pattern in order to assess frequency.
   b. Increasing frequency can result from a variety of conditions—such as infection and diseases of urinary tract, metabolic disease, hypertension, medications (diuretics).

5 Urgency (strong desire to urinate)—due to inflammatory lesions in bladder,

    prostate or urethra, acute bacterial infections, chronic prostatitis in men and chronic posterior urethrotrigonitis in women.

6 Burning upon urination—as seen in urethral irritation or bladder infections.

7 Enuresis (involuntary micturition during sleep)—may be physiological to age 3; after this may be functional or symptomatic of obstructive disease (usually of lower urinary tract).

8 Nocturia (micturition at night)—may indicate renal disease with decrease of functioning renal parenchyma and loss of concentrating power, obstructed bladder, systemic disease (congestive heart failure, diabetes).

9 Strangury (slow and painful urination); only small amounts of urine micturated; blood staining may be noted—seen in severe cystitis.

10 Incontinence (involuntary loss of urine)—may be due to injury to external urinary sphincter, acquired neurogenic disease, severe urgency, etc.

11 Stress incontinence (intermittent leakage of urine due to sudden strain)—indicates weakness of sphincteric mechanism.

12 Polyuria (large volume of urine micturated in given time)—demonstrated in diabetes mellitus, diabetes insipidus.

13 Oliguria (small volume of urine micturated in given time)—may result from acute renal failure, shock, dehydration, fluid–ion imbalance.

14 Anuria (no urine in bladder)—due to acute renal failure and bilateral ureteral obstruction.

15 Pneumaturia (passage of gas in urine during micturition)—caused by fistulous connection between bowel and bladder, rectosigmoid cancer, regional ileitis, sigmoid diverticulitis (most common) and gas-forming urinary tract infections.

Gastrointestinal Symptoms Related to Urological Disease

1 Gastrointestinal symptoms may occur with urological conditions because of:
    a. Renal–intestinal reflexes.
    b. Anatomic relation of right kidney to colon (hepatic flexure), duodenum, head of pancreas, common bile duct, liver and gallbladder.
    c. Anatomic relation of left kidney to colon (splenic flexure), stomach, pancreas, spleen.
    d. Peritoneal irritation—anterior surface of kidneys covered by peritoneum, which is affected by renal inflammation.

2 Gastrointestinal symptoms related to urological conditions include nausea, vomiting, diarrhoea, abdominal discomfort, paralytic ileus, gastrointestinal haemorrhage with uraemia.

3 Gastrointestinal upsets and recurrent fever in young children may be manifestations of urinary tract infection.

4 Appendicitis may present with urinary symptoms.

DIAGNOSTIC INVESTIGATIONS FOR UROLOGICAL DISEASE

Radiography

X-ray

Flat plate (x-ray of kidney, ureter, bladder) is used to delineate size, shape and position of kidneys, but includes organs up to the level of symphysis pubis.

1   Gives a baseline reference for subsequent films.
2   Shows the position, number and size of radiopaque objects suspected of being urinary tract calculi (stones).

Infusion Drip Pyelography

An intravenous infusion of a large volume of dilute solution of contrast material to produce opacification of the renal parenchyma and complete filling of urinary tract. Films taken at intervals to demonstrate the filled and distended collecting system.

1   Patient preparation is same as for excretory urography *except that the patient is not dehydrated* (see below).
2   Infusion drip pyelography has almost replaced standard intravenous pyelography; it is used when regular urographic techniques fail to show drainage structures satisfactorily.

Excretory Urography (intravenous urogram or intravenous pyelogram)

Introduction intravenously of a radiopaque contrast material which concentrates in the urine and thus visualizes the kidneys, ureter and bladder. The contrast media is cleared from the bloodstream by renal excretion.

1   Excretory urography is used in:
   a. Initial investigation of any suspected urological problem, especially in diagnosis of lesions in kidneys and ureters.
   b. To provide a rough estimate of renal function.
2   Patient preparation.
   a. See that patient is not overhydrated—will dilute contrast material and thus cause inadequate visualization.
   b. Remove obstructing intestinal content if possible so as to minimize intestinal gas; enemas are not usually given. Give laxative the night before the test to eliminate faeces and gas in the intestinal tract, e.g., 30 ml castor oil or Dulcolax tablets.
   c. It is customary to take no liquids for 6 hours before this test, although good films are often obtained in the hydrated patient.

Nursing Alert: Elderly patients with poor renal reserve may not tolerate dehydrating procedures and should be given water to drink. Fluids should not be restricted if the patient has myeloma, diabetes or renal failure.

   d. A light, dry breakfast (e.g., lightly buttered toast) may be given on the morning of the examination.
   e. Whenever possible, the patient should be kept ambulant to minimize gaseous shadows in the bowel.
   f. Of necessity emergency intravenous urography is performed without any preparation.
   g. Ascertain if patient has history of allergies—to find the high-risk patient.
      (1) Evaluate for anaphylactoid reaction (rare) to intravenous dosage of contrast material. (No contrast medium is completely innocuous.)
      (2) Watch patient during procedure so that reactions are recognized immediately.
         (a) Mild reaction (relatively common)—flushing, metallic taste, nausea,

vomiting, faintness, tingling—may be due to osmotic or chemical character of contrast medium.

(b) Severe reaction—urticaria, oedema, asthma, hypotension, convulsions, cyanosis, shock and cardiac arrest—due to allergic response to contrast medium.

(3) Have emergency drugs (adrenalin, vasopressors, corticosteroids, etc.), oxygen and tracheostomy equipment ready to restore cardiac activity and maintain adequate respiration and blood pressure. Have equipment available to treat cardiac arrest.

Retrograde Pyelography

Injection of opaque material through ureteral catheters which have been passed up ureters into renal pelvis by means of cystoscopic manipulation. The opaque solution is introduced by gravity or syringe.

1 Retrograde pyelography usually done when nonfunctioning kidney is suspected or if patient is allergic to intravenous contrast material.
2 Performed with decreasing frequency due to improvement of IVU (intravenous urogram) techniques.

Cystourethrogram

Visualization of urethra and bladder either by retrograde injection or by micturition of contrast material.

Micturition Cystourethrogram

1 Bladder is filled with radiopaque medium and patient then micturates while rapid spot films are taken.
2 With the image intensifier, the presence or absence of vesicoureteric reflux and/or congenital abnormalities in the lower urinary tract can be demonstrated. Also used to investigate difficulty in bladder emptying and incontinence.

Cystometrogram

Graphic recording of the pressures exerted at varying phases of filling of the urinary bladder. Intermittent filling of the bladder can be recorded and compared with changes in intravesical pressure.

1 Patient is requested to micturate. Doctor observes the time it takes to initiate micturition; size, force and continuity of urinary stream; degree of straining, hesitancy, intermittency of urination, presence of terminal dribbling.
2 Patient is then placed in lithotomy position and a retention catheter is placed through urethra and into bladder. The residual urinary volume is measured, and the catheter is left in place.
3 The urethral catheter is connected to a water manometer and water is allowed to flow into bladder, usually at the rate of 1 ml/s.
a. Patient informs examiner when he feels the first desire to micturate and again when the bladder feels full. The degree of bladder filling at these points is recorded.
b. The pressures above the zero level at the symphysis pubis are measured and the pressures and volumes within the bladder are plotted and recorded.

Nephrotomogram

Body section x-rays which bring into focus the different layers of the kidney and the diffuse structures in that layer; done also as part of intravenous urogram study.

Ultrasonic Scan (echogram, sonography)

Scanning by ultrasound is a noninvasive technique for investigation of renal disease. The kidneys produce a characteristic ultrasonic pattern making abnormalities readily identifiable. Distinguishes cystic from solid disease.

Radioisotope Studies of Urinary Tract (renogram)

Delineate structure and function of kidneys without disturbing their normal physiological processes.

1 Intravenous radioiodine (Hippuran ^{131}I) is given.
2 Sites over both kidneys are monitored with scintillation counters to reveal differences between the two kidneys with respect to blood flow, tubular function and excretion.

Isotopic Localization of Renal Pathology (renoscan)

Delineates the kidney anatomy by external scanning.

1 A radioisotope is given intravenously. A lesion (tumour, infarct) is detected by absence of radioactivity in the involved area and resultant defect in scan.
2 Technetium scan for renal blood flow can be used to show vascular malformations.

Renal Angiography

Visualization of renal arterial supply. Contrast material is injected through a catheter (which is placed under fluoroscopic control) via the femoral or axillary artery.

1 Useful in diagnosing renovascular abnormalities and in differentiating renal masses, primarily renal cyst from renal tumour.
2 *Nursing responsibilities before procedure:*
    a. Give aperient or enema as prescribed to eliminate faecal material from colon and to ensure unobstructed radiographs.
    b. Shave proposed injection sites: groin (for femoral approach) or axilla (for axillary approach).
    c. Locate and mark peripheral pulses to facilitate postprocedure nursing evaluation.
    d. Inform patient what to expect during procedure:
      (1) Procedure is done under local anaesthesia; patient will probably be given preoperative medication.
      (2) The procedure may take from 30 min to 2 hours.
      (3) There may be a transient feeling of heat along the course of the vessel upon injection of contrast material.
3 *Nursing responsibilities following procedure:*
    a. Take vital signs until stabilized; take blood pressure on opposite arm if axillary artery was punctured.
    b. Apply cold compresses to puncture site—to decrease oedema and pain.

c. Assess puncture site for swelling and development of haematoma.
d. Palpate peripheral pulses (radial, femoral, dorsalis pedis).
e. Note colour and temperature of involved extremity, comparing it with the uninvolved extremity.

Computed Tomography

A computer measures small changes in x-ray absorption and magnifies the differences from tissue to tissue so a display can be made and read. No preparation needed; noninvasive.

Cystoscopic Examination

A *cystoscopic examination* involves visualization of the urethra, prostatic urethra and bladder by means of a tubular lighted telescopic lens.

Uses

1 To inspect bladder wall directly for tumour, stone, ulcer and to inspect urethra, especially the prostatic urethra prior to surgery.
2 To allow insertion of catheters into the ureters in order to obtain a separate specimen from each kidney and evaluate renal function separately.
3 To see configuration and position of ureteral orifices.
4 To remove calculi from urethra, bladder and ureter.
5 To treat lesions of bladder, urethra and prostate.

Patient Preparation

1 Preparation depends on type of anaesthesia to be used (general or local).
2 Give prescribed oral fluids and preoperative medication.

Nursing Support Following Procedure

1 Expect patient to have some burning upon micturition, blood-tinged urine and urinary frequency from trauma to mucous membrane.
2 Watch patients with prostatic hypertrophy for urinary retention due to oedema from instrumentation.
3 Give warm baths or apply heat to abdomen for pain relief and promotion of muscle relaxation.
4 Utilize indwelling catheter if urinary retention persists.

Complications Following Cystoscopy

Usually occur only in those patients with obstructive pathology.

1 Urinary retention.
2 Urinary tract haemorrhage.
3 Infection within prostate or bladder.

Needle Biopsy of Kidney

Needle biopsy of the kidney is performed by needle biopsy through renal tissue or by open biopsy through a small flank incision (Fig. 5.1). It is useful in assessing the course of renal disease.

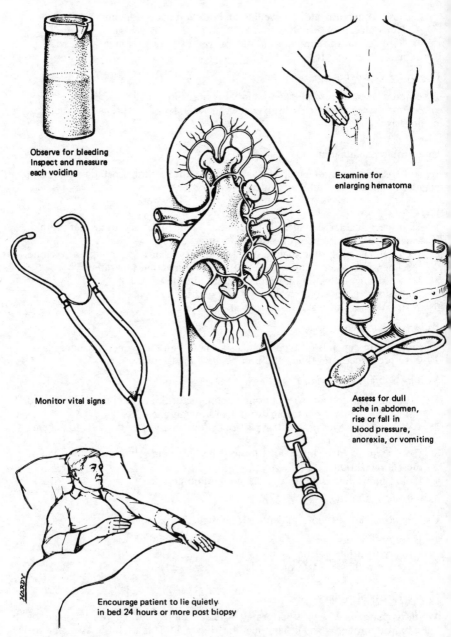

Observe for bleeding
Inspect and measure
each voiding

Examine for
enlarging hematoma

Monitor vital signs

Assess for dull
ache in abdomen,
rise or fall in
blood pressure,
anorexia, or vomiting

Encourage patient to lie quietly
in bed 24 hours or more post biopsy

Figure 5.1. Nursing support of the patient undergoing needle biopsy of the kidney.

Prebiopsy Management

1   Haemoglobin, bleeding, clotting and prothrombin times (including partial thromboplastin time), platelet count and blood urea nitrogren levels are assessed before the biopsy.
2   A plain film or excretory urography precedes the biopsy to accurately locate kidney as a guide for needle insertion. Ultrasonography is useful in locating the kidney as the biopsy is being performed.
3   Have patient lie in a prone position with a firm support under his abdomen. Instruct him to take several deep breaths and then hold a deep breath during inspiration—this prepares the patient for what will be expected of him during the biopsy procedure.

Postbiopsy Nursing Management

Objective

To observe patient for evidences of bleeding.

1   Place patient prone for at least 1 hour after procedure; the patient is to remain on bed rest for 24 hours.
2   Take the vital signs every 5–15 min for first hour and then with decreasing frequency if stable to assess for haemorhage, which is a major complication, i.e.:
    a. Watch for rise or fall in blood pressure, anorexia, vomiting, or development of a dull, aching discomfort in abdomen.
    b. Assess for flank pain or a colicky pain.
    c. Persistent bleeding may be suspected when there is an enlarging haematoma which is palpable.
    d. If perirenal bleeding develops, avoid palpating or manipulating the abdomen after the first examination has determined that a haematoma exists.
3   Inspect and measure each micturition for bleeding; save urine for laboratory examination if indicated.
4   Assess for any patient complaints, especially frequency and urgency.
5   Keep the fluid level at 3000 ml daily if tolerated, unless the patient has renal insufficiency.
6   A haematocrit and haemoglobin study may be done within 8 hours to assess for anaemia.
7   Prepare for transfusion and surgical intervention for control of haemorrhage, which may necessitate surgical drainage or nephrectomy (removal of kidney).

Discharge Planning and Patient Teaching

Instruct the patient as follows:

1   Avoid strenuous activity, strenuous sports and heavy lifting for at least 2 weeks.
2   Notify doctor if any of the following occur: flank pain, haematuria, light-headedness and fainting, rapid pulse or any other signs and symptoms of haemorrhage.

Tests of Renal Function

General Information

1 There is no single test of renal function. Best results are obtained by combining a number of clinical tests.
2 Renal function is variable from time to time, and serial assessments may be necessary.

Renal Concentration Tests

1 Assess the ability of kidneys to concentrate solutes in the urine.
2 Concentration ability is lost early in kidney disease; hence this test detects early defects in renal function.
3 Procedures:
   a. Most common techniques used in concentration tests are those measuring specific gravity, refractive index or osmolality of the urine.
   b. Fluids may be withheld 12–24 hours to assess the concentrating ability of the tubules under controlled conditions. Specific gravity measurements of urine are taken at specific times to determine urine concentration.

Blood Urea

1 Serves as an index of renal excretory capacity.
2 Normal range 2.5–7.5 mmol/l (15–45 mg/100 ml) of blood.
   a. Increase in acute and chronic renal failure, congestive heart failure, obstructive uropathy.
   b. Also increased by nonrenal conditions such as gastrointestinal bleeding and dehydration, and by administration of urea as a medication.

Creatinine Clearance Test

1 A test of renal efficiency which is more sensitive to impairment of renal function than blood urea.
2 Procedure:
   a. Instruct patient to empty bladder. Record time.
   b. Collect all subsequent urine passed for 24 hours, at which time the bladder is emptied again, and this volume is included in the collection.
   c. A 10 ml sample of clotted blood is taken during this time.
3 The result is the measure of the volume of blood cleared of creatinine in 1 min. Normally this is 70–130 ml/min. In severe renal failure the creatinine clearance may fall to 5 ml/min.

Urine Examination

Factors Affecting Composition of the Urine

1 Nutritional status.
2 Metabolic processes.
3 Status of kidney function.

Amount

1   1000–2000 ml/24 hours; less than 600 ml is considered oliguria.
2   Day volume two to three times more than night volume.

Odour

1   Normal—faint aromatic odour.
2   Characteristic odours produced by ingestion of asparagus, thymol.
3   Cloudy urine with ammonia odour—urea-splitting bacteria such as *Proteus*, causing urinary tract infections.
4   Offensive odour—bacterial action in presence of pus.

Colour

1   Colour depends on degree of concentration of chromogen excreted in the volume of fluid.
2   Normal urine is yellow-amber—due to pigment urochrome.
3   Colour varies with specific gravity:
    a. Dilute urine is straw-coloured.
    b. Concentrated urine is highly coloured.
4   Abnormally coloured urine:
    a. Turbid or smoky coloured—may be from haematuria, spermatozoa, prostatic fluid, fat droplets, chyle.
    b. Red or red-brown—is due to blood pigments, porphyria, transfusion reaction, bleeding lesions in urogenital tract, some drugs.
    c. Yellow-brown or green-brown—may reveal obstructive lesion of bile duct system or obstructive jaundice.
    d. Orange-red or orange-brown—from urobilin or from Pyridium (phenazopyridine hydrochloride) a urinary analgesic.
    e. Dark brown or black—due to malignant melanoma, leukaemia.

Appearance

1   Normal urine is clear.
2   Abnormally cloudy urine—due to pus, blood, epithelial cells, bacteria, fat, colloidal particles, phosphate, urates.
3   Turbid urine is not always pathological. Normal urine may develop turbidity on refrigeration or from standing at room temperature; bacteria ferment urine quickly at room temperature.

Reaction (pH)

1   Reflects the ability of kidney to maintain normal hydrogen ion concentration in plasma and extracellular fluid; indicates *acidity* or *alkalinity* of urine.
2   The pH should be measured in fresh urine since the breakdown of urine to ammonia causes urine to become alkaline.
3   Normal pH is around 6 (acid); may normally vary from 4.6 to 7.5.
4   Urine acidity or alkalinity has relatively little clinical significance unless patient is on special diet or is being treated for renal calculous disease.
5   Alkaline urine is often cloudy due to phosphate crystals.

Specific Gravity

1   Measures weight or density of particles in urine; reflects concentrating and diluting power of kidneys; may reflect degree of hydration or dehydration.
2   Normal specific gravity ranges from 1.005 to 1.025.
3   Specific gravity is fixed at 1.010 in chronic renal failure. A dilute urine will have a specific gravity of 1.001–1.010, whereas a concentrated urine will have a specific gravity of 1.025–1.030.

Osmolality

1   Osmolality is an indication of the amount of osmotically active particles in urine (specifically, it is the number of particles per unit volume of *water*). It is similar to specific gravity, but is considered a more precise test; it is also easy to do—only 1–2 ml of urine are required.
2   The unit of osmotic measure is the osmole.
   Average values:
      Females: 300–1090 mOsm/kg   Males: 390–1090 mOsm/kg

Abnormal Urine Constituents

1   *Proteinuria* (albuminuria)—characteristically seen in all forms of acute and chronic renal disease.
   a. Normal urine does not have persistent protein in significant quantities.
   b. Proteinuria also occurs in systemic diseases where there are varying degrees of renal anoxia, cardiac decompensation, diabetic glomerulosclerosis, etc.
2   *Glycosuria*—glucose in the urine; seen most frequently in diabetes mellitus.
3   *Ketonuria*—the presence of ketone bodies (acetone, acetoacetic acid and beta-hydroxybutyric acid).
   Ketonuria is indicative of incomplete fat metabolism (diabetic ketoacidosis), dehydration, starvation; also seen after aspirin ingestion.
4   *Haematuria*—red blood cells in the urine.

Dipstick Tests (Reagent Tests)

Strips that have been impregnated with chemicals are dipped quickly in urine and 'read' as a means of testing urine.

1   When dipped in urine, the chemicals react with abnormal substances in the urine by changing colour.
2   Some dipsticks can test for only one substance whereas others can test several substances simultaneously.
   Billi-labstix—Ames Company, Division of Miles Laboratories, Stoke Poges, Slough, England.

Basic Principles for Collecting Urine Specimens

1   The first morning urine specimen is most concentrated—it reveals sediment abnormalities.
2   Urine should not be left standing at room temperature since it becomes alkaline due to contamination of urea-splitting bacteria from the environment.

3   Microscopic examination should be done within ½ hour after collection—standing causes dissolution of cellular elements and casts and bacterial overgrowth unless obtained under sterile conditions.

4   Urine specimens should be collected from the patient by means of the clean-catch midstream technique (see below) or by careful catheterization.

5   Collection of 24-hour specimen:

a. Ensure that the patient understands the procedure. *All* urine must be collected within a 24-hour period.

b. Have patient empty the bladder at specified time (example: 8:00 a.m.). *Discard urine.*

c. Collect all urine micturated during the next 24 hours.

d. Collect last specimen at 8:00 a.m. on following day (or 24 hours after collection was started).

e. Keep collected urine in the refrigerator in a clean bottle; a suitable preservative may be required.

f. Start with an empty bladder and finish with an empty bladder.

GUIDELINES: Technique for Obtaining Clean-catch Midstream Specimen of Urine

A *clean-catch midstream specimen* is the best clinically effective method of securing a micturated specimen for urinalysis. It is not a simple procedure and requires patient education and active assistance of the female patient.

Equipment

Liquid soap solution
Water
4 × 4 gauze swabs

Disposable gloves for nurse assisting female patient
Sterile specimen container

Procedure

Nursing Action	Reason
Male Patient	
1 Instruct the patient to expose glans penis and cleanse area around meatus. Wash area with liquid soap. *Rinse thoroughly.*	1 The urethral orifice is colonized by bacteria. Urine readily becomes contaminated during micturition. Rinse soap solution thoroughly because these agents can inhibit bacterial growth in a urine culture.
2 Allow the initial urinary flow to escape.	2 The first portion of urine washes out the urethra.
3 Collect the midstream urine specimen in a sterile container.	
4 Avoid collecting the last few drops of urine.	4 Prostatic secretions may be introduced into urine at the end of the urinary stream.

Nursing Action	Reason

5 Send specimen to laboratory immediately.

Female Patient

1 Ask the patient to separate her labia to expose the urethral orifice.

If no one is available to assist the patient she may sit backwards on the toilet seat facing the water tank or sit on (straddle) the wide part of the bedpan.

1 Keeping the labia separated prevents labial or vaginal contamination of the urine specimen. By straddling the toilet seat/bedpan, the patient's labia are spread apart for cleansing.

2 Cleanse the area around the urinary meatus with gauze swabs soaked with soap solution. Rinse thoroughly.

2 The urethral orifice is colonized by bacteria. Urine readily becomes contaminated during micturition.

3 While the patient keeps the labia separated (Fig. 5.2), instruct her to micturate forcibly.

3 This helps wash away urethral contaminants.

4 Allow initial urinary flow to drain into bedpan (toilet) and then catch the midstream specimen in a sterile container.

4 The first portion of urine washes out the urethra.

5 Send the specimen to the laboratory immediately.

5 Too long an interval between collection and analysis produces unreliable results.

CATHETERIZATION

GUIDELINES: Catheterization of the Urinary Bladder

Purposes

1 To empty contents of bladder.
2 To obtain a sterile urine specimen.
3 To determine amount of residual urine in bladder after micturition.
4 To allow irrigation of the bladder.
5 To bypass an obstruction.

Equipment

Sterile gloves
Disposable sterile catheter set with water soluble lubricant for different types of catheters (Fig. 5.3)
Solution for periurethral cleansing (sterile), e.g., Savlon
Sterile container for culture
Sheet for draping
Anglepoise lamp if necessary
Lignocaine gel for male catheterization

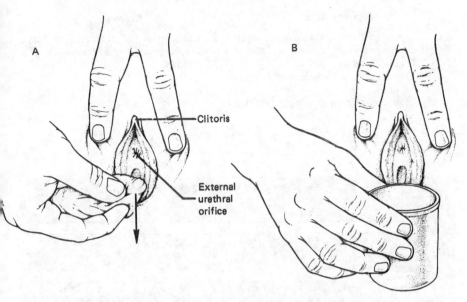

Figure 5.2. Obtaining a clean-catch midstream urine specimen in the female. a. Instruct the patient to hold the labia apart and wash from high up front towards the back with gauze soaked in soap. Then repeat with wet swab. b. The collection cup is held so that it does not touch the body and the sample is obtained only while the patient is micturating with the labia held apart.

Collection of Urine Specimens for Cytology

Urine specimens are sent for cytological examination so that the cells that have been shed from the urinary tract can be examined microscopically. It is therefore important that the specimen sent contains the highest number of cells. Most cells come either at the beginning or end of the stream. A midstream specimen contains the *least* number of cells and therefore should *not* be used for cytological examination. It is also important that cells should be examined quickly before they degenerate. An early morning specimen is not usually suitable as the cells will have been lying in the urine for several hours before being examined. Send specimens immediately to the laboratory.

Procedure for Catheterizing Female Patient (Fig. 5.4)

Nursing Action	Reason
Preparatory Phase	
1 Place patient at ease. Wash vulval area.	1 Patient will feel reassured if the procedure is explained and if she is handled gently and considerately.

Nursing Action	Reason
2 Open catheter pack using aseptic technique. Place waste receptacle in accessible place.	2 Catheterization requires the same aseptic precautions as a surgical procedure.
3 Direct light for visualization of genital area.	
4 Place patient in a supine position	

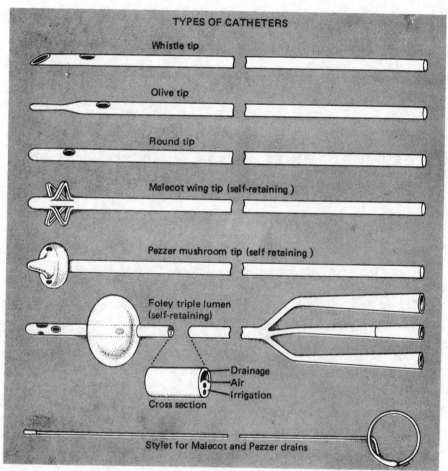

Figure 5.3. Types of catheters.

Nursing Action	**Reason**
with knees bent, hips flexed, and feet resting on bed. Drape the patient.	
5 Position moisture-proof pad under patient's buttocks.	
6 Wash hands. Put on sterile gloves.	

Performance Phase

1 Separate labia minora so that urethral meatus is visualized; one hand is to maintain separation of the labia until catheterization is finished.	1 This manoeuvre helps prevent labial contamination of the catheter (Fig. 5.4).
2 Cleanse around the urethral meatus with Savlon. Dispose of swab after each use.	2 Micro-organisms inhabiting the distal urethra may be introduced into the bladder during or immediately after catheter insertion. Inadequate preparation of the urethral meatus is a major cause of infection.

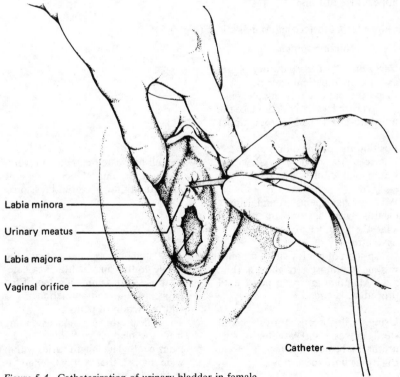

Labia minora

Urinary meatus

Labia majora

Vaginal orifice

Catheter

Figure 5.4. Catheterization of urinary bladder in female.

Nursing Action	Reason
3 Introduce well-lubricated catheter 5–7.5 cm (2–3 in) in an upwards and backwards direction into urethral meatus using strict aseptic technique. **a.** Avoid contaminating surface of catheter. **b.** Ensure that catheter is not too large or too tight at urethral meatus. 4 Remove catheter gently when urinary flow ceases.	3 A well-lubricated catheter reduces friction and trauma to the meatus. The female urethra is a relatively short canal measuring 3.0–4 cm in length. **b.** Too large a catheter may cause painful distension of the meatus.

Follow-up Phase

1 Make patient comfortable; dry area.
2 Measure urine and dispose of equipment.
3 Send specimen to lab as indicated.
4 Record time, procedure, amount and appearance of urine.

Procedure for Catheterizing Male Patient (Fig. 5.5)

Nursing Action	Reason
1 Carry out all of 'preparatory phase' as for female patient except:	
2 Place the patient in a supine position with legs extended. Place the moisture-proof pad across upper thighs.	
3 Position the perineal drape.	
4 Lubricate the catheter well with a water soluble lubricant.	4 A well-lubricated catheter prevents urethral trauma (decreasing the opportunity for bacterial invasion).
5 Wash off glans penis around urinary meatus with Savlon. Insert local anaesthetic and leave for 2 min to have effect.	
6 Grasp shaft of penis (with left hand) raising it almost straight up (Fig. 5.5). Maintain grasp on penis until procedure is ended.	6 This manoeuvre straightens the penile urethra and facilitates catheterization. Maintaining a grasp of the penis prevents contamination and retraction of penis.
7 Using sterile forceps, or fresh pair of sterile gloves, insert catheter into the urethra; advance catheter 15–25 cm (6–10 in) until urine flows.	7 The male urethra is a canal extending from the bladder to the end of the glans penis. The length varies within wide limits; the average length is about 21 cm.

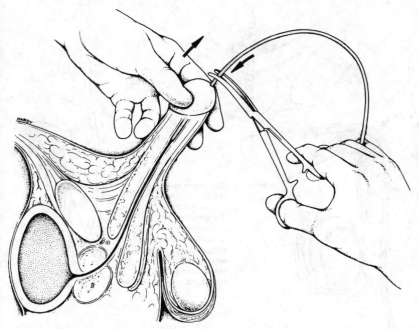

Figure 5.5. Technique for catheterization in male.

8   If resistance is felt at the external sphincter, slightly increase the traction on the penis and apply steady, gentle pressure on the catheter.
    Ask patient to strain gently (as if passing urine) to help relax sphincter.

9   When urine begins to flow, advance the catheter another 2.5 cm (1 in).

8   Some resistance may be due to spasm of external sphincter. Inability to pass the catheter may mean that a urethral stricture or other forms of urethral pathology exist. The urethra may have to be dilated with sounds by a urologist.

9   Advancing the catheter ensures its position in the bladder.

For Indwelling Catheter

1   Advance catheter almost to its bifurcation.

2   Inflate the balloon according to manufacturer's directions.
    a. Be sure catheter is draining properly before inflating balloon.

3   Withdraw catheter slightly and connect to drainage system.

1   This prevents the balloon from becoming trapped in urethra.

    a. Inadvertent inflation of the balloon within the urethra is painful and causes urethral trauma.

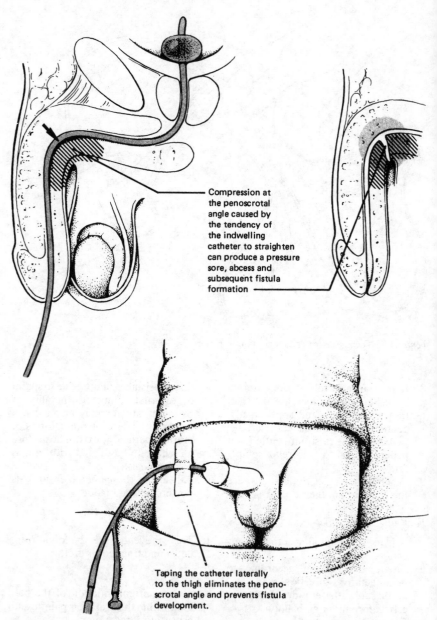

Compression at the penoscrotal angle caused by the tendency of the indwelling catheter to straighten can produce a pressure sore, abcess and subsequent fistula formation

Taping the catheter laterally to the thigh eliminates the penoscrotal angle and prevents fistula development.

Figure 5.6.   Tape the penis laterally (or on the abdomen) to smooth out urethral curve and eliminate pressure on the penoscrotal angle which is a source of infection, periurethral abscesses and urethra fistula formation.

Nursing Action	Reason
4 Anchor the indwelling catheter. Do not pull it tight.	
a. *Female:* Tape the catheter and drainage tubing to the thigh.	**a.** This prevents traction and tension on the bladder.
b. *Male:* Tape the catheter laterally to the thigh (Fig. 5.6) or on the abdomen.	**b.** This smooths out urethral curve and eliminates pressure on the penoscrotal junction which can eventually lead to the formation of a fistula (Fig. 5.6).
c. Tape the tubing (not the catheter) to shaved inner aspect of thigh.	**c.** Taping the tubing to the thigh prevents tension and traction on the bladder.
5 Reduce (or reposition) the foreskin.	5 Paraphimosis (retraction and constriction of the foreskin behind the glans penis), secondary to catheterization, may occur if the foreskin is not reduced.

Follow-up Phase

Same as for female patient.

GUIDELINES: Management of the Patient with an Indwelling Catheter and Closed Drainage System

Purpose

1 To empty urine from the bladder.
2 To clear an obstructed catheter.
3 To rinse the bladder with a continuous solution of an antiseptic or antibiotic solution to prevent infection (less common use).

Equipment

Use a completely closed system (see Fig. 5.7)
Catheter tray with triple lumen catheter
Drainage solution as prescribed
Gauze squares
Iodophor solution (or other antibiotic agent)
Antiseptic soap solution

Procedure

Nursing Action	Reason

Performance Phase

1 Catheterize the patient (p. 232) and attach catheter to drainage apparatus.

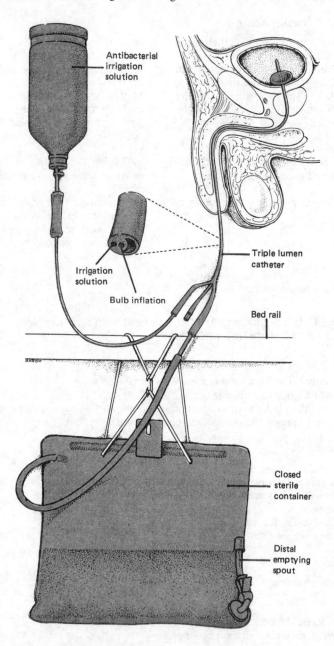

Figure 5.7. Closed sterile drainage system.

Nursing Action	Reason
2 Prevent introduction of organisms where catheter enters urethral meatus. **a.** Cleanse around the meatus at least twice daily with an antiseptic soap, e.g., Savlon. **b.** An antibiotic ointment, e.g., Hibitane cream, may be applied to the meatus.	2 Suppurative drainage and encrustation occur at the exit of any tube. Catheter care helps prevent exudate from entering urethra. Encrustations arising from urinary salts may enter bladder when catheter is removed and may serve as nuclei for stone formation. The catheter must be cleansed of blood or pus to maintain antibacterial protection.
3 Wash the perineal area with soap and water several times daily.	3 Avoid using powders and sprays on the perineal area.
4 Prevent introduction of organisms through the lumen of the catheter. Avoid separating connecting tube and catheter. Obtain a urine specimen without disrupting the closed system.	4 A needle with attached syringe is used to aspirate specimen from special part of the catheter.
5 Prevent introduction of organisms through the distal end of the drainage system: **a.** Do not allow drainage tube to contact urine in the collecting bag. Utilize a drip chamber. **b.** Do not disconnect tubing from drainage bag; use a distal emptying valve to empty bag. Clamp the valve immediately after draining the collecting bag. **c.** Keep the collecting bag below the bladder level; never allow it to touch the floor. **d.** Check the drainage system for kinks and other mechanical causes of obstruction if the catheter is plugged and not draining. **e.** Gentle 'milking' of the drainage tubing will frequently unplug the catheter.	5 Maintain an unobstructed flow at all times. Closed sterile drainage with indwelling catheter is effective in reducing infection. **b.** Empty bag every 8 hours or more often if need be. Avoid holding the bag upside down when emptying.

Management of Continuous Irrigating System

A Three-way (or Triple Lumen) Catheter (Fig. 5.3)

1 One lumen—inflates the bag holding the catheter in place.
2 Second lumen—for outflow of urine and outflow of drainage solution.
3 Third lumen—for inflow of irrigating solution (antiseptic) into bladder.

Flow of Irrigating Solutions

1 For continuous irrigation:
   a. If drainage is bright red, allow. irrigating solution to run in rapidly until drainage becomes lighter.
   b. If drainage is clear, allow irrigating solution to run at rate of 40–60 drops/min.

Other Measures to Prevent Infection

1 Ensure fluid intake, e.g., 3 l in 24 hours—to produce mechanical flushing and to dilute urinary elements producing encrustation.
2 Keep the urine acid—to prevent tube obstruction and encrustation of urinary sand and calculous deposits.

Measures to Prevent Cross-contamination

1 Wash hands thoroughly between patients.
2 Know the patients at risk—female, elderly, debilitated, critically ill.
   There appears to be a greater risk of microbial transmission between catheterized patients.

GUIDELINES: Assisting the Patient Undergoing Suprapubic Drainage (Cystostomy)

Purpose

1 To drain the bladder via a tube placed in the bladder through the suprapubic area.
2 To divert the flow of urine from the urethra.

Clinical Usefulness

1 Injuries to the urethra—stricture, trauma.
2 Following gynaecological procedures (vaginal hysterectomy; vaginal repair —rare.
3 Following bladder surgery.
4 Open prostatectomy.
5 Neurogenic bladder.

Equipment

Sterile suprapubic drainage system package (disposable)
Skin germicide for suprapubic skin preparation
Local anaesthetic agent if needed

Procedure

Nursing Action	Reason

Preparatory Phase

1 Place patient in a dorsal recumbent position with one pillow under head.
2 Expose the abdomen.

Nursing Action	Reason

Performance Phase (by doctor)

3 The bladder is distended with 300–500 ml of sterile saline via a urethral catheter which is removed. (Or the patient may be given water to drink before the procedure.)

3 Makes it easier to locate bladder.

4 The suprapubic area is surgically prepared. After the skin is dried the needle entry point is located.

4 The needle entry point is approximately 5 cm (2 in) above the symphysis.

5 The procedure may be performed in several ways:
a. By open operation.
b. By puncture with needle or trocar.
(1) The catheter is threaded through the needle or trocar well into the bladder.
(2) The needle or trocar is withdrawn, leaving the catheter in place.
(3) The catheter is secured with sutures or tape.

(3) Aseptic technique is employed in the area around the cystostomy tube.

(4) Cover the area around the catheter with a sterile dressing.
(5) Attach the drainage tubing to a closed sterile system.

6 Secure drainage tubing to lateral abdomen with tape (Fig. 5.8).

6 Prevents undue tension on the catheter.

7 If it is necessary to disconnect the collecting system, be sure there is a column of urine in the catheter.

7 The cystostomy tube acts as a siphon and must be kept full of fluid.

8 If the catheter is not draining properly, withdraw the catheter 2.5 cm (1 in) at a time until urine begins to flow. Do not dislodge catheter from bladder.

9 The drainage is maintained continuously for several days.

10 If a 'trial of micturition' is ordered the catheter is clamped for 4 hours.
a. Have the patient attempt to micmicturate while the catheter clamped.
b. After the patient micturates, unclamp the catheter and measure residual urine.

10 Usually, patients will micturate earlier after surgery with suprapubic drainage than the indwelling catheters.

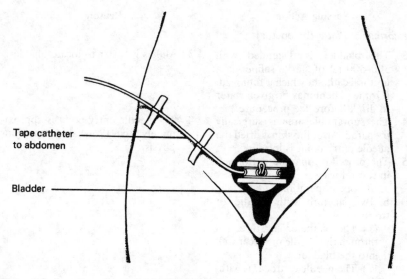

Figure 5.8. Location of suprapubic bladder drain.

c. Usually, if the amount of residual urine is less than 100 ml on two separate occasions (a.m. and p.m.), the catheter may be removed.

d. If the patient complains of pain or discomfort, or if the residual urine is over the prescribed amount, the catheter is usually left open.

11 The catheter is removed upon order and a sterile dressing is left over the needle, trocar or stab site.

11 Suprapubic drainage is considered more comfortable than an indwelling urethral catheter; it allows greater patient mobility and there is less risk of bladder infection.

URINE RETENTION

Urinary retention is the inability to urinate despite a desire to do so. Retention may be acute or chronic. Chronic retention will often lead to overflow incontinence.

Aetiology

Males

1 Benign prostatic hypertrophy.

Females

1 Urethral obstruction secondary to stricture, stones, vaginal cysts, carcinoma, oedema.

Males	Females
2 Stricture of urethra, calculus or foreign body in urethra, urethritis, tumour.	2 Retroverted uterus.
3 Phimosis.	

Either Male or Female

1 Following any operation, particularly on anal or perineal region—due to reflex spasm of sphincters.
2 Trauma.
3 Neurogenic bladder dysfunction—spinal cord tumour, trauma, herniated intervertebral disc, multiple sclerosis.
4 Certain drugs (anticholinergics, antihistamines).
5 Faecal impaction.
6 Psychogenic urinary retention.

Clinical Features (see Fig. 5.9)

1 History of not micturating or frequent passing of small amounts of urine without relief.
2 Progressive slowing of urinary stream; hesitancy.
3 Lower abdominal discomfort and distress; severe pain.
   Patient may have little or no discomfort if bladder distends slowly.
4 Oval-shaped mass is palpable over bladder.
5 Dullness to percussion above symphysis pubis (residual urine below 130 ml is not usually percussible).
6 Visualization of a rounded swelling arising out of the pelvis.
7 Urine-stained clothing.

Treatment and Nursing Management

Objectives

To treat underlying cause.
To prevent overdistension of the bladder with resultant infection.

1 Utilize measures to help patient pass urine.
   a. Transport patient to bathroom (or bedside commode) or allow to stand beside bed if possible—many patients are unable to micturate while lying in bed.
   b. Use warmth to relax sphincters—bath, warm shower.
   c. Give hot tea to drink.
   d. Have patient listen to sound of running water; place hands in warm water.
   e. Administer bethanechol chloride (Urecholine) only if directed.
   f. Give psychological reassurance and support.
2 Give prescribed analgesic medication postoperatively.
   a. Micturition may be difficult because of pain in incisional area, especially in anterior vaginal operations.
   b. Sphincter spasm is generally present in patients with acute urinary retention.
3 Decompress bladder before overdistension occurs—bladder mucosa which has been stretched from urinary retention is readily infected.
   a. Utilize indwelling catheter and closed drainage.

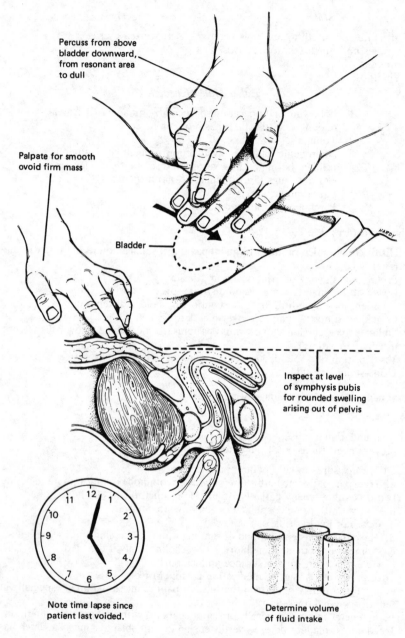

Percuss from above
bladder downward,
from resonant area
to dull

Palpate for smooth
ovoid firm mass

Bladder

Inspect at level
of symphysis pubis
for rounded swelling
arising out of pelvis

Note time lapse since
patient last voided.

Determine volume
of fluid intake

Figure 5.9. Nursing assessment for urinary retention.

(1) It may be advisable to decompress the bladder gradually if patient is elderly or hypertensive or has diminished renal reserve, or if retention of large amounts of urine has persisted for several weeks.

(2) Call urologist if unable to pass catheter easily; he will use special instruments (or operation may be necessary).

(3) Blood pressure may fluctuate and renal function decline the first few days after bladder drainage is instituted.

   b. Suprapubic cystostomy may be required if it is impossible to pass urethral catheter (p. 240).

4   Blood urea tests and other renal function tests are carried out.

5   Assist in carrying out diagnostic tests if obstructive uropathy (pathologic change in urinary tract from obstruction) is suspected.

NURSING ASSESSMENT FOR FLUID AND ELECTROLYTE IMBALANCE

The following signs and symptoms tend to occur in patients with renal disease.

Clinical Manifestations

Signs and Symptoms	Possible Indication
Acute weight loss (in excess of 5%), drop in body temperature, dry skin and mucous membranes, longitudinal wrinkles or furrows of tongue, oliguria or anuria	Volume deficit of extracellular fluid
Acute weight gain (in excess of 5%), oedema, moist râles in lungs, puffy eyelids, shortness of breath	Volume excess of extracellular fluid
Abdominal cramps, apprehension, convulsions, oliguria or anuria	Sodium deficit of extracellular fluid
Dry sticky mucous membranes, flushed skin, oliguria or anuria, thirst, rough and dry tongue	Sodium excess of extracellular fluid
Anorexia, gaseous distension of intestines, silent intestinal ileus, weakness, soft, flabby muscles	Potassium deficit of extracellular fluid
Diarrhoea, intestinal colic, irritability, nausea	Potassium excess of extracellular fluid
Abdominal cramps, carpopedal spasm, muscle cramps, tetany, tingling of ends of fingers	Calcium deficit of extracellular fluid
Deep bony pain, flank pain, and muscle hypotonicity	Calcium excess of extracellular fluid
Deep rapid breathing (Kussmaul), shortness of breath on exertion, stupor, weakness	Primary base bicarbonate deficit of extracellular fluid
Depressed respiration, muscle hypertonicity, tetany	Primary base bicarbonate excess of extracellular fluid

Signs and Symptoms	*Possible Indications*
Chronic weight loss, emotional depression, pallor, ready fatigue, soft, flabby muscles	Protein deficit of extracellular fluid
Positive Chvostek's sign, convulsions, disorientation, hyperactive deep re-reflexes, tremor	Magnesium deficit of extracellular fluid

Nursing Responsibilities

1 Observe the clinical course of the patient; record the data collected.
2 Keep an accurate intake and output record.
3 Check the vital signs every 4 hours. Weight the patient daily.
4 Give psychological support to the patient having repeated blood examinations for the surveillance of electrolyte balance.

ACUTE RENAL FAILURE

Acute renal failure is a sudden and almost complete loss of kidney function caused by failure of the renal circulation or by glomerular or tubular damage. The substances normally eliminated in the urine accumulate in the body fluids. Renal failure is a total body disease.

Precipitating Factors

1 Reduction in blood volume (shock).
2 Trauma.
3 Septicaemia.
4 Dehydration.
5 Hypersensitivity (allergic disorders).
6 Kidney stones.
7 Obstruction of renal vessels (embolism, thrombosis).
8 Nephrotoxic agents (bacterial toxins, drugs).
9 Mismatched blood transfusion.

Altered Physiology

Hypotension or nephrotoxins → decrease in renal flow → decreased glomerular filtration rate → renal ischaemia → tubular necrosis → tubular obstruction → oliguria.

Preventive Measures

1 Initiate adequate hydration before surgical procedures during and after operation.
2 Correct blood, fluid and electrolyte losses, especially in traumatized or surgical patients.
3 Avoid exposure to various nephrotoxins. Be aware that the majority of drugs or their metabolites are excreted by the kidneys.
4 Monitor urinary output hourly in sick patients to detect onset of renal failure at

the earliest moment. Frusemide (Lasix), mannitol, etc., may be given if necessary to maintain output around 60 ml/hour.
5 Treat hypotensive states promptly with steroids, fluid, blood, antibiotics, etc.
6 Schedule diagnostic studies requiring dehydration so that there are 'rest days', especially in aged who may not have adequate renal reserve.
7 Avoid infections which may produce progressive renal damage.
8 Serial renal function tests while taking nephrotoxic antibiotics for prolonged periods (kanamycin, colistin, cephaloridine, tetracycline) may be taken.

Clinical Phases

1 Period of oliguria (urine volume less than 400–600 ml/24 hours). (However, there can be decrease in renal function with increasing nitrogen retention even when the patient is excreting more than 1 litre of urine daily—calle high output failure.)
   a. Accompanied by rise in serum concentration of elements usually excreted by kidney (urea, creatinine, uric acid, organic acids and the intracellular cations—potassium and magnesium).
   b. Clinical manifestations—scant, bloody urine, lethargy, nausea.
   c. Lasts about 8–16 days.
2 Period of diuresis—gradually increasing urinary output reaching at least 2 l or more daily.
3 Period of convalescence—restoration of renal function may take 6–12 months.

Objectives of Treatment and Nursing Management

To restore the normal homoeostatic environment.

To Remove the Cause of Renal Failure if Possible

1 Rule out and treat urinary tract obstruction.
   a. Plain film of abdomen.
   b. Intravenous urogram to demonstrate kidney size, morphology, patency and configuration of lower urinary tract.
   c. Cystoscopy and retrograde study if necessary.
   d. Angiogram or radioisotope renogram or renoscan to evaluate arterial blood supply and detect kidney masses.
2 Stop drugs that may be nephrotoxic.

To Prepare for Peritoneal Dialysis or Haemodialysis to Prevent Metabolic Deterioration (see pp. 251–258).

1 Dialysis produces a more sustained correction of biochemical abnormalities.
2 Allows for liberalization of fluid, protein and sodium intake; helps wound healing; diminishes bleeding tendencies and predisposition to infection.

To Restore Adequate Blood Flow to the Kidneys

1 Give intravenous fluids and medications as directed to improve renal plasma flow, decrease intrarenal vascular resistance and increase renal blood flow to the renal cortex.
   a. Administer frusemide mannitol or ethacrynic acid as directed to initiate diuresis and prevent or minimize subsequent development of renal failure.

b. Give albumin infusion (for volume expansion) when hypovolaemia is associated with hypoproteinaemia.
2 Restore circulating blood volume.
3 Control shock.
4 Manage local or systemic infections.
5 Debride necrotic tissue.

To Maintain Fluid and Electrolyte Balance
1 Biochemical studies are carried out. (Electrolyte administration is guided by serial measurements of central venous pressure, serum and urine electrolyte concentrations, fluid losses and the clinical status of the patient.)
2 Give only enough fluids to replace current losses during oliguric phase (usually 400–500 ml/24 hours plus measured fluid losses associated with gastrointestinal drainage, fever, surgical drainage or other routes).
3 Weigh the patient daily to provide an index of fluid balance—expected weight loss 0.2–0.5 kg (0.5–1 lb) daily.
4 Monitor the urinary output and urine specific gravity.
   Measure and record intake and output (include urine, gastric suction, stools, wound drainage, perspiration, etc.).
5 Observe fluid excess by assessing patient's clinical status—dyspnoea, tachycardia, distended neck veins, peripheral oedema, pulmonary oedema.
6 Limit dietary protein during oliguric phase to minimize protein breakdown and to prevent rises in blood urea nitrogen.
   a. Give high-calorie foods since carbohydrates have a greater protein-sparing power. Calories may be temporarily supplied via the intravenous route.
   b. Chewing gum will stimulate saliva flow and lessen thirst.
   c. Give multivitamin supplements.
7 Measure and replace sodium losses, especially if large losses occur from the gastrointestinal tract via suction, vomiting or diarrhoea.
8 Control potassium balance (protein catabolism causes release of cellular potassium into body fluids, resulting in serious potassium intoxication).
   a. Sources of potassium are diet, tissue breakdown, blood in the gastrointestinal tract, blood transfusion, other sources (intravenous infusions, potassium penicillin) and extracellular shift in response to metabolic acidosis.
   b. Assess for hyperkalaemia (potassium intoxication) by serum potassium levels correlated with ECG changes and notify medical officer.
   c. Give ion exchange resins—Resonium A; provides for more prolonged correction of elevated potassium.
       (1) Orally (laxative may be given concurrently to avoid faecal impaction).
       (2) By retention enema since the colon is the principal site for potassium exchange.
          (a) Use catheter with balloon to facilitate retention if necessary.
          (b) Assist the patient to retain the resin 30–45 min to remove the potassium.
          (3) Sorbitol (induces water loss in gastrointestinal tract) may be given orally or as enema with Resonium A.
   d. Intravenous glucose and insulin or calcium gluconate sometimes used as emergency (and temporary) measure for potassium intoxication; causes potassium to enter cells.

e. Give intravenous hypertonic sodium bicarbonate as directed—promotes elevation of plasma pH; when available sodium ions are provided, there is a migration of potassium into the cell and a lowering of potassium in the plasma; this is short-term therapy and is used with other long-term measures.

f. Be prepared for cardiac arrest since increased potassium elevations lead to cardiac arrhythmias.

9 Watch for signs of dehydration or hypovolaemia during the diuretic phase (reduction in body weight, decreasing skin turgor, dryness of mucous membranes, hypotension, tachycardia).

To Prevent Infection

1 Utilize environmental asepsis.
2 Pay special attention to draining wounds, burns, etc., which may develop sepsis.
3 Avoid use of indwelling urethral catheters if possible.
   a. Give meticulous catheter care to prevent cystitis and ascending pyelonephritis (p. 237). Obstructed catheter may lead to pyelonephritis.
   b. Utilize three-way closed bladder irrigation system to decrease incidence of systemic infection if patient has to have indwelling catheter.
4 Turn, cough and exercise the patient to prevent pulmonary infections.
5 Be aware of the danger of aspiration of gastric contents in stuporous patients.

To Anticipate and Forestall Complications

1 Infection.
2 Potassium intoxication.
3 Acidosis.
4 Circulatory overload (dyspnoea, orthopnoea, pulmonary congestion, pulmonary oedema).
5 Hypertension, hypertensive crisis, convulsions.

CHRONIC RENAL FAILURE

Chronic renal failure is a progressive deterioration of renal function which ends fatally in uraemia (an excess of urea and other nitrogenous wastes in the blood) and its complications, unless haemodialysis or a kidney transplant is performed.

Reversible Causes

1 Urinary tract obstruction and infection.
2 Infectious diseases which cause increased catabolism with retention of metabolites and hyperkalaemia.
3 Hypertension.
4 Metabolic disease.
5 Nephrotoxic (poisonous to kidney cells) agents.

Clinical Manifestations

1 Gastrointestinal manifestations—anorexia, nausea, vomiting, hiccoughs, ulceration of gastrointestinal tract and haemorrhage.
2 Cardiopulmonary manifestations—hypertension, fibrinous pericarditis, pleuritis.

3   Nervous system manifestations—anxiety, irritability, delusions, hallucinations, drowsiness, muscle twitching, convulsions, coma.
4   Anaemia.
5   Skin discoloration (from retained urinary chromogen).
6   Uraemic frost on face (late).
7   Ammonia odour on breath.

Diagnosis

1   Anaemia (a characteristic sign).
2   Elevated serum creatinine or blood urea.
3   Elevated serum phosphate.
4   Decreased serum calcium.
5   Low serum proteins, especially albumin.
6   Usually low CO_2 and acidosis (low blood pH).

Treatment and Nursing Management

Objectives

To make the best possible use of remaining renal function.
To reduce the metabolic load.
To preserve the patient's extrarenal health.

1   Reversible causes of chronic renal failure will be treated (see above).
2   Offer diet according to blood chemistry levels and clinical status of the patient.
    a. Reduce protein intake according to impairment of renal function since metabolites that accumulate in the blood derive almost entirely from protein catabolism.
        (1) Protein should be of high biological value (dairy products, eggs, meat) so that patient does not rely on tissue catabolism for essential amino acids.
        (2) As renal function declines, protein intake may be restricted proportionately.
        (3) Protein may be increased if patient is on dialysis programme.
    b. Ensure high calorie intake—essential to spare protein for its own work and to provide energy.
        Encourage intake of sweets, jellies, etc.
    c. Give additional amino acids and supplementary vitamins as needed.
3   Prevent water and electrolyte disturbances.
    a. Weigh patient daily to assess fluid overload or depletion—weight should not increase or decrease over 0.45 kg (1 lb) per day.
    b. Treat acidosis if patient is symptomatic; acidosis commonly appears in chronic renal failure.
        (1) Assess patient for stupor, deep, rapid breathing of Kussmaul type, shortness of breath on exertion, weakness, unconsciousness.
        (2) Replace bicarbonate stores by infusion or oral administration of sodium bicarbonate.
        (3) Give daily sodium requirements as ordered (determined by sodium balance studies and daily weights)—patients with chronic renal disease are sensitive to salt depletion.

    c. Restrict or supplement potassium intake to prevent hyperkalaemia or hypokalaemia—excessive amounts of potassium can be lost or retained.

    d. The following treatment may or may not be employed:

        (1) Decrease intestinal phosphate absorption by dietary and pharmacologic means—phosphate retention contributes to development of secondary hyperparathyroidism.

        (2) Increase intestinal calcium absorption by dietary and pharmacological means. Patients with renal failure tend to be hypocalcaemic and may have osteomalacic changes.

    e. Give fluids to maintain adequate urinary volume and avoid dehydration.

        (1) Fluid restriction is not usually initiated until renal function is quite low.

        (2) Fluid allowance should be distributed throughout the day.

        (3) Avoid restricting fluids for prolonged periods for laboratory and radiological examinations since dehydrating procedures are hazardous to those patients who cannot concentrate urine.

4   Associated cardiac conditions will be treated with digitalis, diuretics and antiarrhythmic agents to reverse congestive heart failure and to improve renal haemodynamics.

    a. Patients with chronic renal failure may also have a variety of other conditions—hypertension, neuropathy, bone disease, infection, anaemia—that require pharmacological therapy.

    b. Patients with renal failure have increased sensitivity to drugs due to impaired metabolism and renal excretion.

Nursing Alert: Patients with impaired renal function may require major adjustments of common therapeutic agents. Give medications with caution.

5   Monitor blood pressure. Hypertension increases rate of renal deterioration and adversely affects the vascular system.

6   Prepare the patient for an intermittent dialysis programme and ultimately a kidney transplant (if he is a candidate for this type of therapy).

7   Treat patient's discomforts symptomatically (itching, thirst, etc.).

8   Observe for complications.

    a. Anaemia—has many causes and is invariably found in patients with advanced renal failure.

    b. Renal osteodystrophy—uraemia is associated with abnormal calcium metabolism causing bone pathology.

    c. Pericarditis, severe resistant hypertension, increasing oedema, heart failure.

    d. Infection.

    e. Paresthesias.

9   Give attention to 'little things' since these chronically ill individuals become weary, discouraged and despondent.

GUIDELINES: Assisting the Patient Undergoing Short-Term Peritoneal Dialysis

Peritoneal dialysis is a substitute for kidney function during renal failure. The peritoneum is used as a dialysing membrane.

Purposes

1   To aid in the removal of toxic substances and metabolic wastes.
2   To remove excessive body fluid.
3   To assist in regulating the fluid balance of the body.
4   To control blood pressure.

Equipment

Dialysis administration set (disposable, closed system)
Peritoneal dialysis solution as ordered
Supplemental drugs as ordered
Local anaesthesia, syringe, needles
(Central venous pressure monitoring equipment—if required)

Peritoneal catheter
ECG may be taken
Skin antiseptic, e.g., Savlon, proviodine
Sterile peritoneal set (contains forceps, swabs, towels, suturing equipment)
Sterile gown and gloves

Procedure (Fig. 5.10)

Nursing Action	Reason
Preparatory Phase	
1 Prepare the patient emotionally and physically for the procedure.	1 Nursing support is offered by explaining procedure mechanics, providing opportunities for the patient to ask questions, allowing him to verbalize his feelings and giving expert physical care.
2 See that the consent form has been signed (see local policy).	
3 Weigh the patient before dialysis and every 24 hours thereafter (preferably on an in-bed scale).	3 The weight at the beginning of the procedure serves as a baseline of information. Daily weight is helpful in assessing the state of hydration.
4 Take temperature, pulse, respiration and blood pressure readings prior to dialysis.	4 A knowledge of vital signs at the beginning of dialysis is necessary for comparing subsequent changes in vital signs.
5 Have the patient empty his bladder.	5 If the bladder is empty there is less likelihood of perforating it when the trocar is introduced into the peritoneum.
6 If necessary assist with insertion of central venous pressure catheter. ECG monitoring may also be employed.	6 Central venous pressure measurements may be carried out to assess fluid volume changes. Cardiac arrhythmias may occur due to serum potassium changes and vagal stimulation.

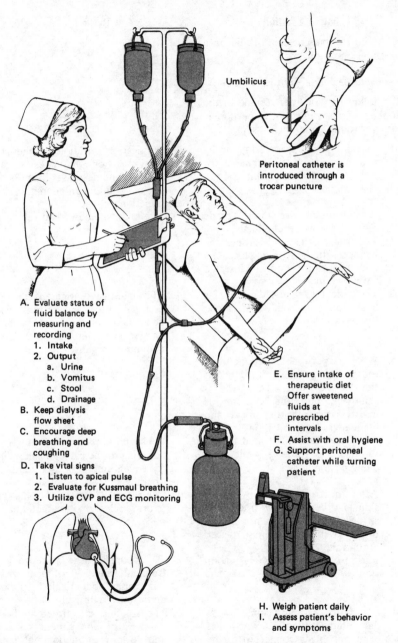

Umbilicus

Peritoneal catheter is
introduced through a
trocar puncture

A. Evaluate status of
   fluid balance by
   measuring and
   recording
   1. Intake
   2. Output
      a. Urine
      b. Vomitus
      c. Stool
      d. Drainage
B. Keep dialysis
   flow sheet
C. Encourage deep
   breathing and
   coughing
D. Take vital signs
   1. Listen to apical pulse
   2. Evaluate for Kussmaul breathing
   3. Utilize CVP and ECG monitoring

E. Ensure intake of
   therapeutic diet
   Offer sweetened
   fluids at
   prescribed
   intervals
F. Assist with oral hygiene
G. Support peritoneal
   catheter while turning
   patient

H. Weigh patient daily
I. Assess patient's behavior
    and symptoms

Figure 5.10. Nursing management of patient undergoing peritoneal dialysis.

Nursing Action	Reason

7   Make the patient comfortable in a supine position.

Performance Phase (by the doctor)

The following is a brief résumé of the method of insertion of the peritoneal catheter (done under strict asepsis).

1   The abdomen is prepared surgically and the skin and subcutaneous tissues are infiltrated with a local anaesthetic.

    1   Surgical preparation of the skin minimizes or eliminates surface bacteria and decreases the possibility of wound contamination and infection.

2   A small midline stab wound is made 3–5 cm below the umbilicus.

    2   The midline area is relatively avascular.

3   The trocar is inserted through the incision with the stylet in place, or a thin stylet cannula may be inserted percutaneously.

4   The patient is requested to raise his head from the pillow after the trocar is introduced.

    4   This manoeuvre tightens the abdominal muscles and permits easier penetration of the trocar without danger of injury to the intra-abdominal organs.

5   When the peritoneum is punctured, the trocar is directed toward the left side of the pelvis. The stylet is removed, and the catheter is inserted through the trocar and manoeuvred into position.

    Dialysis fluid is allowed to run through the catheter while it is being positioned.

    This prevents the omentum from adhering to the catheter, impeding its advancement or occluding its opening.

6   After the trocar is removed, the skin may be closed with a purse-string suture. (This is not always done.) A sterile dressing is placed around the catheter.

    6   The catheter is attached to the skin to prevent loss of the catheter in the abdomen.

7   Flush the tubing with dialysis solution.

    7   The tubing is flushed to prevent air from entering the peritoneal cavity. Air causes abdominal discomfort and drainage difficulties.

8   Attach the catheter connector to the administration set which has been previously connected to the container of dialysis solution

    8   The solution is warmed to body temperature for patient comfort and to prevent abdominal pain. Heating also causes dilation of the

Nursing Action	Reason
(warmed to body temperature, 37°C).	peritoneal vessels and increases urea clearance.
9 Drugs (heparin, etc.) are added in advance.	9 The addition of heparin prevents fibrin clots from occluding the catheter. Potassium chloride may be added on order unless the patient has hyperkalaemia.
10 Permit the dialysing solution to flow unrestricted into the peritoneal cavity (usually takes 5–10 min for completion).	10 The inflow solution should flow in a steady stream. If the fluid flows in too slowly the catheter may need to be repositioned since its tip may be buried in the omentum, or it may be occluded by a blood clot.
11 Allow the fluid to remain in the peritoneal cavity for the prescribed time period (15–30 min). Prepare the next exchange while the fluid is in the peritonal cavity.	11 In order for potassium, urea and other waste materials to be removed, the solution must remain in the peritoneal cavity for the prescribed time (dwell or equilibration time). The maximum concentration gradient takes place in the first 5–10 min and this is the most effective dwell time.
12 Unclamp the outflow tube. Drainage should take approximately 10 min or more, although the time varies with each patient.	12 The abdomen is drained by a siphon effect through the closed system. Gravity drainage should occur fairly rapidly, and steady streams of fluid should be observed entering the drainage container. The drainage is usually straw-coloured.
13 If the fluid is not draining properly, move the patient from side to side to facilitate the removal of peritoneal drainage. The head of the bed may also be elevated. Ascertain if the catheter is patent.	13 If the drainage stops, or starts to drip before the dialysing fluid has run out, it may indicate that the catheter tip is buried in the omentum. Rotating the patient may be helpful (or it may be necessary for the doctor to reposition the catheter).
14 When the outflow drainage ceases to run, clamp off the drainage tube and infuse the next exchange using strict aseptic technique.	
15 Take blood pressure and pulse every 15 min during the first exchange and every hour thereafter. Monitor the heart rate for signs of arrhythmia.	15 A drop in blood pressure may indicate excessive fluid loss from the glucose concentrations of the dialysing solutions. Changes in the vital signs may indicate impending shock or overhydration.

Nursing Action	Reason
16 Take patient's temperature every 4 hours (especially after catheter removal).	16 An infection is more apt to become evident after dialysis has been discontinued.
17 The procedure is repeated until the blood chemistry levels improve. The usual time is 12–36 hours; depending on the patient's condition, he will receive 24–48 exchanges.	17 The duration of dialysis depends on the severity of the condition and on the size and weight of the patient. Patients requiring only a few peritoneal dialysis treatments may have a plastic T-shaped button (Dean's prosthesis) placed in the catheter tract between dialyses to avoid need to repuncture the abdomen for catheter insertion. Patients requiring prolonged peritoneal dialysis should have implanted silastic catheters used with closed automated dialysis systems.
18 Keep an exact record of the patient's fluid balance during the treatment. **a.** Know the status of the patient's loss or gain of fluid at the end of each exchange. **b.** The fluid balance should be about even or should show slight fluid loss.	18 Complications (circulatory overload, hypertension, congestive heart failure) may occur if most of the fluid is not recovered.
19 Promote patient comfort during dialysis. **a.** Frequent care of pressure areas. **b.** Rotate from side to side. **c.** Elevate head of bed at intervals. **d.** Allow patient to sit in chair for brief periods if condition permits.	19 The dialysis period is lengthy, and the patient becomes fatigued.
20 Observe for the following: **a.** Respiratory difficulty. (1) Slow the inflow rate. (2) Make sure tubing is not kinked. (3) Prevent air from entering peritoneum by keeping drip chamber of tubing three-quarters full of fluid. (4) Elevate head of bed; encourage coughing and breathing exercises.	20 **a.** This is caused by pressure from the fluid in the peritoneal cavity and the upward displacement of the diaphragm—producing shallow respirations. (3) In severe respiratory difficulty, the fluid from the peritoneal cavity should be drained immediately and the doctor notified.

Nursing Action	**Reason**
(5) Turn patient from side to side.	
b. Abdominal pain. Encourage patient to move about.	**b.** Pain may be caused by the dialysing solution's not being at body temperature, incomplete drainage of the solution, chemical irritation, irritation by the catheter, peritonitis.
c. Leakage. (1) Change the dressings frequently. (2) Use sterile plastic drapes to prevent contamination.	**c.** Leakage around the catheter predisposes to peritonitis.

21 Keep accurate records:
   a. Exact time of beginning and ending of each exchange; starting and finishing time of drainage.
   b. Amount of solution infused and recovered.
   c. Fluid balance.
   d. Number of exchanges.
   e. Medications added to dialysing solution.
   f. Pre- and postdialysis weight.
   g. Level of responsiveness at beginning, throughout and at end of treatment.
   h. Assessment of vital signs and patient's condition.

Complications

1 Peritonitis.
   a. Watch for abdominal pain, tenderness, rigidity, cloudy dialysate return.
   b. Send specimen of dialysate for smear and culture.

1 Peritonitis is the most common complication. Antibiotics may be added to dialysate and also given systemically.

2 Bleeding.

2 A small amount of bleeding around the catheter is not significant if it does not persist. During the first few exchanges, blood-tinged fluid from subcutaneous bleeding is not uncommon. Small amounts of heparin may be added to inflow solution to prevent the catheter from becoming clogged.

3 Shock.

3 Symptoms of shock may occur due to excessive fluid loss.

Nursing Action	Reason
4 Protein loss.	4 There may be a significant protein loss, because most serum proteins pass through the peritoneal membrane during dialysis. Serum albumin determinations are made throughout the treatment.

Haemodialysis

Haemodialysis is a process of cleansing the blood of accumulated waste products. It is used for patients with end-stage renal failure.

Objectives

To extract toxic nitrogenous substances from the blood.
To remove excess water.

Underlying Principles

1   Heparinized blood passes down a concentration gradient through a semipermeable membrane (by dialysis) to the dialysate fluid.
2   The dialysate is composed of all of the important electrolytes in their ideal concentrations in extracellular space.
3   Through the process of diffusion, the blood components equilibrate with those in the dialysate. By appropriate adjustment of the dialysate bath composition, noxious substances (urea, creatinine, uric acid, phosphate and other metabolites) are transferred from the blood into the dialysate so that they can be discarded. Small pores of the membrane hold back desirable blood components.
4   Excess water is removed from the blood (ultrafiltration).
5   The body buffer system is maintained by the addition and diffusion of acetate from the dialysate into the patient; it is metabolized to form bicarbonate.
6   Purified blood is returned to the body through a vein of the patient.
7   At the end of the treatment the majority of poisonous wastes have been removed, electrolyte and water balances have been restored, and the buffer system has been replenished.

Requirements for Haemodialysis

1   Access to the patient's circulation.
2   Dialyser with semipermeable membrane.
3   Appropriate dialysate bath.

Time—4–12 hours, three times weekly, depending on the type of artificial kidney used.
Place—home (if feasible) or at a dialysis centre.

Methods of Access to Patient's Circulation

1   Arteriovenous fistula—can be created wherever a vein and artery are close together.

a. Usually radial artery and adjacent vein are anastomosed; arterialization of the vein makes it stronger and more readily accessible to repeated venepuncture.
b. Arterial end is used for arterial flow and distal end for reinfusion of dialysed blood.
c. Arteriovenous fistula may also be created in leg.
d. *Problems:*
  (1) Arteriovenous fistula—may be site of potential infection.
  (2) Occasionally, high blood flow through fistula may overload heart.
  (3) Disadvantage of being stuck with large-bore needles before each dialysis treatment.
2 External arteriovenous shunts.
a. Teflon-silastic catheter sewn into radial artery and a forearm vein. The two are connected by a teflon bridge.
b. During dialysis the bridge is removed and the arterial and venous ends are connected to the flow lines of the artificial kidney.
c. Shunts may also be placed in the legs.
d. *Problems:*
  (1) Limited shunt life—must be surgically revised every few months.
  (2) Clotting and infection.
  (3) Permanent reminder to patient of his disability.
3 Saphenous vein autografts.
4 Bovine arterial heterografts.
5 Direct cannulation of vessels.

Types of Dialysers

Many varieties of artificial kidneys have been described, but most conform to one of the following types:

1 Coil dialyser.
2 Flat plate or parallel flow dialyser.
3 Hollow-fibre kidney.

Monitoring During Dialysis*

The following parameters are monitored during haemodialysis:†

1 Chemical composition of dialysis fluid.
2 Temperature of dialysis fluid.
3 Pressure within the blood circuit.
4 Continuity of the blood column in the return line.
5 Blood flow through the dialyser.
6 Dialysis fluid flow rate.
7 Dialysis fluid pressure.
8 Presence of blood in dialysis fluid.

---

* The management of the patient on the dialyser is a complex subject beyond the scope of this discussion. The reader is referred to the written protocol of the particular machine being used.

† Kerr, D N S (1974) Dialysis for renal failure. In Wells, C, Kyle, J and Dunphy, J E (Eds) Scientific Foundations of Surgery, W B Saunders, pp. 645–652.

9   Pressure in the arterial line.
10   Blood clotting time.
11   Temperature, pulse and respiration of patient.

Dietary Management of Patient on Long-term Haemodialysis

1   The individual patient's dietary regime is modulated according to the extent of his residual renal function.
2   Dietary management involves restriction or adjustment of protein, sodium, potassium and/or fluid intake.
   a. Protein—protein of highest biological quality is given to maintain positive nitrogen balance and replace amino acids lost during each dialysis.
      (1) Usually 1 g of protein per kg of ideal body weight is given.
      (2) Carbohydrates and fats are supplied in generous amounts to provide energy and to spare tissue protein breakdown.
   b. Sodium.
      (1) Patient may not excrete the necessary amount of sodium to maintain balance.
      (2) Observe for fluid overload—hypertension, oedema.
      (3) Or patient may be a 'salt loser', unable to conserve salt; he thus loses large amounts of sodium in the urine and will require sodium replacement by pharmacological and dietary means.
   c. Potassium—potassium is a mineral found in the body cells.
      (1) Ability to eliminate excessive amounts of potassium is decreased in chronic renal failure.
      (2) Accumulation of potassium in body can be toxic to heart and cause serious arrhythmias.
      (3) Potassium is found in practically all foods—fruit juices, salt substitutes, bananas, chocolate and baked potatoes are rich sources of potassium.
   d. Fluid limitations.
      (1) Fluid limitations placed on some patients (overhydrated, cardiac or hypertensive patients).
      (2) Patient should be able to adjust his fluid intake according to the weight he has gained between dialysis treatments.

Health Teaching

Instruct the patient as follows:

1   Avoid eating frequently in places where salt-free cooking cannot be assured.
2   Read food labels carefully; avoid commercially prepared foods which have added sodium.
3   Avoid 'salt substitutes'—may contain potassium chloride which should be avoided.
4   Eat fresh vegetables and fruits within dietary prescription.

Pharmacologic Management

1   Phosphate-binding gels (Aludrox, Basojel).
   a. Phosphorus tends to accumulate, resulting in hyperparathyroidism and osteodystrophy.

b. These medications bind phosphate in the intestine and may help maintain proper calcium and phosphorus levels in the blood.
2   Potassium-binders—bind potassium in intestine to prevent dangerous elevations in blood.
3   Multivitamins and iron supplements.
   a. These medications necessary because of significant nutrient losses during dialysis (especially of ascorbic acid and folic acid).
   b. Iron deficiency due to loss of blood in dialyser coil is correctable.

Medical Problems of Patients on Long-term Haemodialysis

Although haemodialysis can prolong life indefinitely, it does not completely control uraemia or halt the natural course of the underlying kidney disease.

1   Arteriosclerotic cardiovascular disease—leading cause of death and major factor limiting long-term survival.
   a. Disturbances of lipid metabolism (hypertriglyceridaemia) appear to be accentuated by haemodialysis.
   b. Congestive heart failure, coronary heart disease with anginal pain, stroke, peripheral vascular insufficiency may incapacitate patient.
2   Intercurrent infection—patient has reduced resistance to infection.
   a. Exposure of blood to blood products and foreign material—may cause infection and gram-negative and gram-positive bacteraemia.
   b. Local infection of shunt site and in fistulas.
   c. Haemodialysis-associated hepatitis (serum hepatitis).
3   Anaemia and fatigue—may be caused by accelerated red cell loss (from haemolysis and bleeding) and impaired erythropoietin production.
   a. Sleeplessness, fatigue and malaise may be persistent.
   b. Diminution of physical and emotional well-being—lack of energy, drive, loss of interest.
4   Bleeding.
   a. Bleeding from heparin rebound.
   b. Gastrointestinal bleeding.
   c. Subdural haematoma.
   d. Haemorrhagic pericarditis.
   e. Menorrhagia.
5   Disordered calcium metabolism.
   a. Renal osteodystrophy (leading to bone pain and fractures)—pathogenesis obscure but excessive parathyroid hormone secretion and vitamin D resistance may be causal factors.
   b. Aseptic necrosis of hip.
   c. Vascular calcification.
   d. Intractable pruritus (itching).
6   Chronic ascites—may be due to fluid overload associated with congestive heart failure, malnutrition (hypoalbuminaemia) and inadequate dialysis.
7   Disequilibrium syndrome—from rapid fluid and electrolyte changes.
      May produce hypertension, headache, vomiting, convulsions, coma and psychiatric problems.

Psychosocial Problems

Long-term haemodialysis has unpredictable and uneven results. The impact of renal disease and its treatment can be destructive to the ego and can place its victims under severe mental and emotional stress.

1 Depression—an expected occurrence; most common psychological manifestation seen in patients on haemodialysis.

Depression occurs from multiple causes—losses of bodily functions, working capability and sexual drive; impotence, other physical complications, chronic illness, feelings of deprivation from diet and fluid restriction, limited capacity to compete, fear of death and dying, unpredictable medical status.

2 Dependence–independence conflict.
a. Although patient is dependent on the machine, personnel and treatment regime, he is at the same time encouraged to be independent, work and lead a 'normal' life.
b. Dependence may create aggressive feelings which cannot be expressed.
c. May repress hostility toward medical and nursing staff.

3 Anxiety—a normal reaction to stress and threat.
a. Patient anxious because of constant changes in his clinical status and unpredictability of his health.
b. May use denial, fantasy, repression, rejection, etc., as defence mechanisms to deal with anxiety.

4 Suicidal behaviour—usually an act that stems from depression.
a. Allow patient to express his feelings about self-destruction.
b. Point out his positive coping mechanisms and emphasize his capabilities.
c. Psychiatric referral may be necessary.

5 Denial—a common response to a shift in health status.
a. Denial may be protective and useful to a certain extent—may protect patient from emotional decompensation (denial has both adaptive and maladaptive functions).
b. Failure of this defence may lead to depression.

Impact of Dialysis on Family

1 Altered family life style.
a. Social activities may be decreased due to large amount of time spent on dialysis.
b. Close confinement to home (if patient on home dialysis)—may create conflicts, frustration and depression in some families.
c. Patient and family may impose unnecessary limitations on their own activities.

2 Decreasing sexual activity—may lead to marital problems.

3 Feelings of resentment (revealed or hidden)—due to personal sacrifices made by family.

4 Feeling that patient is a 'marginal' person with limited life expectancy—can be transmitted to patient.

5 Difficulties in communication between patient and spouse—difficult to express anger, negative feelings and fear of death.
a. Fear that expressed anger will cause something to happen to patient.
b. Expressions of anger may be displaced or covered up by anxiety.

Health Teaching

1 Encourage patient to assume the management and control of his therapeutic regime.
   a. Determine patient's value system and ego strengths; use these to help him adapt to a different life style.
   b. Emphasize his capabilities.
   c. Teach patient about his condition and treatment in 'small doses'.
   d. Discourage the patient's image of himself as 'sick'.
   e. Help him to develop a sense of independence from the machine.
   f. Encourage patient to interact with his surroundings during dialysis.
2 Encourage patient to set realistic goals.
   a. Work activities should be introduced gradually—returning to work may not be a realistic goal for some patients.
   b. Modify attitudes in direction of permissiveness in area of productivity.
3 Encourage patient to express his angry feelings (pain, discomfort, frustration)—helps to reduce level of emotional tension and will help prevent depression.
4 Let family have an opportunity (away from patient) to express their feelings of anger, helplessness, etc.
   a. Help family to accept their negative feelings.
   b. Teach family what is involved in chronic haemodialysis.

KIDNEY TRANSPLANTATION

Kidney transplantation is the transplantation of a kidney from a living donor or human cadaver donor to a recipient with end-stage renal failure who requires support from dialysis in order to maintain life.
   Kidney transplants from well-matched related living donors are more successful than those from cadaver donors.

Potential Problems

1 Infection—leading cause of death after transplant.
2 Possibility of recurrence of original disease in the graft.
      Example: rapidly progressive glomerulonephritis.
3 Renal graft failure and renal graft rejection.
      Except when the donor is a twin, the immunological defence of the recipient tends to reject (and destroy) a foreign substance, e.g., the kidney graft.
4 Death from complications.

Operative Procedures Done Before Transplantation

Surgical operations on all recipients before transplantation may or may not include:

1 Bilateral nephrectomy—for uncontrolled hypertension (renin variety), for removal of potential source of infection, if present, and for patients with obstructed kidneys or vesicoureteral reflux, rapidly progressive glomerulonephritis, polycystic renal disease.
2 Splenectomy—reported to decrease the amount of antibody-producing tissues of

the host; permits the administration of larger doses of immunosuppressive drugs with less suppression of the leucocytes (leucopenia).
  a. Role of splenectomy in kidney transplantation still controversial.
  b. Procedure limited to selected patients.
3 Vagotomy/pyloroplasty—may be done as a prophylactic measure for patients with history of gastrointestinal bleeding or duodenal ulcer.

Surgical procedure:

1 The donor kidney is transplanted retroperitoneally in either iliac fossa.
2 The ureter of the newly transplanted kidney is transplanted into the bladder or anastomosed to the ureter of the recipient.

Preoperative Medical and Nursing Management Before Transplantation

Objective

To bring patient's metabolic state as close to normal as possible.

1 Tissue typing done to determine histocompatibility of donor and recipient.
2 Antibody screening for red and white cell antibodies.
3 Immunosuppressive drugs given in order to minimize or overcome body's defence mechanism:
    Azathioprine (Imuran) and prednisone are usually begun 48 hours preoperatively on a scheduled transplant patient.
4 Blood transfusion (if necessary)—should be washed, packed or frozen red cells to decrease exposure to leucocyte antigens.
5 Blood counts, chemistries, coagulation profiles, liver function tests, required cultures, ECG, state of hydration, blood pressure, temperature, pulse rate and weight are corrected and documented.
6 Haemodialysis (p. 258) is usually done the day before the scheduled transplant.
7 Preoperative skin preparation is meticulous to decrease bacterial count on the skin.
8 Avoid pulmonary complications by:
    a. Cessation of cigarette smoking 2 weeks prior to surgery.
    b. Instruction and practise in deep breathing, coughing and leg and ankle exercises.
9 Routine bacteriological cultures may be taken from recipients before operation, e.g., throat and nasal swabs.
10 All patients being considered for transplantation should have a recent Australia antigen test. A positive test means no transplant.

Postoperative Objectives of Surgical and Nursing Management

Objective

To maintain homoeostasis until kidney transplant is functioning well. (Many facets of care are similar to those of patients having renal and vascular surgery.)

To Anticipate at the Earliest Moment any Evidence of Threatened Rejection

1 Maintain surveillance for abnormal changes in blood chemistry tests and for

oliguria, oedema, fever, increasing blood pressure, apprehension, weight gain, swelling or tenderness over graft.

a. Combinations of immunosuppressive drugs (Azathioprine (Imuran)), prednisone or antilymphocytic globulin (ALG), or combination(s) of cyclophosphamide, prednisone, ALG are given as directed.

b. Doses are gradually tapered; therapy is continued indefinitely.

c. Renal graft failure and rejection may be early (first 24–72 hours), delayed (3–14 days) or late (after 3 weeks).

(1) Transplanted kidney is removed when rejection is inevitable or when excessive immunosuppression is required to maintain kidney.

(2) Patient placed back on maintenance dialysis; will require understanding and supportive emotional care.

2　Leucocyte and platelet counts are monitored—immunosuppression depresses formation of leucocytes which may produce agranulocytosis; resistance to infection is lowered and lethal sepsis may develop.

To Anticipate and Avoid all Possible Complications

1　Monitor and protect patient from infection—kidney recipient is susceptible to faulty healing and infection due both to immunosuppressive therapy, which suppresses the immune response, and to complications of renal failure.

a. Infection may be masked or confused with symptoms of rejection since impaired renal function and fever are evidences of both infection and rejection.

b. Immunosuppressive drugs render the transplant recipient more vulnerable to infection, permitting opportunistic infections to occur (moniliasis, cytomegalic virus disease, *Pneumocystis carinii* pneumonia.

2　Carry out protective isolation as required; health team members and family may wear masks until immunosuppressive drug dosages are lowered.

3　Give aseptic care to wounds and puncture sites (central venous pressure lines, intravenous lines, draining sites, etc.).

a. Wound healing may be delayed due to effects of renal disease and immunosuppressive drugs.

b. Change dressings promptly if drainage is present—drainage is an excellent culture medium for bacteria.

c. Bacteriological testing of urine and all exit wounds are carried out. Catheter and drain tips are cultured on removal.

(1) Before removing catheter, disinfect skin around entry site of catheter (or drain). Remove.

(2) Using aseptic technique, cut off tip of catheter or drain and place in sterile container for lab culture.

4　Monitor vascular access to haemodialysis to ensure patency and watch for evidences of infection.

5　Give oral nystatin mouthwash—to prevent mucosal candidiasis (fungal colonization occurs secondarily to steroid and antibiotic administration).

6　Give regular skin hygiene.

To Keep an Accurate Fluid and Electrolyte Balance

After kidney transplant the following may occur:

1   A few donor kidneys function immediately after grafting.
   a. May produce large quantities of dilute urine (10–15 l in first 24 hours)—due partly to tubular dysfunction or overhydrated state found in some dialysed patients.
   Intravenous fluid replacement to balance losses, is given.
   b. Cadaver kidney (due to period of ischaemia following donor's death) may undergo tubular necrosis and not function for 2–3 weeks.
   Fluid intake is restricted—usually approximately 600 ml/24 hours plus amount of fluid losses from drainage, etc.
   c. Or kidney may produce amounts of urine varying from extremes of no urine to large volumes of urine.
2   Monitor central venous pressure, ECG and skin temperature frequently to guard against blood volume depletion and electrolyte imbalance.
   a. Central venous pressure readings observed and recorded hourly or more frequently as necessary.
   b. Avoid using dialysis access extremity for intravenous or intra-arterial monitoring.
3   Monitor output from indwelling catheter which has been connected to a closed drainage system.
   a. Measure urine every 30 min–1 hour.
   b. Irrigate catheter only on direct order.
   c. Palpate bladder to detect presence of distension.
   d. Instruct patient to micturate frequently after catheter removal to avoid stressing the bladder closure.
4   Serum and urine electrolytes are monitored to determine patient's chemical balance.
   a. Anticipate adjustment of fluid replacement.
   b. Intravenous fluids are given according to urine volume and serum electrolyte levels; serum and urine chemistries are measured at specified intervals.
   c. Notify doctor immediately if arrhythmias or other cardiac symptoms develop.
5   Prepare for haemodialysis in postoperative period until transplanted kidney is functioning well.

To be Alert for Other Complications

1   Gastrointestinal complications
   a. Incidence of gastrointestinal ulceration and bleeding is high (steroid-induced).
      (1) Steroids mask symptoms of ulceration.
      (2) Gastrointestinal haemorrhage associated with high mortality rate.
      (3) Give antacids frequently as directed until steroid doses are lowered—as a means of protection against gastrointestinal ulceration.
   b. Fungal colonization of gastrointestinal tract—occurs secondarily to steroid and antibiotic administration.
   c. Faecal impaction—decrease in colonic motility may occur from steroid effect.
2   *Other complications:*
   a. From steroids—infection, diabetes, gastrointestinal bleeding, thrombosis, osteoporosis, psychosis, disorders of calcium metabolism, cushingoid facies, glaucoma, cataracts, acne.

b. From immunosuppressive therapy—bone marrow depression.
c. Vascular complications—haemorrhage and thrombosis.
d. Grafted ureter—stricture, fistula (fistula of bladder also).
e. Serum hepatitis.
f. Cancer—persons on long-term immunosuppressive therapy develop cancer more frequently than the general population.

To Give Continuing Psychological Support

1 Keep the patient informed of his progress, proposed treatment plans and short- and long-term goals.
2 Observe for changes in behaviour, altered thought and feeling processes.
3 See p. 263 for other aspects of psychological suuport.

Discharge Planning and Health Teaching

1 The hospitalization period for a kidney transplant may be 6 weeks or longer.
2 The patient receives individualized instruction about the following:
   a. Diet.
   b. Medications.
   c. Fluids.
   d. Daily weight.
   e. Daily measurement of urine.
   f. Management of intake and output.
   g. Prevention of infection.
   h. Resumption of activity.
3 Instruct patient to report to the doctor immediately if any of the following occur:

   a. Decrease in urinary output.
   b. Weight gain.
   c. Malaise.
   d. Changes in blood pressure readings.
   e. Fever.
   f. Respiratory distress.
   g. Tenderness over graft.
   h. Anxiety, depresssion, changes in eating, drinking or other habit patterns.
4 Advise patient to avoid strenuous contact sports after surgery.
5 Patient should know that follow-up care after transplantation is a lifelong necessity.

NURSING MANAGEMENT OF THE PATIENT UNDERGOING RENAL/UROLOGICAL SURGERY

Preoperative Nursing Care

Objective

To restore the patient to as normal a physiological state as possible with as little psychological trauma and physical morbidity as possible.

To Recognize the Fear and Anxiety of the Patient Concerning the Threat of Impending Surgery

1 Keep in mind that most patients entering the hospital with urological conditions have pain, fever, haematuria, difficulty in micturating, etc.
2 Encourage the patient to recognize and express his feelings of anxiety.
3 Obtain patient's confidence by establishing a relationship of trust and by giving gentle and considerate care.
4 Increase the patient's understanding of what to expect during the pre- and postoperative periods.
5 Assess for alertness, appetite and general well-being of the patient.
6 Avoid physical inactivity.
7 Give preoperative medications as prescribed to allay worry and fear.

To Assess Anatomic and Functional Status of Urinary Tract and Kidneys

1 Diagnostic studies:
   a. Serum electrolyte studies.
   b. Blood urea.
   c. Creatinine clearance test.
   d. Intravenous urogram and other x-ray studies.
   e. Radioisotope renography.
2 Give antibacterial agents as indicated before surgery, especially in following instances:
   a. Prostatic operations.
   b. Surgery on infected kidneys, ureters, bladder.

To Assess Cardiopulmonary Status of the Patient

1 Determine history of patient's ability to engage in physical activity without distress.
   Observe for dyspnoea, productive cough, other cardiac symptoms.
2 An electrocardiogram is done on all patients over 50. The preoperative cardiogram also serves as a baseline reference in event of postoperative cardiopulmonary complications.
3 A chest x-ray is taken.
4 Ensure that the blood volume is as normal as possible.
   a. Total blood volume determination is carried out preoperatively when indicated.
   b. Transfusions of whole blood, packed red cells, plasma are given when indicated.
5 Assess status of vascular system of lower extremities (especially varicosities).
   a. Elevate patient's legs and apply elastic stockings to minimise stasis in superficial veins.
   b. Encourage patient to do leg exercises.
6 Inquire if patient has any bleeding tendencies.
7 Teach the patient deep-breathing exercises and an effective cough routine.
8 Manage coexisting diseases (diabetes, congestive heart failure).

To Discover and Correct any Abnormalities of Fluid and Electrolyte Balance

1 Weigh patient daily to determine status of fluid balance.

2   Assess status of mucous membranes and skin turgor.
3   Measure and record intake and output as an index of hydration.

To Determine the Drug and Allergy History of the Patient so that Therpeutic Corrections can be Made if Necessary

1   Antihypertensives and tranquillizers—predispose to refractory hypotension during general anaesthesia.
2   Anticoagulants—depress prothrombin activity; can produce haemorrhagic complications especially in prostatic surgery and operations on retroperitoneal area.
3   Adrenal cortical steroids—may produce adrenal insufficiency during periods of stress.
4   Anticholinergics and antihistamines—may impair emptying of bladder.
5   Alcohol—previous overuse may precipitate onset of delirium tremens.

Postoperative Nursing Care

Objective

To reduce factors that contribute to postoperative complications.

To Promote the Safety and Comfort of the Patient

1   Employ frequent and close observation of blood pressure, pulse and respiration in order to recognize symptoms of shock, haemorrhage and early atelectasis.
2   Give postoperative sedation and pain control on an individual basis to reduce respiratory embarrassment and to permit coughing.
3   Be alert for symptoms of postoperative ileus (fairly common following renal surgery).
    a. Assess for abdominal distension, pain and lack of intestinal peristalsis (determined by stethoscope auscultation).
    b. Avoid oral intake for patient until active bowel sounds are heard (auscultation) or passage of flatus is noted.
    c. Give adequate and appropriate fluid replacement intravenously.
    d. Give enema or rectal tube; administer neostigmine methylsulphate (Prostigmin) if patient is uncomfortable from gas (rectal tube may be contraindicated in prostatism); encourage moving and turning.
    e. Encourage patient to use bedside commode as soon as possible.
4   Weigh patient daily to determine status of fluid balance; adjust fluid intake to maintain patient's weight within 2% of preoperative level.
5   Give inhalation therapy to encourage deep respiratory movements and aid in expectoration of tracheobronchial secretions.
6   Give antibiotics as prescribed on the basis of culture identification of causative organism.
7   Employ early ambulation techniques as an aid in preventing thromboembolic episodes.
    a. Ambulation contraindicated in prostatic patients with bleeding and with some types of plastic reconstruction surgery.
    b. Encourage patient to do leg exercises in bed.
8   Make certain that drainage tubes are functioning since almost all urological patients have drains, tubes or catheters.

    a. Make sure indwelling catheter is dependent and draining.
     (1) Tape tubing to thigh to relieve traction on bladder. In supine male patient tape catheter to abdomen.
     (2) Give meticulous catheter care (see p. 239).
    b. Change dressings as indicated when patient has profuse drainage.
    c. Observe patients with prostatic drainage since they have a tendency to bleed.
     (1) Irrigate catheter as often as every 30 min to flush out clots, or use continuous bladder irrigation at sufficiently rapid rate to keep drainage clear.
     (2) Institute straight drainage as soon as drainage is clear.
    d. Employ care with patient with nephrostomy tube drainage (intubation of kidney used as a method of temporary or rarely permanent diversion of urine).
     (1) Purpose of nephrostomy drainage:
      (a) To provide drainage from kidney after surgery.
      (b) To conserve and permit physiological restoration of renal tissue that has been traumatized by obstructive disease.
      (c) To provide drainage when ureter is no longer functioning.
     (2) Assess for bleeding from nephrostomy site (main complication of nephrostomy).
     (3) Do not clamp the nephrostomy tube.
     (4) Irrigate nephrostomy tube only by direct order of doctor.
    e. Assess patient with indwelling ureteral catheter (utilized to permit drainage from affected kidney).
     (1) Ureteral catheters are inserted through a cystoscope and left in place for a period of time; they are taped to indwelling urethral catheter to hold them in place.
     (2) Tape catheter to thigh to reduce pulling on catheter.
     (3) Make notation on nursing care plan that catheter is a *ureteral* catheter.
     (4) Do not irrigate a ureteral catheter; this is done by the urologist.

To Assess Patient Constantly for Complications

1 Haemorrhage (and shock)—chief danger during renal surgery.
    a. Assess for haemorhage in patients who have had prostatic surgery, cystectomy or renal surgery.
    b. Adequate blood transfusion therapy is employed before surgery, if necessary.
    c. Blood loss is replaced with fresh whole blood.
2 Acute renal failure.
    a. Watch patients who have prolonged surgery, shock or arterial hypotension for a period of time.
    b. Measure urinary volume to determine if oliguria is present.
    c. See p. 249 for treatment of renal failure.
3 Wound infection—take smear and culture for offending organism.
4 Postoperative atelectasis.
    a. Utilize preventive techniques of deep breathing, exercise and coughing.
    b. Stimulate coughing by tracheal suctioning if necessary to dislodge mucus plug.
    c. Prepare for bronchoscopic aspiration if necessary.
5 Pulmonary embolism.
    a. Prevent embolic episodes by early ambulation, passive and active leg exercises, elastic stockings and low-dose heparin as prescribed.

    b. Examine and measure circumference of calves of legs daily.
    c. Examine for positive Homan's sign—pain in calf on dorsiflexion of the foot.
    d. Assess patient for low grade fever and elevation of pulse rate.
6 Paralytic ileus—more common after operations in which there is manipulation of
   the intestines.
    a. Usually transient.
    b. Oral feedings resumed after bowel sounds are heard.

INFECTIONS OF THE URINARY TRACT

A *urinary tract infection* (UTI) is caused by the presence of pathogenic micro-
organisms in the urinary tract with or without signs and symptoms (Fig. 5.11).
Infection may predominate at the bladder (cystitis); urethra (urethritis); prostate
(prostatitis); or kidney (pyelonephritis). Unfortunately, noninfectious conditions
may generate symptoms which mimic those of urinary tract infection.

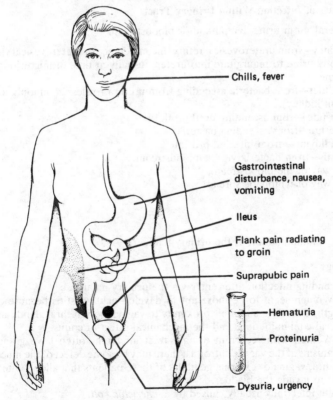

Chills, fever

Gastrointestinal
disturbance, nausea,
vomiting

Ileus

Flank pain radiating
to groin

Suprapubic pain

Hematuria

Proteinuria

Dysuria, urgency

Figure 5.11. Assessment of patient with infection of genitourinary tract.

Bacteriuria refers to the presence of bacteria in the urine. (The normal urinary tract is sterile except near the urethral.orifice.)

Colony count of at least 100 000 colonies/ml of urine on a clean midstream or catheterized specimen implies infection.

Nursing Alert: Infections in any part of the urinary tract may persist for months or years without symptoms and eventually cause serious kidney damage.

Predisposing Factors

1 Urinary stasis and obstruction—slowing of urinary flow causes kidney to be more susceptible to bacterial infection; obstruction is primary predisposing factor.
2 Presence of foreign body—indwelling catheter, stone.
3 Neurogenic bladder dysfunctions—impair effective drainage.
4 Disease of blood vessels—(arteriosclerosis).
5 Lowered body resistance.
6 Certain underlying conditions—pregnancy, sickle-cell trait, hypertension, diabetes mellitus.

Pathways of Infection Within Urinary Tract

In general, from urine, lymph and/or bloodstream.

1 Kidney—from ureterovesical reflux (incompetence of ureterovesical valve which allows urine to regurgitate into ureters, usually at time of micturition); bloodborne.
2 Bladder—from bacteria ascending from urethra (or less commonly descending from kidney).
3 Prostate—from ascending urethral flora.
4 Urethra—from ascending bacteria.
5 Epididymis—from infected prostate.
6 Testis—from bacteria via the bloodstream.
7 By way of the bloodstream.
8 By way of lymphatic spread.

Cystitis

Cystitis is inflammation of the urinary bladder.

Aetiology

1 Ascending infection after entry via the urinary meatus.
   a. Women seem to be more apt to develop acute cystitis because of shorter length of urethra, anatomic proximity to vagina, periurethral glands and rectum (faecal contamination) and the mechanical effect of coitus.
   b. Women with recurrent urinary tract infections often have gram-negative organisms at the vaginal introitus; there may be some defect of the mucosa of the urethra, vagina or external genitalia of these patients that allows enteric organisms to invade the bladder.
2 Acute infections usually caused by *Escherichia coli*.
3 Upper urinary tract disease may occasionally cause recurrent bladder infection.

Clinical Manifestations

1 Frequency and urgency.
2 Burning in the urethra.
3 Suprapubic tenderness; pain in region of the bladder.
4 Changes in the composition of urine (pus and blood).

Treatment and Nursing Management

Objectives

To eradicate the causative pathogens.
To prevent recurrences.
To preserve renal function.

1 Obtain uncontaminated urine specimen for smears, culture and sensitivity studies (p 229) to determine pathogen so that appropriate drug may be selected.
   a. Urine culture may be repeated several times during therapy and 7–10 days after completion of treatment to ensure elimination of infection.
   b. Patients with recurring infections should have periodic urine cultures since most recurrences are new infections with different organisms.
2 Assist with evaluation studies to determine if infection is secondary to a functional or structural abnormality (x-rays, intravenous urogram, cystoscopy).
   a. Take careful history for previous symptoms of urinary tract disease.
   b. Obtain detailed description of present illness (example: frequency).
     (1) How often does patient micturate?
     (2) How much urine is passed at each micturition?
     (3) How much fluid is taken? What types of fluid?
     (4) Relationship between micturition and other symptoms.
   c. Obtain similar detailed information about dysuria, nocturia, urgency, incontinence, changes in appearance of urine, urinary stream, pain.
   d. Assist with physical examination.
3 Remove the contributing cause(s) and source of obstruction if found (neoplasm of kidney, bladder calculus, prostatism, stricture).
4 Give prescribed antibiotic medication since urinary infections usually respond to drugs that are excreted in the urine in high concentrations; a potentially effective drug should rapidly sterilize the urine and thus relieve the patient's symptoms.
5 Maintain an appropriate urine pH—efficacy of certain antibiotic drugs is affected by the reaction (pH) of the urine.
   a. Aminoglycoside antibiotics (streptomycin, kanamycin, neomycin and gentamicin) are more active with an alkaline pH.
     Sodium bicarbonate alkalinizes urine.
   b. The tetracyclines, and lexamine mandelate (Mandelamine) are more active with an acid pH.
     Ascorbic acid acidifies urine.
6 Attempt to enhance body's normal defence mechanism.
   a. Encourage patient to drink sufficient fluids to promote renal blood flow and to flush out bacteria in urinary tract.
   b. Encourage patient to micturate frequently (every 2–3 hours) and to empty

bladder completely since this enhances bacterial clearance, reduces urine stasis and prevents reinfection.

7　Promote patient comfort.

a. Encourage bed rest during the acute phase.

b. Give analgesics, antispasmodics, and heat to perineum to relieve pain, spasm and urgency.

Discharge Planning and Health Teaching

1　Encourage patient to have follow-up urine studies for at least 2 years or more to determine if asymptomatic infection is present—*there is a marked tendency for infection to recur.*

2　Instruct patients who have had urinary tract infections during pregnancy to have follow-up studies.

3　For women with repeated urinary tract infections give the following instructions:

a. Reduce vaginal introital concentration of pathogens by hygienic measures.

(1) Wash in shower or while standing in bathtub—bacteria in bath water may gain entrance into urethra.

(2) Cleanse around the perineum and urethral meatus after each bowel movement.

b. Drink liberal amounts of fluid to flush out bacteria.

c. Micturate every 2–3 hours during day and completely empty bladder.

d. In certain women sexual intercourse is the initiating event for the development of bacteriuria.

(1) A single dose of an oral antibiotic agent may be ordered following sexual intercourse.

(2) Micturate immediately after sexual intercourse.

e. An antibiotic vaginal suppository may be ordered to reduce concentration of bacteria in introitus.

f. Apply antibiotic ointment around urinary meatus as directed.

g. Patients with persistent bacteria may require long-term antibiotic therapy to prevent colonization of periurethral area and recurrence of urinary tract infection.

Take drug the last thing at night after emptying bladder to ensure adequate concentration of drug during overnight period since low rates of urine flow and infrequent bladder emptying predispose to multiplication of bacteria.

Pyelonephritis

Pyelonephritis is an infection of the renal pelvis, tubules and interstitial tissue of one or both kidneys with variable manifestations. (Pyelonephritis may be acute or chronic.)

Causes

1　Secondary to ureterovesical reflux (incompetence of ureterovesical valve which allows urine to regurgitate into ureters, usually at time of micturition).

2　Urinary obstruction.

3　Enteric bacteria.

4 Blood-borne infection.
5 Renal disease.
6 Trauma.
7 Pregnancy.
8 Metabolic disorders.

Altered Physiology

Swelling of renal parenchyma → patchy distribution of acute infectious processes throughout kidney → swelling and scarring → kidney atrophy → renal failure.

Complications

1 Hypertension.
2 Chronic infection (usually silent).
3 Renal insufficiency and renal failure unilateral or bilateral.

Clinical Manifestation

1 Symptoms vary from none to severe.
2 The patient may be asymptomatic for many years although renal damage may be extensive.
3 Scarring of kidneys may follow each acute infection, causing the kidney to become atrophied.

Acute Pyelonephritis (an active infection)	*Chronic Pyelonephritis* (results from scarring effects of previous bacterial infection; it is a silent disease until it produces renal insufficiency)
1 Frequency, dysuria, burning on urination.	1 Fatigue, malaise.
2 Chills and fever with aching and malaise.	2 Headache, anorexia.
3 Dull aching in back or pain over costovertebral angle.	3 Polyuria, excessive thirst.
4 Pyuria and bacteriuria and casts in the urine sediment.	4 Weight loss.
	5 Proteinuria; symptoms of chronic renal insufficiency.

Objectives of Treatment and Nursing Management

To Determine if Obstruction is Present and to Locate it Precisely

1 Carry out intravenous urogram and other diagnostic tests—relief of obstructions is essential to save kidney from rapid destruction.

To Find and Treat Conditions Known to Cause Urinary Tract Infection

To Obtain Permanent Eradication of Bacteria from Urinary Tract by Eliminating the Obstruction.

1 Obtain urine specimen for culture and sensitivity studies (under aseptic conditions) since choice of drug is based on sensitivity studies.
2 Give organism-specific antibiotic therapy. Antibacterial agent is maintained in urine for a long enough period to prevent reseeding of residual foci of infection.
  a. Acute pyelonephritis usually caused by *E. coli*, which is sensitive to many antibiotic drugs.
  b. The patient should improve in 24–48 hours.
3 Obtain urine for repeated cultures to determine patient's response to treatment and to search for secondary organisms.

If Patient has Chronic or Recurring Infections

Objectives

To prevent progressive parenchymal damage.
To preserve renal function.
To locate and relieve the obstruction causing the infections.

1 Employ continuous treatment with urine-sterilizing agents after initial antibiotic treatment has been employed.
2 Advise patient to keep up this regimen for months to years until (i) there is no evidence of inflammation, (ii) causative factors have been treated or controlled and (iii) there is evidence of stability of renal function.
3 Emphasize to patient that serial urine cultures and evaluation studies must be done for an indefinite period of time.
4 Encourage patient to have blood counts and serum creatinine determinations if he is on long-term therapy.

Health Teaching

See p. 274

Tuberculosis of the Kidney

Tuberculosis of the kidney (and urinary tract) is caused by the organism *Mycobacterium tuberculosis* and is usually disseminated from the lungs via the bloodstream to one or both of the kidneys and to other organs of the genitourinary tract.

Clinical Manifestations

1 Haematuria (microscopic or gross).
2 Bladder irritation—burning on urination, frequency, nocturia.
3 Manifestations from infection of prostate and epididymis.

Diagnosis

1 Urine culture for tubercle bacilli (smears of urinary sediment also stained for acid-fast bacilli).
2 Excretory urogram—to reveal renal and ureteral lesions.
3 Cystoscopic examination—to determine extent of bladder involvement, for biopsy purposes and for ureteral catherization of each kidney to determine if one or both kidneys are affected.

4   Acid urine with persistent symptoms of cystitis and pyuria may yield a negative 'routine' culture; it may take special culture media and up to 6 weeks to grow acid-fast bacillus.

Nursing Alert: A search for tuberculosis elsewhere in the body must be conducted when tuberculosis of the kidney or urinary tract is found.
Be alert for patient who has had previous contact with tuberculosis.

Treatment

Objective

To eradicate the offending organism.

1   Multiple drug regime appears to delay the emergence of resistant organisms.
2   One of these combinations is usually given:
   a. Cycloserine, sodium aminosalicylic acid (PAS), isoniazid (INH).
   b. Cycloserine, ethambutol, isoniazid.
   c. Rifampicin, ethambutol, isoniazid.
3   The multiple drug combinations are given for 12–18 months.
4   All medications may be given together in a single daily dose; certain patients may have to divide cycloserine.
5   General health of patient should be promoted since renal tuberculosis is a manifestation of a systemic disease.
   a. Adequate rest.
   b. Nutritious diet.
   c. Avoidance of excessive exertion.
6   Surgical intervention may be necessary to prevent obstructive problems and to remove severely infected organ. However, emphasis is on medical treatment.

Discharge Planning and Health Teaching

Instruct the patient as follows:

1   Follow-up examinations are necessary for a prolonged period—to detect reactivation of disease.
2   Have periodic urine examination and cultures.
3   Report for cystoscopic examination as directed—to detect urethral stricture formation which is a complication of genitourinary tuberculosis.
4   Undergo excretory urograms as indicated.
5   For other aspects of health teaching, see p. 274.

ACUTE GLOMERULONEPHRITIS

Acute glomerulonephritis is an inflammatory disease involving the renal glomeruli of both kidneys. It is thought to involve an antigen–antibody reaction which produces damage to the glomerular capillaries.

Aetiology

1   Antecedent infection of pharynx and tonsils due to beta-haemolytic streptococci—certain strains are nephritogenic (capable of initiating nephritis).

2   May follow pneumococcal or staphylococcal infection.
3   Pyoderma (impetigo) is a common antecedent in children under 6.

Altered Physiology

Inflammation and swelling of glomeruli → narrowing of glomerular tufts → obstruction of blood flow through capillaries → interference with glomerular filtration → atrophy and disappearance of nephrons → renal failure.

Clinical Manifestations

1   The disease may be so mild that it is discovered accidentally through a routine urinalysis.
2   History of preceding pharyngitis or tonsillitis with fever (7–20 days previously).
3   Scant smoky or bloody urine.
4   Facial oedema and oedema of extremities.
5   Fatigue and anorexia.
6   Mild hypertension.
7   Tenderness at costovertebral angle.
8   Anaemia—from nitrogen retention in blood.

Diagnosis

1   Urinalysis—haematuria (microscopic or gross), proteinuria (2+ to 4+), red cell casts, white cells, renal epithelial cells and various casts in the sediment.
2   Blood—elevated blood urea nitrogen and serum creatinine, low total serum protein level, Antistreptolysin O (ASO) and CRP (C-reactive protein) titre rises during course of disease.
3   Needle biopsy—reveals obstruction of glomerular capillaries from proliferation of endothelial cells.

Clinical Course

1   Diuresis usually starts 1–2 weeks after onset of symptoms.
   a. Renal clearances and blood urea concentration return to normal.
   b. Oedema decreases and hypertension lessens.
   c. Microscopic proteinuria or haematuria may persist many months.
2   Recovery is usual in children and young adults; in older person the disease may progress to chronic glomerulonephritis.

Objectives of Treatment and Nursing Management

To Protect the Poorly Functioning Kidneys

1   Encourage bed rest during the acute phase. (Rest also facilitates diuresis.)
   a. Keep patient at rest until urine clears and blood pressure is normal.
   b. Restrict normal activities until proteinuria and haematuria clear since increasing activity may increase urinary abnormalities.
   c. Allow patient to resume activity on a gradual basis.
2   Restrict dietary protein moderately if there is oliguria.
   a. Give carbohydrates liberally to provide energy and reduce catabolism of protein.

b. Restrict protein more drastically if acute renal failure develops (see p. 246).
c. Restrict sodium intake in presence of oedema or signs of congestive heart failure.
3 Measure and record intake and output.
4 Give fluids according to patient's urinary output and daily body weight.

To Recognize and Treat Complications Promptly

1 Explain to patient that he must have follow-up evaluations of blood pressure and urinary protein to determine if there is exacerbation of disease activity.
2 Recognize and treat intercurrent infections promptly.
  Long-term penicillin therapy may be required to prevent recurrent streptococcal infections.
3 Watch for symptoms of renal failure—oliguria, acidosis, etc. (see p. 246).
4 Observe patient for:
  a. Hypertensive encephalopathy.
  b. Cardiac failure and pulmonary oedema.
5 Dialysis may be considered if uraemia and fluid retention cannot be controlled.

Discharge Planning and Health Teaching

Instruct the patient as follows:

1 Avoid exertion until abnormalities in blood and urine have subsided.
2 Treat any infection promptly.
3 Dizziness and flushing are not infrequent during convalescence.

NEPHROTIC SYNDROME

Nephrotic syndrome is a clinical disorder characterized by (i) marked proteinuria, (ii) hypoalbuminaemia, (iii) oedema and (iv) hypercholesterolaemia.

Aetiology

Seen in any condition that seriously damages the glomerular capillary membrane.

1 Chronic glomerulonephritis.
2 Diabetes mellitus (intercapillary glomerulosclerosis).
3 Amyloidosis of kidney.
4 Systemic lupus erythematosus.
5 Toxins.
6 Renal vein thrombosis.
7 Primary lipoid nephrosis in children.
8 Possible early symptom of malignant disease.

Clinical Manifestations

1 Insidious onset of oedema; easily pitting oedema.
2 Proteinuria (4–5 g daily).
3 Extensive depletion of body proteins (hypoalbuminaemia) from extensive urinary protein losses.
4 Hypercholesterolaemia (high blood cholesterol level).

Diagnosis

1 Needle biopsy of kidney—for histological examination of renal tissue to confirm diagnosis.
2 Serum electrolyte evaluations (protein, albumin, etc.).
3 Triglyceride profile—to evaluate degree of hyperlipaemia.
4 Urinary tests—for microscopic haematuria, granular and epithelial cell casts.
5 Renal function tests.

Treatment and Nursing Management

Objective

To preserve renal function.

1 Keep on bed rest for a few days—to mobilize oedema.
2 Utilize dietary treatment—to replace protein losses.
   a. Low sodium diet—to control severe oedema.
   b. High protein diet—to replenish wasted tissues and restore body proteins.
   c. High calorie diet (25–50 cal/kg body weight/day).
3 Give diuretics—if renal insufficiency is not severe.
4 Give adrenocorticosteroids (prednisone)—to reduce oedema and proteinuria.
5 Immunosuppressive agents may be effective when nephrosis is associated with autoimmune disease.
6 Protect patient from infection—causes exacerbation of symptoms.
7 See p. 277 for nursing the patient with acute glomerulonephritis, and p. 249 for care of patient with chronic renal failure.

HYDRONEPHROSIS

Hydronephrosis is distension of the pelvis and calyces of one or both kidneys with resulting thinning of renal parenchyma due to obstruction of urinary flow. (A partial block may occur at any level in the urinary tract.)

Causes

1 Congenital causes—stenosis of ureteropelvic junction, urethral valves.
2 Progressive changes in bladder, ureters and kidneys from obstruction anywhere in urinary tract.
   a. Obstruction from enlarged prostate.
   b. Obstructing calculus.
   c. Malignant lesion (cancer of prostate, bladder or cervix).
   d. Obstruction of ureter—from calculus, stricture, etc.
3 Neurogenic causes.
4 Vesicoureteral reflux.

Altered Physiology

Interference with passage of urine from kidney → chronic infection → increasing pressure → distension of renal pelvis and calyces → atrophy of renal parenchyma (as one kidney undergoes gradual destruction, the contralateral kidney gradually enlarges (compensatory hypertrophy)).

Clinical Manifestations

1 Often asymptomatic and insidious onset.
2 Aching in flank and back (present with acute obstruction).
3 Bladder irritability—fever and dysuria if infection is present.
4 Gastrointestinal disturbances.
5 Chills, fever, tenderness, pyuria—from infection.
6 Haematuria—hydronephrotic kidney may bleed from congestion.
7 Uraemia—if condition is bilateral and advanced.
8 Failure to thrive—in children.

Diagnosis

Complete urographic survey:

1 Excretory urography—gives information regarding cause, duration and reversibility of hydronephrosis.
2 Total creatinine clearance.
3 Isotope renography.
4 Renal scan.
5 Retrograde pyelography (done occasionally).

Treatment and Nursing Management

Objectives

To achieve complete relief of urinary stasis.
To treat the patient's infection.
To restore and conserve renal function.

1 Relieve obstruction, etc.
   Urine may have to be diverted by nephrostomy or other types of diversion.
   Place ureteral catheter to decompress kidney—if patient is having severe flank pain.
   See p. 270 for care of patient having a nephrostomy.
2 Eradicate infection since residual urine in calyces produces infection and pyelonephritis.
3 Prepare for surgical intervention to correct obstruction.
   a. Nephrectomy—if one kidney is severely damaged.
   b. Operations to improve drainage of kidney, such as pyeloplasty—plastic operation to remove and correct results of obstruction at ureteropelvic junction.
   c. See p. 267 for care of patient having renal surgery.

NEPHROPTOSIS

Nephroptosis refers to the downward displacement or falling of the kidney.

Causes

1 Congenital defects.

2   Loss of fatty support of the kidney, often after dieting.
3   Traumatic dislocation.

Clinical Manifestations

1   Pain; dull, dragging pain in lumbar area; however, nephroptosis is a rare cause of backache.
   a. May be acute or chronic.
   b. Severe pain as a result of kinking of ureter or torsion of renal pedicle.
2   Fatigue.
3   Gastrointestinal disturbances.
4   Hypertension.
5   Urinary tract infection.

Diagnosis

1   History and physical examination.
2   Retrograde pyelography—to determine degree of renal mobility and rotation and presence of distortions of ureters and pelvis.
3   Supine and upright intravenous urogram or ^{131}I renogram.

Treatment and Nursing Management

1   Exercises to improve posture and strengthen abdominal muscles.
2   Use of a supporting kidney belt or pantigirdle (helpful to some, of questionable value to others).
   a. Adjust belt with patient lying down with hips elevated.
   b. Tighten belt from below and then upwards.
3   Rest in bed with foot of bed elevated during painful episodes.
4   Surgical intervention: nephropexy—surgical elevation and fixation of a ptosed (fallen) kidney.
5   See p. 267 for nursing management of patient following renal surgery.

UROLITHIASIS

Urolithiasis refers to the presence of stones in the urinary system.

Factors Favouring Stone Formation

1   Obstruction and urinary stasis facilitating precipitation of salts from the urine.
2   Infection—particularly of urea-splitting organisms (*Proteus vulgaris*).
3   Dehydration and urine concentration—encourages precipitation of solids.
4   Immobilization—produces slowing of renal drainage and altered calcium metabolism.
5   Hypercalcaemia (abnormally high concentration of blood calcium compounds) and hypercalciuria (abnormally large amounts of calcium in urine).
   a. Hyperparathyroidism.

    b. Excessive intake of vitamin D.

    c. Excessive intake of milk and alkali.

    d. Myeloproliferative disease (unusual proliferation of blood cells derived from bone marrow—leukaemia, polycythaemia vera).

6 Excessive excretion of uric acid.

7 Vitamin deficiency (especially vitamin A).

8 Foreign bodies in urinary tract.

9 Small bowel disease or surgical rearrangement.

10 Heredity plays a part in calcium oxalate stones (most common type).

11 Idiopathic—no cause can be found.

Clinical Features

1 The problem occurs predominantly in the third to fifth decade, affecting men more than women.

2 The majority of stones contain calcium or magnesium in combination with phosphorus or oxalate.

3 Infection and obstruction may cause destruction of renal tissue; large stones may cause serious kidney damage from ischaemia and necrosis.

4 Most renal stones migrate downwards (causing severe, colicky pain) and are discovered in the lower ureter.

5 People who have had two stones tend to have more stones.

Clinical Manifestations

Dependent on presence of obstruction, infection, oedema.

1 Pain.

    a. Discomfort anywhere along course of ureter with sudden sharp pain radiating down ureter.

    b. Renal colic—severe pain caused by obstruction or passage of stone in the renal pelvis or ureter.

    c. Pain may be referred to testicle in male and radiate to vulva in female.

2 Gastrointestinal symptoms.

    a. Due to renal–intestinal reflexes and anatomic relation of kidneys to stomach, pancreas, colon, etc.

    b. Include nausea, vomiting, diarrhoea, abdominal discomfort.

3 Haematuria (microscopic or gross).

4 Symptoms of urinary tract infection—chills, fever, dysuria.

Diagnosis

1 X-rays of entire urinary tract—the majority of stones are radiopaque.

2 Cystoscopy may be required to allow relief of pain by bypassing stone with a catheter or withdrawing the stone by stone manipulation.

3 Serum protein concentration; blood urea; serum concentrations of calcium, phosphorus, chloride; carbon dioxide combining power; alkaline phosphatase; uric acid.

4 Urinalysis for:

    a. Red cells.

b. Gram stain of sediment—for evidence of infection and to determine predominant crystals.

c. Urine culture—to identify bacteria and to provide spectrum of sensitivity to antibiotic agents.

d. Urinary pH—to determine acidity or alkalinity.

5 Urinary excretory studies for calcium, phosphorus, uric acid, cystine and oxalate.

Treatment and Nursing Management

Objectives

To eradicate the stone.
To determine the stone type.
To prevent nephron destruction.

1 Encourage patient to maintain a high round-the-clock fluid intake (at least 3000 ml/daily) to reduce concentration of urinary crystalloids and to ensure a high urinary output (2000 ml/day output).

2 Strain all urine to obtain the crystals or calculus for x-ray diffraction or crystallographic analysis—to establish the type of stone formation. (Knowledge of the composition of the stone is helpful in planning effective treatment.)

3 Give specific treatment as ordered (magnesium oxide, phosphates, d-penicillamine, allopurinol, orthophosphate salts, thiazide diuretics)—the drug given depends on the stone type.

4 Maintain proper urine reaction (pH); give appropriate drugs to acidify or alkalinize urine (depending on stone type).

    a. Phosphate, oxalate and carbonate stones form in alkaline urine.

    (1) Drugs used to acidify urine include ammonium chloride and hexamine mandelate (Mandelamine).

    b. Uric acid, urate and cystine stones form in acid urine.

    (1) Drugs used for alkalinizing the urine include potassium acetate or citrate, sodium bicarbonate.

5 Employ principles of diet therapy if stone composition is known—to control urine pH, supply proper vitamins and eliminate stone-forming substances (see Table 5.1).

6 Treat infection (if present) with appropriate drugs—infection may accelerate stone growth and be difficult to eradicate.

7 Correct obstructive process to prevent impairment of tubular function, atrophy of nephrons, reduced renal blood flow and increased susceptibility to infection.

8 Treat and correct metabolic problems (hyperparathyroidism, renal tubular acidosis).

9 Prepare for surgical intervention if patient's condition indicates that:

    a. Stone is too large to pass, or is

    b. Producing enough obstruction to cause renal atrophy and/or uraemia, or that

    c. Patient is having repeated episodes of pain.

Surgical Procedures

Objective

To remove stone with a minimum of trauma to the kidney.

Table 5.1. Moderately Reduced Calcium and Phosphorus Diet
(This diet will contain from 500–700 mg of calcium and from 1000–1200 mg of phosphorus*)

Foods Allowed	Foods to be Avoided
Beverages	
Coffee, Postum, tea, ginger ale	Carbonated 'soft' drinks; cocoa
Milk	
Limited to 1 cup (½ pint) a day. Cream may be substituted for part of the milk	
Cheese	
Cottage cheese only. Limited to 2 oz	All except cottage cheese
Fats	
As desired	
Eggs	
Limited to one a day; egg whites as desired	
Meat, fish, fowl	
Limited to 4 oz daily of beef, lamb, pork, veal, chicken, turkey, fish. See those to be avoided	Brains, heart, liver, kidney, sweetbreads. Game (pheasant, rabbit, deer, grouse). Sardines, fish roe
Soups and broths	
All. Cream soups made with milk allowance only	
Vegetables	
At least three servings besides potato. One or two servings of deep green or deep yellow vegetables to be included daily	Beet greens, spinach, turnip greens. Dried beans, peas, lentils, soyabeans
Fruits	
All except rhubarb. Include citrus fruit daily	Rhubarb
Breads, cereals, macaroni products	
White, enriched bread, rolls and crackers except those made from self-raising white flour. Cornflakes, corn meal, rice, Rice Krispies, Puffed Rice. Macaroni, spaghetti, noodles	Whole-grain breads, cereals and crackers. Rye bread. All breads made with self-raising flour. Oatmeal, brown and wild rice. Bran, Bran Flakes, wheat germ. All dry cereals except those allowed
Desserts	
Fruit pies, fruit cobblers, fruit ices, gelatin. Puddings made with allowed milk and egg. Angel food cake. (Do not use packaged mixes)	All except those allowed
Condiments	*Miscellaneous*
Sugar, jellies, honey, salt, pepper, spices	Nuts, peanut butter, chocolate, cocoa. Condiments having calcium of a phosphate base. (Read labels)

* Adapted from Mitchell, H S et al (1976) Nutrition in Health and Disease, 16th edition, Philadelphia, J B Lippincott.

1 Cystoscopic—for stone extraction from distal ureter or to bypass obstruction with a catheter.
2 Ureterolithotomy—removal of a stone lodged in the ureter.
3 Pyelolithotomy—removal of a stone from kidney pelvis.
4 Nephrolithotomy—incision into kidney for removal of stone.
5 Nephrectomy—removal of kidney, indicated when kidney is extensively and irreparably damaged and is no longer a functioning organ.
6 Cystolithotomy—removal of stone from bladder.
7 See pp. 267–271 for nursing management of patient undergoing renal surgery.

Discharge Planning and Health Teaching

Instruct the patient as follows:

1 Maintain a high fluid intake over a 24-hour period since stones form more readily in concentrated urine.
   a. Drink at least 3000 ml daily if you are a stone former.
   b. Drink larger amounts if you perspire freely.
2 Avoid prolonged periods of recumbency.
3 Avoid excessive ingestion of vitamins and minerals, especially vitamin D.
4 Test urine pH with a pH indicator if urine reaction is a factor in causing your type of stones.
5 Stay on prescribed diet; take vitamin A if prescribed (see Table 5.1).

Diet Therapy for Kidney Stones

Since over 90% of kidney stones contain calcium combined with phosphate or other substance, the diet selected for these patients is a moderately reduced calcium and phosphorus diet.

TUMOURS OF THE KIDNEY

Types of Kidney Tumours

1 Tumours of the renal parenchyma.
2 Tumours of the renal pelvis.
3 Tumours of the renal parenchyma of children; usually embryonic in origin (Wilms' tumour).

General Considerations

1 All renal tumours should be considered malignant until proven otherwise.
2 Renal cell carcinoma is the most common malignant renal tumour and occurs more frequently in males; more than one-third present as metastatic disease.
3 Many renal tumours produce no symptoms and are discovered on routine physical examination as an abdominal mass.

Clinical Manifestations

1 Classic triad (late symptoms).

a. Flank pain.
b. Palpable mass in flank.
c. Haematuria (intermittent, microscopic or gross)—may be initial, terminal or total depending on location of tumour.
2 Low-grade fever, anaemia, weight loss—systemic effects common to most tumours.
3 Gastrointestinal symptoms—due to reflex action or encroachment on intraperitoneal organs.
4 Metastatic manifestations may be first indication—metastasis most frequently involves the liver, lungs, long bones and regional lymph nodes.

Diagnosis

1 Plain film of abdomen—often shows kidney enlargement.
2 Intravenous urography and intravenous drip nephrotomogram.
3 Cystoscopic examination—for visualization of tumour by retrograde pyelography—possible location of site of bleeding.
4 Exfoliative cytology of urinary sediment for exfoliated cells (tumours of renal pelvis).
5 Assessment of urinary lactic dehydrogenase activity; this enzyme may be elevated in carcinoma of the kidney, bladder, prostate, in infection, etc.
6 Ultrasonography—helpful in differentiating renal cyst from renal tumour.
7 Renal angiogram—definitive study.

Treatment

Objective

To eradicate the tumour and prevent metastasis.

1 Radical nephrectomy (removal of kidney), perirenal tissue, lymph nodes and adjacent organs if involved (spleen, bowel, tail of pancreas) and if tumour is operable. (See p. 269 for nursing management following renal surgery.)
2 Radiation therapy if tumour is radiosensitive, or as palliative measure for patients with inoperable tumour. (See Nursing Management of Patient with Cancer.)
3 Chemotherapy or regional chemotherapy—chemotherapeutic agent injected in patients with tumours of solitary kidney or inoperable neoplasms; wide variety of chemotherapeutic agents in use.
4 Hormone therapy.

INJURIES TO THE KIDNEY

Blunt trauma to abdomen and lower chest may produce renal injury. Suspicion of renal injury is high in a patient with multiple injuries.

Types of Injuries

1 Simple bruising and ecchymosis (contusion).
2 Lacerations of kidney.
3 Rupture or renal vascular pedicle injury—produces massive bleeding.

Major Problems Following Kidney Trauma

1 Control of haemorrhage—may be persistent or recurring.
2 Injuries to other organs.
3 Injuries vary from contusion to complete avulsion (tearing away).

Clinical Manifestations

1 Pain—costovertebral, flank, upper abdomen.
2 Haematuria—may be gross.
3 Nausea, vomiting, abdominal rigidity—from ileus (seen when there is retroperitoneal bleeding).
4 Shock, if injury is severe.

Diagnosis

1 History of injury—determine if injury caused by blunt trauma/stab/gunshot wounds.
2 Serial urine studies for haematuria using unspun urine examined under low power objective.
3 Plain film of abdomen—to determine presence of other fractures (pelvis, ribs, transverse processes of lumbar vertebrae).
4 Excretory urograms—to define extent of injury of involved kidney and establish location and condition of contralateral kidney.
5 Renal scanning—to evaluate renal blood flow and tubular function.
6 Renal angiography—to assess vascular integrity, outline renal parenchyma.

Complications

1 Haemorrhage.
2 Perirenal infection.
3 Hypertension.
4 Stone formation.
5 Loss of renal function.

Nursing Alert: Excessive bleeding may occur several days after renal injury. Perirenal abscess or infection may occur 2–4 weeks following injury.

Treatment and Nursing Management

Objectives

To control haemorrhage, pain and infection.
To preserve and restore renal function.
To maintain urinary drainage.

1 Place patient on bed rest.
2 Monitor blood pressure and pulse—to assess for bleeding and impending shock.
3 Save, inspect and compare each urine specimen—to follow the course and degree of haematuria.
4 Serial haematocrit and haemoglobin determinations will be carried out to assess degree of anaemia since progressive anaemia indicates haemorrhage.

5 Assess the patient frequently during the first few days following injury.
   a. Assess for flank and abdominal pain, muscle spasm and swelling over flank.
   b. Examine renal area for development of bruising and/or swelling.
   c. Watch for any *sudden* change in patient's condition. This may indicate haemorrhage and require surgical intervention.
6 Avoid narcotic analgesia—may mask accompanying abdominal symptoms.
7 Prepare for surgical exploration if patient has increasing pulse rate, hypotension or shock (drainage of kidney region, repair of kidney, nephrectomy).
8 Give antibiotics as directed to discourage infection—from perirenal haematoma and/or urinoma (cyst containing urine).

Discharge Planning and Health Teaching

Encourage patient to have follow-up examinations after discharge—to detect late-developing complications (post-traumatic hypertension, decreasing renal function).

NEUROGENIC BLADDER

Neurogenic bladder is any bladder disturbance due to a lesion of the nervous system.

Normal Physiology

1 Normal bladder action depends on intact sensory and motor nerve supply.
2 The bladder fills to approximately 300–500 ml—triggers an emptying reflex.
3 This reflex initiates a contraction of the musculature inside the bladder wall which forces urine out through the urethra until the bladder is empty.

Causes

1 Spinal cord injury.
2 Disease—multiple sclerosis, tabes dorsalis, diabetes mellitus, syphilis.
3 Spinal cord tumour or herniated intervertebral disc.
4 Certain congenital anomalies (spina bifida, myelomeningocele).
5 Infection.

Types of Neurogenic Bladder

Spastic (Reflex or Automatic)

1 A bladder disorder caused by any lesion of the cord above the micturition reflex arc (upper motor neuron lesion).
2 Most common type.
3 There is loss of conscious sensations and cerebral motor control.
4 Patient has reduced bladder capacity and marked hypertrophy of bladder wall.
5 Bladder behaves in reflex fashion with minimal or no controlling influence to regulate its activity (spontaneous uncontrolled micturitions).

Flaccid (Atonic, Nonreflex or Areflexic or Autonomous)

1 A bladder disease caused by lower motor neuron lesion.
2 Bladder continues to fill until it becomes greatly distended—bladder musculature does not contract forcefully at any time.

3   When pressure reaches a breakthrough point, small amounts of urine dribble from urethra as bladder continues to fill (overflow incontinence).
4   Sensory loss may accompany flaccid bladder; patient is not aware of discomfort.
5   Extensive distension causes damage to bladder musculature, infection of stagnant urine and infection of kidneys by back pressure of urine.

Mixed

Complications

1   *Infection*—bladder cannot empty itself; catheterization produces infection.
2   *Hydronephrosis*—hypertrophy of bladder wall leads ultimately to vesicoureteral reflux.
3   *Calculus*—from demineralization of bone from bed rest; urinary stasis and infection.
4   *Renal failure*—major cause of death of patients with neurological impairment of the bladder.

Treatment

Objectives

To prevent overdistension of the bladder.
To empty bladder regularly and completely.
To maintain urine sterility with no stone formation.
To maintain adequate bladder capacity without ureterovesical reflux.

Initial Treatment

Following spinal cord injury, the syndrome of spinal shock is reflected in the bladder; it usually cannot contract and empty itself, and its outlet is obstructed. The bladder must be decompressed either by intermittent or continuous catheterization.

1   Intermittent catheterization.
    Bladder catheterized at designated intervals (4, 6 or 8 hours) with a small calibre catheter; this intermittent emptying approximates physiological bladder function; circumvents complications usually seen with indwelling catheter.
    (1) Hourly fluid intake and output record is kept to help assess individual output patterns.
    (2) Catheterization technique requires strict asepsis and skilled personnel.
    (3) Patients with upper extremity function may be taught to catheterize themselves.
2   Continuous catheterization.
    Bladder is catheterized using continuous drainage and irrigation system (p. 237) to avoid overdistension and risk of contracture from being constantly empty.
    (1) Tape catheter to abdomen (male) to remove sharp angulation and pressure at penoscrotal angle (Fig. 5.6).
    (2) Maintain a high fluid intake.

3 Encourage liberal fluid intake—there is reduction in urinary bacterial count with increase in urine flow; hydration reduces statis and decreases concentration of calcium in urine, minimizing precipitation of urinary crystals and stone formation.

4 Keep patient as mobile as possible—to reduce incidence of calculosis (presence of calculi).
   a. Turn, move and exercise patient.
   b. Get patient up on tilt-table or in wheelchair as soon as possible.
   c. Give low calcium diet—to prevent calculosis.
   Avoid dairy products.

5 Evaluation studies (as soon as patient's condition permits)—to assess for bladder and bladder neck problems. Do initial studies early to provide a baseline against which later changes can be measured.
   a. Serial studies of blood urea, serum creatinine, creatinine clearance are carried out to determine status of renal function.
   b. Cystogram—to determine presence of vesicoureteral reflux.
   c. Urethrogram—for presence of urethral complications.
   d. Intravenous urogram—to outline upper urinary tract.
   e. Pressure and flow studies.
   f. Cystoscopy—to assess for loss of muscle fibres and elastic tissues; gives opportunity for biopsy.

Treatment for Chronic Phase

Each person with neurogenic bladder disease has a particular type of problem(s); it is difficult to assess what the rehabilitation potential and eventual urological disability may be.

Objective

To develop effective spontaneous reflex micturition.

1 Have patient drink a measured amount of fluid from 8 a.m.–10 p.m.; no fluids (except sips) taken after 10 p.m. to avoid bladder overdistension.

2 At specified time, patient attempts to micturate using pressure over bladder, abdominal tapping or digital stretch of anal sphincter to trigger the bladder.

3 Palpate the bladder at repeated intervals to determine if bladder is being emptied (Fig. 5.9).

4 Immediately following micturition attempt, catheterize the patient to determine urine residual.
   a. Measure all urine, micturated and catheterized.
   b. Avoid *overdistension* of bladder.
   c. Caution patient to be alert for any sign that his bladder is full—perspiration, coldness of hands or feet, feelings of anxiety, etc.

5 *Intervals between catheterizations.*
   Catheterization intervals are increased and programme is moved forward as urine residuals become less and less; catheterization checks usually are discontinued when the patient's residual urine is at an acceptable level, compatible with urine sterility and the upper urinary tract appears normal on radiological examination.

Treatment for Flaccid Bladder

1   Patient may be placed on bladder routine (outlined above); the fluid intake and output are adjusted to prevent bladder overdistension.
    Patient may be given orally-administered doses of parasympathomimetic drugs (bethanechol chloride). This is sometimes very effective, especially for a condition of hypotonic bladder without significant bladder outlet obstruction.
2   *Or* if no reflex or only a partial reflex can be induced, the patient is maintained on intermittent catheterization until he develops spontaneous reflex micturition; or surgical intervention may be required.
3   Male patient—may use condom collecting device if bladder empties well and no residual remains.
4   Female patient—may use pads, waterproof pants; or urinary diversion procedure may be required.
5   Surgical intervention may be carried out to correct bladder neck contractures, correct vesicoureteral reflux or perform urinary diversion procedures (p. 297).

Health Teaching

Instruct the patient to do vaginal and rectal contractions to strengthen periurethral tissue.

1   Tighten the rectum or vaginal vault.
2   Hold the contraction while counting slowly to 6; relax.
3   Continue relaxing and tightening for a 5-min period.
4   Perform these exercises twice daily for 5 min over a 6- to 8-week period—success or failure of exercise programme is then evaluated.

GUIDELINES: Intermittent Self-Catheterization; Clean (Nonsterile) Technique

Intermittent self-catheterization is the periodic drainage of urine from the bladder by the patient via catheterization; it is necessitated by temporary or permanent inability to empty the bladder (vesical dysfunction, neurogenic disease, obstructive uropathy, decompensated bladder).

Underlying Considerations

1   Intermittent catheterization is the treatment of choice following spinal cord injury. It is done under aseptic conditions by qualified health professionals until the patient is able to catheterize himself. After discharge from the hospital the patient may be able to use a 'clean' (nonsterile) technique.
2   The patient should be medically followed at regular intervals to prevent complications—reflux, hydronephrosis, external sphincter spasm.
3   Advantages of self-catheterization: Better patient acceptance; promotes independence; fewer complications; permits more normal sexual relations.
4   *Objective*: to decrease morbidity associated with long-term use of indwelling catheter and to achieve a catheter-free status, if possible.

Equipment

14 Fr. catheter (several to be kept in reserve); lubricant

Mirror (female patient)
Shallow pan
Clear plastic bag or case—for carrying catheter

Procedure

Action (by patient)	Reason
1 The patient must understand the importance of frequent catheterization and emptying of bladder at prescribed time regardless of circumstances.	1 An overdistended bladder slows the circulation of blood through the bladder walls and weakens its resistance to infection.
2 Wash hands with soap and water.	2 Do not forgo catheterization if soap and water are not available.
3 Try to micturate before catheterizing self using reflex triggering mechanisms—pressure on abdomen, thigh stroking, etc.	3 This may help to develop voluntary micturition without catheterization.

Female

1 Position mirror in line of vision with urinary meatus. Assume modified dorsal recumbent position with feet on bed, legs flexed and knees apart; later, patient may sit on toilet seat if physical conditions permits.	1 This position helps to expose the urethral meatus.
The nurse points out the location of the clitoris, urethral meatus and vaginal outlet (in the mirror).	The patient is taught to confirm the position of the clitoris, urethral meatus and vaginal outlet by palpation so that eventually mirror will not be necessary.
2 Lubricate the catheter with water or water-soluble jelly. Hold the catheter 7.5 cm (3 in) from its tip and insert it 5–7.5 cm (2–3 in) in a downwards and backwards direction into the urethra. Allow urine to flow into a shallow pan/toilet.	
3 Remove catheter when urine stops flowing.	3 Measure or estimate volume of residual urine.

Male Patient

1 Assume sitting position until technique is learned.	
2 Lubricate the catheter.	2 A well-lubricated catheter is particularly necessary in the male to avoid traumatic urethritis.

Action (by patient)	Reason
3 Retract foreskin of penis with left hand; then grasp penis and hold it at right angle to body.	3 This manoeuvre straightens the urethra and facilitates ease of catheter insertion.
4 Grasp the catheter and insert it 15–25 cm (6–10 in) until urine begins to flow.	
5 Then advance catheter about 2.5 cm (1 in more) and allow urine to flow into shallow pan/toilet. When urine stops flowing, remove catheter.	5 Measure or estimate volume of residual urine.

Follow-up Phase

1 Wash catheter in warm, soapy water.
2 Rinse. Rinse inside of catheter using syringe.
3 Wrap catheter in clean towel/paper towel.

3 The catheter may be carried in a clean plastic bag or case. The emphasis should be on availability and cleanliness.

INJURIES TO THE BLADDER (AND URETHRA)

Types of Bladder Injuries

1 Contusion of bladder.
2 Intraperitoneal rupture } or combination of both.
3 Extraperitoneal rupture }
4 Injury to urethra.

Problems Associated with Bladder Injury

1 Injuries to the bladder and urethra are commonly associated with multiple trauma. Certain surgical procedures (hysterectomy, surgery of lower colon and rectum) also carry a risk to the bladder.
2 With injury there is rise in intravesical (within bladder) pressure which produces extravasation of urine into the peritoneal cavity or perivesical space.
3 Rupture of the bladder requires immediate treatment.
4 Pelvic bone fracture may be accompanied by injury to urethra.

Clinical Manifestations

1 Shock and haemorrhage—pallor, rapid and increasing pulse rate.
2 Suprapubic pain and soreness.
3 Rigid abdomen—indicates intraperitoneal rupture.
4 Gross haematuria.
5 Failure to micturate.

Diagnosis

1   Urethrogram—to detect any rupture of urethra. *Do first* (before catheterization).
2   Cystogram—to detect and localize perforation of urinary bladder.
3   Plain film of abdomen—may show associated pelvic fracture.
4   Excretory urogram—to survey the kidneys for injury.

Treatment

1   Catheterize patient only after urethrogram is done.
   a. Indwelling catheter serves as a means of continuous urinary drainage.
   b. Catheter also serves as a splint to urethra if urethra has been injured but it may complete a partial rupture if urethral injury is not recognized with a urethrogram.
2   Treat for shock and haemorrhage.
3   Prepare for surgical intervention if bladder rupture has occurred.
   a. Bladder tears will be sutured; urethral repairs may be postponed.
   b. Extravasated blood and urine will be drained and urine diverted with suprapubic cystostomy and indwelling catheter.
4   Observe drainage systems after surgery.
   a. Suprapubic cystostomy drainage—until healing of bladder is complete (p. 240).
   b. Indwelling urethral catheter drainage—to divert urine drainage and permit suprapubic incision to heal.
   c. Perivesical areas drained with Penrose drain (will be brought out through suprapubic incision).
5   Obtain urine specimens for bacteriological examination.

Nursing Management

See p. 267 for nursing management of patient with urological surgery.

CANCER OF THE BLADDER

Aetiology

It appears that multiple agents are responsible for the development of cancer of the bladder. The specific aetiology is unknown.

1   Cigarette smoking.
2   Prolonged exposure to aromatic amines or their metabolites—generally dyes manufactured by the chemical industry and used by other industries.
3   Causal relationship may exist between excessive coffee drinking and consumption of excessive amounts of analgesics and bladder cancer.
4   Bladder schistosomiasis (rare in UK).
5   Secondary metastasis from prostate, colon, rectum (males) and lower gynaecological tract (females).

Clinical Features

1   Bladder tumours comprise 2% of all malignancies and account for 3% of all cancer deaths.

2 They are seen three times more frequently in males (more men exposed to urinary carcinogens); occur after the fifth decade.
3 Large numbers of these tumours occur in the lateral and posterior bladder wall and near the trigone.
4 Metastases appear in vesical, hypogastric, common iliac and lumbar lymph nodes; in liver, lungs, vertebrae, pelvis.
5 Recurrences may occur years after last known tumour was treated; carcinogen's effect persists.
6 Small bladder tumours are seeded from tumours of renal pelvis.

Clinical Manifestations

1 Painless haematuria, either gross or microscopic—most characteristic sign.
2 Dysuria, frequency, urgency—symptoms of bladder irritation.
3 Flank pain, chills, fever—from progressive tumour growth, infiltration of bladder wall, obstruction to ureteral orifice and bladder infection.
4 Pelvic or back pain—from distant metastasis.

Diagnosis

1 Cystourethroscopy—for visualization and biopsy of lesion.
2 Bimanual examination of pelvis—to determine degree of mobility, fixation of tumour and degree of extravesical extension.
3 Intravenous urography—to rule out ureteral obstruction or presence of renal pelvic tumour.
4 Retrograde pyelography—to define presence/absence of upper urinary tract pathology.
5 Urinalysis (three-glass test)—for blood and bacteria.
6 Cytology study of fresh urinary sediment to assess for malignant transitional cells shed from tumour.
7 Enzyme studies—urinary lactic dehydrogenase and alkaline phosphatase which may or may not be elevated (a nonspecific test).
8 Chest x-ray and bone survey—to demonstrate distant metastases.
9 Bone scan.

Treatment

Underlying Rationale

1 There is no single effective method of treatment. The surgical procedure of choice depends on the characteristics of the tumour and whether or not bladder wall infiltration and local or distant metastasis has occurred. The patient's age and physical, mental and emotional status are considered.
2 The patient is usually considered incurable if gross extension of the tumour beyond the bladder wall has occurred; in such cases radiotherapy and chemotherapy may be somewhat palliative.

Modalities of Treatment

1 Transurethral and transvesical electroexcision—for simple papillomas.
2 Chemotherapy—may be effective as topical therapy for multiple very superficial bladder tumours.

3 Intravesical application of radium or implantation of radioactive materials into the tumour.
4 External radiation for undifferentiated types of tumours—may be used with operative treatment or for control of disease in nonsurgical candidates.
5 Segmental resection of bladder (partial resection)—used in highly selected patients.
6 Urinary diversion procedures to relieve frequency and reduce haemorrhage in patients with inoperable disease.
7 Cystectomy (removal of bladder) or radical cystectomy for invasive and poorly differentiated tumours; requires urinary diversion.
   a. Radical cystectomy in male—removal of bladder, pelvic peritoneum, prostate, seminal vesicles and urethra, with regional node dissection.
   b. Radical cystectomy in female—removal of bladder, pelvic peritoneum, urethra, uterus, broad ligaments, vagina, tubes and ovaries, and regional lymphadenectomy (iliac and pelvic nodes).
   c. Cystectomy requires diversion of the urinary stream (anastomosing the ureters in an isolated loop of ileum which is brought out through the abdominal wall as an ileostomy, or to similar segment of colon).
   d. Complications include wound infection (wound dehiscence or evisceration), peritonitis, pyelonephritis, adynamic ileus, atelectasis, disturbances of vascularization of ileal loop, urinary leakage, postoperative haemorrhage, intestinal obstruction.
   e. See below for nursing management of patient with a urinary diversion procedure.

URINARY DIVERSION

Urinary diversion refers to diverting the urinary stream from the bladder so that it exits via a new avenue.

Clinical Conditions Requiring Urinary Diversion

1 Malignancy of bladder or ureters; pelvic malignancy.
2 Birth defects.
3 Stricture and trauma to ureters and urethra.
4 Neurogenic bladder.
5 Severe ureteral and renal damage due to vesicoureteral reflux or chronic infection.
6 Injuries.

Methods of Urinary Diversion

1 *Cutaneous ureterostomy*—anastomosis of ureters to the skin, usually high on the abdominal wall, slightly medial to the spinous process of ilium.
2 *Ileal conduit (ureteroileostomy)*—implantation of ureters to a section of the terminal ileum, one end of which is brought to the abdominal wall as an ileostomy opening. The loop of ileum acts as a conduit (passageway) for urine.
3 *Ureterosigmoidostomy*—diversion of the ureter(s) into the sigmoid colon. This allows urine to flow through the colon and out of the rectum. The patient should have adequate control of the anal sphincter.

4   *Nephrostomy*—insertion of catheter into renal pelvis via incision in the flank (see p. 267).
5   *Cystostomy (vesicostomy)*—opening of bladder and drainage of catheter through an abdominal wound.

Preoperative Considerations for Patients Having Intestinal Urinary Diversion Procedures (Ileal Conduit and Ureterosigmoidostomy)

1   See p. 267 for patient undergoing renal surgery for general aspects of preoperative care.
2   Pay careful attention to cardiopulmonary status since cardiopulmonary complications account for more than one-third of postoperative morbidity and mortality. (Urinary diversion procedures may be of long duration.)
3   Prepare patient for sigmoidoscopy and barium enema if ureterosigmoidostomy is to be performed.
    a. Enemas are given (increasing in amount) to help develop sphincter control.
    b. Assess patient's ability to retain enema as a means of evaluating adequacy of rectal sphincter.
    c. Assist with renal function studies to determine kidney status and renal reserve.
4   The surgeon selects the prospective stoma site—where the patient can see it, away from bony prominences, scars and skin creases, and where it will not interfere with patient's dress.
    a. Apply several types of skin adhesives or cement to abdomen preoperatively to determine contact allergies and to facilitate management of ostomy appliance postoperatively.
    b. Have patient wear the intended appliance preoperatively.
5   Prepare the bowel for surgical intervention.
    a. Give low residue diet.
    b. Administer antibiotic agents (Neomycin, kanamycin) as directed for bowel disinfection to reduce pathogenic bacterial flora.
    c. Give enemas as directed for mechanical cleansing of lower bowel (usually kept to a minimum).
6   Assist patient undergoing nasogastric intubation on morning of surgery.
7   Employ adequate hydration procedures to ensure urine flow during surgery. Intravenous fluids may be prescribed.
8   Encourage patient to express his feelings about his situation.

Postoperative Nursing Emphasis

Objectives

To preserve and maintain renal function.
To assist patient to adapt to his altered body image and to enjoy a full and satisfying life.

General Considerations

1   See Volume 2 for nursing management of patient following intestinal surgery and p. 269 for nursing management of patient following urological surgery.

2   Watch for any abnormal signs and symptoms (wound infections, leaking at anastomosis site, peritonitis, paralytic ileus, intestinal obstruction, stenosis of stoma). These operations are extremely taxing, and patients have little or no reserve.

3   Assure adequate circulating volume with blood and plasma.

4   Keep nasogastric tube in place until patient passes gas via rectum.

5   Accept the depression of the patient which usually follows any surgery that interferes with body integrity.
   a. Accept the patient's irritability and lack of motivation to learn.
   b. Give the patient extra support until he can cope with is situation.

Following Cutaneous Ureterostomy

1   Patient may have indwelling ureteral catheters for 7–10 days.

2   Following removal of ureteral catheters, uterostomy cups are fastened on the abdominal wall with special cement.
   a. The cemented-on appliance is worn at all times.
   b. Ureteral dilatation with sterile catheter is performed at regular intervals to assure patency and prevent ureteral stricture.

3   See below—nursing considerations for patient having ileal conduit—for general aspects of care.

Following Ureterosigmoidostomy

1   Patient will have rectal tube (or mushroom catheter) draining urine postoperatively—to ensure drainage and prevent reflux of urine into ureters and kidneys.
   a. Tape the tube to the buttocks.
   b. If the tube must be removed for defaecation reinsert the tube approximately 10 cm (4 in) into rectum to prevent trauma to site of ureteral anastomosis.

2   Give special skin care around anus to prevent skin erythema and excoriation.

3   Following removal of the tube (per order) the patient micturates through his rectum.
   a. Encourage patient to empty rectum every 2–3 hours (or more often)—keeps rectal pressure low.
   b. In time the patient will be able to differentiate between the sensation to micturate and the urge to defaecate.
   c. Reinsert the tube (catheter) at night (attached to drainage bottle) to permit uninterrupted sleep.
   d. Do not give enemas or aperients.

4   Give specific diet instructions when patient can tolerate oral intake.
   a. Avoid gas-forming foods since flatus can cause stress incontinence, socially embarrassing offensive odour and discomfort.
   b. Watch for air swallowing (chewing gum, smoking, carbonated beverages) to avoid gas.
   c. Reduce salt intake to prevent hyperchloraemic acidosis.
   d. Increase potassium intake through medication and foods since potassium may be lost in acidosis.

5   Evaluate patient for hyperchloraemic acidosis, potassium loss, pyelonephritis due to bacterial absorption from colon and reflux of bacteria from colon.

Following Ileal Conduit (Fig. 5.12)

1   Patient wears transparent disposable urinary drainage bags until oedema subsides and stoma shrinks to normal size. (Some patients prefer using disposable bags permanently.)

2   The patient with an ileal conduit wears a cemented-on appliance day and night. The ileal bladder drains urine constantly (but not faeces). The appliance has a drain valve for ease of emptying.

3   *Determining stoma size* (for ordering correct ostomy appliance).

   a. The stoma will shrink considerably as oedema subsides   (approximately 6 weeks).

   b. Measure the widest part of the stoma with a ruler.

   c. The inside diameter of the faceplate should be no more than 1/8 in larger than the diameter of the stoma.

   d. The stoma will need to be recalibrated for shrinkage at intervals during the first year postoperatively.

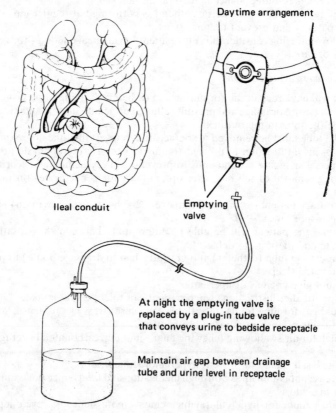

Daytime arrangement

Ileal conduit

Emptying valve

At night the emptying valve is replaced by a plug-in tube valve that conveys urine to bedside receptacle

Maintain air gap between drainage tube and urine level in receptacle

Figure 5.12.   Ileal conduit, Anatomy and appliances.

e. Patient is taught to dilate stoma himself with a finger in a plastic glove (usually weekly).

4 *Appliances in current use:*

a. Reusable or 'permanent' appliance—has a faceplate that is attached to the body with cement or adhesive.

b. Semidisposable appliance—has a reusable faceplate (or gasket) to which disposable pouches are attached.

c. Disposable appliance—discarded after each change.

5 Choice of appliance determined by activity, body build, location of stoma; patient should 'experiment' until he finds an appliance that suits his needs.

6 *Changing the appliance:*

a. Change appliance early in morning—before taking fluids.

b. Assemble all equipment needed for the type used.

c. Moisten the edge of the faceplate with adhesive solvent or soap and water and gently remove it. Adhesive solvent is not used if skin barrier (Stomahesive) is used.

d. Instruct the patient to bend over quickly and remain in that position for a minute to allow conduit to empty before the skin is washed and dried.

e. Clean all cement from the skin with adhesive solvent; use a soft cloth. Wash skin with noncream-based soap and water. Pat dry. *The skin must be dry or appliance will not adhere.*

(1) Inspect skin for signs of irritation.

(2) Keep the skin free from direct contact with urine.

(3) A gauze or tissue wick may be inserted in the stoma to absorb urine while the appliance is being changed.

f. Prepare the appliance according to the manufacturer's directions; the skin of the abdomen should be taut.

g. Centre the appliance directly over the stoma and apply it carefully. Apply gentle pressure around appliance for secure adherence.

h. Apply nonallergic tape in a picture-frame effect around the pouch.

i. The skin under the appliance may be dusted with pure talcum powder and an appliance cover applied to absorb perspiration and eliminate warmth from the pouch.

j. The use of a belt is optional; but follow manufacturer's directions, since an ill-fitting belt can cause abrasion of the stoma.

7 *Odour control:*

a. Instruct the patient to avoid foods and medication that produce strong odours (e.g., asparagus).

b. Drink liberal amounts of fluids to flush the conduit free of mucus and reduce possibility of urinary infection.

c. Introduce a few drops of liquid deodorizer or diluted white vinegar through the drain spout into the bottom of the pouch with a syringe or eye dropper.

8 *Managing the ostomy appliance:*

a. Empty the appliance when it is one-third to half full to prevent weight of urine from loosening adhesive seal—urinary ostomy appliances are closed with a drain valve (spigot) for periodic emptying.

b. Some patients prefer wearing a leg bag attached with an adapter to the drainage apparatus.

    c. Attach outlet on appliance to a collecting bottle with plastic tubing for night-time drainage; have at least 1.5 m (5 ft) of tubing to allow patient to turn in bed.

    The tubing may be threaded down the pyjama leg to prevent kinking.

9 *Securing a urine specimen for culture from a ileal conduit:*

    a. Open catheter set.

    b. Remove the bag from the stoma. Place a 3 × 4 gauze sponge over the stoma to absorb the urine.

    c. Don sterile gloves.

    d. Using sterile surgical forceps and cotton balls, cleanse the area around the stoma from the centre outwards.

    e. Insert a French catheter 5–10 cm (2–4 in) into the stoma and wait for the urine to flow by gravity into the sterile collecting tube. This may take several minutes.

    f. Replace ileal appliance (see no. 6).

10 *Cleaning and deodorizing the appliance:*

    a. Clean faceplate with solvent and remove all adhesive; rinse in clear water.

    b. Clean appliance with a brush and detergent solution; rinse and soak in white vinegar, washing soda solution or any commercial deodorizing solution.

    c. After soaking (5–10 min) hang it up to air-dry.

    d. Discard equipment that can no longer be cleaned adequately.

Discharge Planning and Health Teaching

Objective

To become an expert in the management of your stoma and appliance.

Instruct the patient as follows:

1 Urinary stoma care is not difficult or complicated and should be regarded as part of personal grooming and dressing routine.

2 The stoma is normally red in colour; it may protrude or be flush with the skin. It may bleed if it is bumped or rubbed. Report to your doctor if it continues bleeding for several hours.

3 Mucous shreds in the urine are normal following an ileal conduit operation.

4 Choose an appliance that fits your needs. Successful urinary ostomy requires a well-fitting appliance, meticulous skin care and control of urinary odour.

5 Always carry spare pouches and cement in a small case in handbag or pocket.

6 The wearing time of an appliance varies. Experiment with your appliance; usually an appliance may be worn 5–7 days. See p. 301 for changing, cleaning and management of appliance.

7 Before changing to a new skin adhesive, apply a test patch to the other side of the abdomen or forearm.

8 Wear cotton (rather than nylon) underwear. Avoid a heavy girdle as it may cause chafing of the stoma and leakage from pressure on the pouch.

9 Avoid heavy lifting for 6 weeks. Sexual activities, driving the car, returning to work, etc., may be resumed when energy level increases.

10 Get in touch with local medical supply distributor or stoma therapist.

11 Call your doctor for instructions if skin problems develop or if one or more of

the following symptoms of kidney complications occur: fever, chills, pain, change in colour of urine (cloudy, bloody), diminishing urine output.

12 Contact local ostomy association for visits, reassurance and practical information from ostomy visitor.

13 For further information and valuable periodical materials: Ileostomy Association of Great Britain, 1st Floor, 23 Winchester Road, Basingstoke, Hants RG21 1UE and Urinary Conduit Association, c/o 36 York Road, Denton, Manchester M34 3HL.

PROBLEMS AFFECTING THE URETHRA

Urethral Stricture

Urethral stricture is a narrowing of the lumen and loss of distensibility of the urethra caused by scar tissue formation and contraction.

Aetiology

1 Urethral injury.
   a. Urethral instrumentation—transurethral surgical procedures, indwelling catheters, cystoscopic procedures.
   b. Straddle injuries, automobile accidents, pelvic fractures, direct trauma to urethra.
2 Untreated gonorrhoeal urethritis.
3 Congenital abnormalities.

Clinical Manifestations

1 Diminution in force and size of urinary stream.
2 Urinary infection and retention—dysuria and urgency.
3 Symptoms of complication from stricture—back pressure produces cystitis, prostatitis, pyelonephritis, etc.

Diagnosis

1 Urethrogram and micturating cystogram—to locate site and degree of stricture.
2 Elevated white blood cells and pus and bacteria in urine—if urinary tract infection present.
3 Passing of catheter or sounds (bougies)—to determine the diameter and location of urethral narrowings.
4 Residual urine measurement.

Complications

1 Periurethral abscess, infection of bladder and kidneys.
2 Hydroureter, hydronephrosis and pyelonephritis.
3 Urethrocutaneous fistula.
4 Chronic prostatitis.
5 Incontinence.

Prevention

1 Treat urethral infections promptly.
2 Utilize utmost care in urethral instrumentation (catherization, etc.).
3 Avoid prolonged urethral catheter drainage.

Treatment

1 Dilatation of urethra with urethral sounds.
  a. Sounds of increasing size are used.
  b. Sounds are passed at lengthening intervals (2 weeks, 1 month, 3 months) for an indefinite period depending on how long the strictured lumen is patent.
  c. Hot baths and non-narcotic analgesics—to control pain after instrumentation.
  d. Sulphonamides may be given several days after dilatation—lessens discomfort and minimizes infectious reaction.
2 Surgical excision or urethroplasty may be necessary for severe strictures.
3 Surgery for incontinence.

Urethritis

Urethritis is inflammation of the urethra.

Aetiology

1 Nonspecific—urethritis not caused by gonococcus. However, a large number of cases are sexually transmitted by:
  a. *Chlamydia*—a virus-like intracellular bacterium.
  b. *Trichomonas vaginalis.*
  c. *Herpesvirus hominis,* Type 2.
  d. *Candida.*
  e. Mycoplasms.
  f. Unknown organisms.
2 Nonsexually transmitted:
  a. Bacterial urethritis—may be associated with urinary tract infection.
  b. From trauma—secondary to passage of urethral sounds, repeated cystoscopy, indwelling catheter.
3 Reiter's syndrome—urethritis, conjunctivitis, arthritis of unknown aetiology.

Clinical Manifestations

1 Dysuria and frequency.
2 Urethral discharge; may be scant or profuse; thin, clear or mucoid; or thick and purulent.
3 Itching and burning around area of urethra.
4 Penile pain.

Diagnosis

1 Study of stained urethral smear.
2 Culture for gonorrhoea.

3   Blood test for syphilis.
4   History and physical findings (interview to elicit past history of gonorrhoea).

Treatment

1   Give antibiotic—tetracyclines are usually effective for *Chlamydia* infection.
    a. Give on empty stomach, preferably 1 hour before meals.
    b. Do not take with milk, antacids, iron supplements—reduce absorption of drug.
2   Metronidazone (Flagyl) may be given for *Trichomonas* infection.
3   Treat associated prostatitis (p. 307).

Health Teaching

1   Advise patient to temporarily discontinue sexual activity and ingestion of alcohol—these activities may prolong the acute phase of urethritis.
2   Urge treatment for sexual partner—in event of treatment failure and recurrence.
3   Support and reassure patient—nonspecific urethritis is usually self-limited and is not a serious health threat.

Urethritis from Gonorrhoea

Aetiology

1   *Neisseria gonorrhoeae*—the specific organism.
2   Transmitted through sexual contact.
3   More and more asymptomatic carriers are being recognized.

Clinical Manifestations

Male

1   Urethral discharge: scant and serous to thick, yellowish pus (4–10 days or longer after sexual exposure).
2   Inflammation of meatal orifice; burning on urination.

Female

1   Purulent urethral discharge.
2   Frequency, urgency, nocturia.
3   Red, swollen urinary meatus.
4   Pelvic infection accompanied by abdominal pain.
5   Often is asymptomatic (disease not diagnosed).

Complications (local)

1   Male—periurethritis, prostatitis, epididymitis, urethral stricture, sterility due to vasoepididymal duct obstruction.
2   Female—pelvic infection, abscess of greater vestibular glands (Bartholin's glands), urethral stricture.

Treatment and Health Teaching

1 Give penicillin as directed (or tetracycline if patient is sensitive to penicillin).
2 Instruct patient to refrain from sexual intercourse until after a cure has been verified.
3 Emphasize that patient must return in 1 week to assess results and determine if there is need for further treatment and tests.
4 Urge patients to have their sexual contacts present themselves for treatment.

CONDITIONS OF THE PROSTATE

Benign Prostatic Hyperplasia (Hypertrophy)

Benign prostatic hyperplasia is enlargement of the prostate. The aetiology is unknown but it appears to accompany the ageing process in the male.

Clinical Manifestations

1 In early or gradual prostatic enlargement there may be no symptoms since the bladder can compensate for increased peripheral resistance.
2 Prostatic enlargement is usually a slow but continuous process.
3 Enlargement of the gland causes narrowing of the prostatic urethra.
   a. *Bladder:*
   (1) Symptoms of recurring urinary infection and stasis—frequency, dysuria, nocturia, chills, fever.
      Obstruction of urinary outflow may develop from hypertrophy of bladder neck, formation of benign adenoma of prostate, or a combination of both processes.
   (2) Symptoms of urethral obstruction—hesitancy, decrease in size and force of urinary stream, partial or complete urinary retention, nocturia, haematuria, dribbling.
   b. *Renal* (prolonged obstruction):
   Symptoms of renal complications from retrograde pressure of urine—ureteral dilatation, hydronephrosis, renal infection, uraemia.

Diagnosis

1 Cystoscopic examination—to view degree of prostatic enlargement and subsequent bladder-wall changes.
2 Cystourethrography—to view the posterior urethra and outline of prostate gland.
3 Excretory urogram—to demonstrate complications from back pressure of urine.
4 Catheterization after micturition—to determine amount of residual urine.
5 Cystometrogram—to evaluate the presence of a neurogenic bladder.
6 Rectal examination—allows rough estimate of size of gland.

Treatment and Nursing Management

1 The plan of treatment depends on the cause, the severity of obstruction and the condition of the patient.

2   Prepare patient for prostatectomy if this type of surgery is advised. (See p. 311 for nursing management of patient having a prostatectomy).
3   Conservative treatment.
    a. Prostatic massage—thought to help evacuate the ducts of the gland and decrease inflammation; gives limited improvement.
    b. Urinary antiseptics—to relieve symptoms of infection and frequency.
    c. Advise patient to report every 6 months for re-evaluation.
4   Cystostomy drainage of bladder—for poor-risk patient or one acutely ill with retention uraemia, etc. (see p. 240).

Prostatitis

Prostatitis is an inflammation of the prostate gland.

Aetiology

1   Bacterial invasion of prostate.
    a. From haematogenous (bloodstream) origin (tonsils, gastrointestinal tract, genitourinary tract).
    b. From ascent of bacteria from urethra.
    c. Secondary to urethritis (p. 304).
    d. Secondary to gonorrhoea (p. 305).
2   Descending infection from kidneys.
3   Other infectious agents—viruses, fungi, mycoplasmas, chlamydiae, or trichomonas may create prostatitis.
4   Prostatic urethral and midurethral stricture.
5   Benign prostatic hyperplasia.
6   Stress.
7   Irregular sexual activity.

Clinical Manifestations

From infection and local inflammation.

1   Pain in perineum, rectum, lower back, lower abdomen and penile head.
2   Chills and fever (moderate to high fever).
3   Pain in groin—if seminal vesicles are involved.
4   Bladder irritability—frequency, dysuria, urgency, haematuria.
5   Urethritis and urethral discharge—may or may not be present.

Diagnosis

1   Rectal examination—frequently reveals enlarged, oedematous and painful prostate.
2   Culture and sensitivity tests of urethral and prostatic fluid (often not helpful since prostatic secretion is bacteriostatic).
    By collection of divided urine specimens and prostatic fluid (obtained by prostatic massage) the bacteria (and other causative agents) in each specimen are identified.
3   Urinalysis—for evidences of infection; cystitis is usually also present.

Complications

1   Urinary retention—from swelling of the gland; recurring urinary tract infection.
2   Epididymitis, prostatic abscess.
3   Bacteraemia/septicaemia.
4   Pyelonephritis.

Treatment and Nursing Management

Objective

To avoid complications of abscess formation and septicaemia.

Acute

Treat with antibiotic to which organism causing infection is susceptible.

Intravenous administration of antibiotics may be advisable to achieve high serum and tissue levels; also, patient may be nauseated and vomiting.

Chronic

1   Give specific therapy (trimethoprim-sulphamethoxazole, minocycline); chronic bacterial prostatitis is difficult to treat because many antibacterial agents diffuse poorly into prostatic fluid.
2   Keep patient on bed rest.
3   Promote comfort with:
    a. Analgesics for pain relief.
    b. Antispasmodics and bladder sedatives—to relieve bladder irritability.
    c. Hot baths—to relieve pain and spasm.
    d. Stool softeners.
4   Ensure adequacy of fluid intake. (Avoid 'forcing fluids' since this merely increases urinary frequency.)
5   Watch for urinary retention—due to acute oedema of prostatic tissue.
    a. Suprapubic catheter may be required; may be more comfortable and cause fewer complications than urethral catheter.
    b. For urethral catheterization—use *small* catheter to avoid urethral trauma.

Discharge Planning and Health Teaching

Instruct the patient as follows:

1   Avoid spicy foods, coffee and alcohol—these substances cause prostatic irritation and secondary congestion.
2   Avoid prolonged automobile rides.
3   Avoid sexual intercourse during the period of acute inflammation; sexual intercourse may be beneficial in treatment of chronic prostatitis.
4   Be assured that the causative agent of prostatitis is not the type that causes sexually transmitted (venereal) disease. (This may be an unspoken fear.)
5   Medical follow-up is necessary for at least 6 months to 1 year since recurrence of prostatitis due to the same or different organisms can occur.

Cancer of the Prostate

Cancer of the prostate is a malignant tumour of the prostate gland. It arises from the parenchyma of the prostate, usually in the most posterior part; therefore most prostatic cancers are palpable on rectal examination.

Clinical Features

1 Cancer of the prostate is the third most common cause of death from cancer in men.
2 It spreads into the seminal vesicles and bladder neck and metastasizes to the regional nodes, bony pelvis and spine; late metastasis may involve liver and lungs.
3 Early localized cancer of the prostate does not produce symptoms; the obstructive symptoms occur late in the disease.
4 This cancer tends to be chronic and variable in its course.

Clinical Manifestations

1 Symptoms due to obstruction of urinary flow:
   a. Hesitancy and straining on micturition, frequency, nocturia.
   b. Diminution in size and force of urinary stream.
2 Symptoms due to metastases:
   a. Pain in lumbosacral area radiating to hips and down legs.
   b. Perineal and rectal discomfort.
   c. Anaemia, weight loss, weakness, nausea, oliguria (from uraemia).
   d. Haematuria—from urethral or bladder invasion, or both.

Diagnosis

1 Palpation by rectal examination—reveals 'stony hard' fixed gland if lesion is advanced (there are indurated lumps without fixation if condition is found earlier).
2 Cystoscopy—helps evaluate local extent of disease.
3 Prostatic biopsy.
4 Laboratory studies:
   a. Serum acid phosphatase—frequently increases when cancer extends outside prostatic capsule; this test reveals extent of tumour.
   b. Serum alkaline phosphatase—elevated when there is bony metastasis.
   c. Tests for anaemia—advanced anaemia is present when bone marrow is replaced by bone tumour.
5 Bone scan—to detect metastasis.
6 Skeletal x-rays—to reveal osteoblastic metastases.
7 Bone marrow aspiration for tumour cells.
8 Bone biopsy.
9 X-rays of pelvis, lumbar spine, femoral heads, skull, ribs.
10 Excretory urogram—to demonstrate changes from ureteral obstruction.
11 Urinary function tests—to evaluate degree of urinary obstruction.
12 Lymphangiography—to seek evidence of metastases to pelvic nodes.

Treatment

Objectives

To control tumour spread.
To draw up a rational plan of treatment.

Curative (if performed before metastasis)

1 *Radical prostatectomy*—removal of prostate and its capsule, seminal vesicles and portion of bladder neck; may include regional lymphadenectomy if done by retropubic approach. This procedure may be followed by orchidectomy or oestrogen therapy.
   a. Done by perineal or retropubic approach.
   b. Sexual impotency follows radical procedure, but urinary control is usually normal.
2 See p. 311 for care of patient undergoing prostatectomy.

Palliative

Objective

To provide a longer period of meaningful life.

1 *Radiation therapy* to local lesion or gross tumour extension; may also be used as primary treatment with hope of cure.
   a. Results in decrease in tumour size and regression of obstructive lesions and frequently in relief of bone pain.
   b. Some degree of proctitis, diarrhoea and urinary frequency may be seen towards the end of treatment.
2 *Hormonal manipulation* (endocrine control therapy or antiandrogen therapy)—the aim of endocrine control therapy is to suppress or eliminate the main sources of androgen production (most prostatic cancers are androgen dependent) and thereby to alleviate symptoms and retard progress of disease.
   a. *Bilateral orchidectomy*—removal of testes (major testosterone-producing organ); this removes androgenic hormone upon which growth of malignancy depends.
   b. *Oestrogen therapy* (diethylstilboestrol).
   (1) Long-term therapy with oestrogens has been reported to increase death rate from cardiovascular disease, but many urologists with extensive experience dispute the data and the conclusions.
   (2) Watch for evidences of aggravation of cardiac failure since oestrogen therapy is said to lead to some measure of salt and water retention.
   (3) Patient may experience soreness and enlargement of breasts (gynaecomastia).
   c. Both orchidectomy and oestrogen may be used in treatment.
3 *Interstitial radiation* with ^{198}AU.
4 *Chemotherapy*—cyclophosphamide (Cytoxan) and 5-fluorouracil, etc.
5 *Cryosurgery*—freezing of prostatic tissue via a cryoprobe results in cellular death of obstructive tissue; used in poor-risk patients.
6 *Medical adrenalectomy*—Cortisone (or equivalent drug) may be tried when oestrogen therapy effectiveness diminishes.

7   *Bilateral adrenalectomy hypophysectomy*—may be done for advanced disease in patients with endocrine-resistant neoplasm.

Symptomatic Treatment for Patient with Recurring Symptoms

1   Corticosteroids may give symptomatic relief but do not affect the tumour.
    a. Restrict sodium intake since corticosteroids produce considerable sodium retention.
    b. Add potassium to diet.
2   Transurethral resection to remove obstructing tissue.
3   Suprapubic cystostomy drainage for bladder outlet obstruction when transurethral resection cannot be done.
4   If tumour enlarges and metastasis is widespread the following treatment may be used:
    a. Hypophysectomy or bilateral adrenalectomy.
    Irradiation hypophysectomy—transnasal inoculation of radioactive material into pituitary gland under radiological guidance brings relief of metastatic pain.
    b. Discontinuation of oestrogen.
    c. Discontinuation of steroids.
    d. Testosterone therapy.
    e. Blood transfusions to maintain adequate haemoglobin when bone marrow is replaced by tumour.
    f. Radiation therapy as palliative treatment.
5   See Nursing Management of Patient with Terminal Cancer and Nursing the Dying Patient (Volume 1, Chapter 7).

Management of the Patient Undergoing Prostatic Surgery

Surgical Procedures

Four Approaches for Prostatectomy

1   Transurethral removal of prostatic tissue by an instrument introduced through urethra.
2   Open surgical removal of prostate (procedures used are named for area of incision).
    a. Perineal.
    b. Retropubic.
    c. Suprapubic.

Factors Influencing Choice of Surgical Approach

1   Size of gland and severity of obstruction.
2   Age and condition of patient.
3   Presence of associated disease(s).

Bilateral Vasectomy

May be performed at time of prostatectomy to reduce risk of epididymitis—a complication that frequently follows prostatectomy.

Preoperative Objectives of Nursing Management

To Establish Kidney Function at the Patient's Optimum Level

1 Maintain adequate bladder drainage via indwelling catheter or suprapubic cystostomy—renal function usually improves with re-establishment of drainage.
   a. Introduce indwelling catheter if patient has continuing retention or if residual urine is more than 75–100 ml.
   b. Give antibiotics (according to culture and sensitivity tests) as prescribed to combat and control infection.
   c. Utilize cystostomy if patient cannot tolerate urethral catheter.
   d. Watch patient closely after drainage is instituted—blood pressure fluctuates and renal function may decline first few days after drainage is established.
   e. Ensure adequate hydration—patient is frequently dehydrated from self-limitation of fluids because of frequency.
      (1) Encourage fluid intake of 2500–3000 ml daily (if cardiac reserve is adequate).
      (2) Weigh patient daily and monitor fluid intake and output.
      (3) Give intravenous fluids according to need as indicated by clinical status and serum electrolyte determinations.
2 Carry out prescribed renal function studies—to determine if there is renal impairment from prostatic back pressure and to evaluate renal reserve.

To Ensure that Patient is in Best Possible Condition

Older people have diminishing functional reserves of vital organs and may have coexisting disease.

1 Carry out complete haematological investigation—to ascertain specific clotting defects since haemorrhage is a major postoperative complication.
2 Correct nutritional deficiencies, hypoproteinaemia, vitamin deficiencies and anaemia.
3 Give cardiac supporting drugs when indicated—helps alleviate renal symptoms.
4 Prepare patient with pulmonary emphysema with antibacterial agent, tracheobronchial cleansing and intermittent positive pressure breathing if prescribed. Patient should stop smoking at least 2 days before surgery.
5 Teach active leg exercises; apply below-the-knee elastic stockings to prevent deep vein thrombosis.
6 Blood typing and cross matching for blood transfusion will be carried out.

Postoperative Objectives of Nursing Management (Fig. 5.13)

To Evaluate for Shock and Haemorrhage

1 Watch for evidence of haemorrhage in drainage bottle, on dressings and at incision site.
2 Take blood pressure, pulse and respiration as frequently as clinical condition indicates. Compare with preoperative vital sign readings to assess degree of hypotension present.
   a. Observe for cold, sweating skin, pallor, restlessness, fall in blood pressure, increasing pulse rate.

b. Prepare for surgical intervention if bleeding persists (suturing of bleeders or transurethral coagulation of bleeders).
3 Give blood transfusion as indicated.

To Promote Adequate Drainage of the Bladder

1 A closed sterile gravity system of drainage—three-way system may be used in controlling bleeding; irrigating system keeps clots from forming (does not correct the *cause* of bleeding).
2 Watch drainage for evidence of increased bleeding.
3 Irrigate bladder (amount and time prescribed by urologist) to avoid clot formation in the bladder.
  a. Frequency of bladder irrigation determined by amount of bleeding.
  b. Irrigation is adjusted to keep urine a light pink to straw colour, free of clots and transparent in appearance.
4 Explain again to the patient the purpose of the catheter.
  a. Tell him that the urge to micturate is caused by the presence of the catheter and bladder spasm.
  b. Encourage him to refrain from pulling on catheter—will cause bleeding, clots, plugging of catheter and distension.
  c. Tape catheter to abdomen or laterally (Fig. 5.6) to prevent pressure on penoscrotal junction.
  d. Wash urethral meatus adjacent to catheter with soap and water; rinse and apply an antibacterial ointment several times a day as directed.
5 Be alert for blockage of urinary drainage tube by kinking, mucous plugs and blood clots.
6 Tape the drainage tubing (not the catheter) to shaved inner thigh—to prevent traction on bladder. (However, traction on the catheter by the urologist may control bleeding.)
7 Tape cystostomy catheter to lateral abdomen.
8 Note time and amount of each micturition after removal of catheter.
  a. May be urinary leakage around wound several days after removal of catheter in perineal, suprapubic and retropubic surgery.
  b. Cystostomy tube may be removed before or after removal of urethral catheter.

To Anticipate Postoperative Complications

1 Haemorrhage and shock.
2 Urinary infection.
3 Epididymitis.
4 Pulmonary complications.

To promote Comfort and Rehabilitation of the Patient

1 Keep patient quiet, and comfortable during *immediate* postoperative period to prevent episodes of bleeding.
   When a patient experiences pain following prostatectomy, it may cause him to strain (from bladder irritability); this causes pelvic vein engorgement and promotes venous haemorrhage and clot formation.

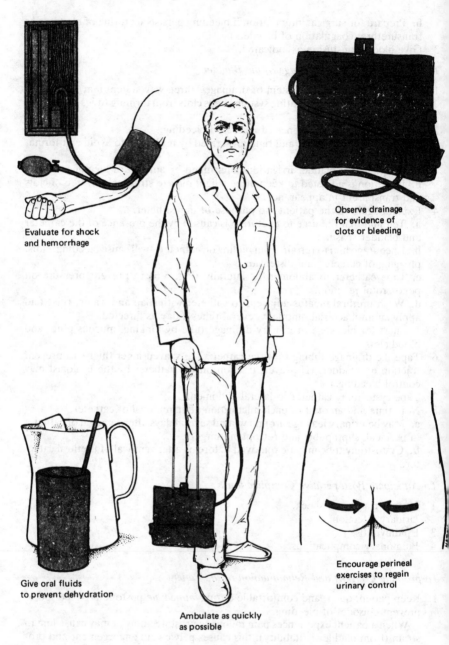

Evaluate for shock
and hemorrhage

Observe drainage
for evidence of
clots or bleeding

Give oral fluids
to prevent dehydration

Ambulate as quickly
as possible

Encourage perineal
exercises to regain
urinary control

Figure 5.13. Nursing management of patient following prostatectomy.

2 Use tranquillizers, sedatives, antispasmodics and appropriate analgesics for pain control.
   a. Elderly patients do not usually tolerate barbiturates.
   b. Take blood pressure before administering tranquillizers and analgesics.
3 Give antibiotics as directed—to promote urinary antisepsis.
4 Avoid rectal temperatures, rectal tubes and enemas following perineal prostatic surgery.
5 Help the patient to ambulate as quickly as possible.
6 Promote the comfort of the patient with perineal sutures.
   a. Wash perineum with surgical soap as directed.
   b. Use heat lamp to perineal area (cover scrotum with towel)—to promote healing.
   c. Assist patient with salt bath as directed—to promote healing.

Discharge Planning and Health Teaching

The major concerns of the patient usually centre on urinary control and sexual competence. Instruct the patient as follows:

Urinary Control

1 After the catheter is removed there may be some burning on urination and/or frequent desire to micturate. These symptoms will disappear in a few weeks.
2 Expect urinary dribbling for a period of time (especially after catheter removal). Urinary incontinence may follow any type of prostatic surgery.
3 Exercises to gain urinary control.
   a. *Perineal exercises.*
   (1) Tense the perineal muscles by pressing the buttocks together. Hold this position as long as possible; relax.
   (2) Perform this exercise 10–20 times each hour.
   (3) Continue with perineal exercises until full urinary control is gained.
   b. *When starting to micturate.*
   (1) Shut off the stream for a few seconds.
   (2) Continue with full micturition.
   (3) Continue this exercise with each urination until control improves; may take many weeks.
4 Urinate as soon as the first desire to do so is felt.
5 The urine may be cloudy for several weeks after surgery. As the prostate area heals, the cloudiness will disappear.
6 Avoid long automobile trips which increase tendency to bleed.
7 Avoid alcohol which increases urinary burning.
8 Drink adequate fluids (8 glasses) since dehydration increases tendency for clot obstruction.
9 Do not take anticholinergics and diuretics unless by direct order of the doctor.

Sexual Potency

1 Prostatectomy does not usually cause impotence.
   Total prostatectomy (removal of entire prostatic contents and capsule) results in impotence since the nerves and muscular tissue surrounding the capsule (which have a function in penile erection) have been severed.

2 In most instances sexual activity may be resumed in 6–8 weeks; this is the time required for healing of the prostatic fossa to take place.
3 Do not be alarmed if no fluid appears on ejaculation; following ejaculation the seminal fluid goes into the bladder and is excreted with the urine. This is not harmful.

Other Considerations

1 Avoid straining and strenuous exercises.
2 Report to the doctor if a decrease in the size of the urinary stream takes place.

HYDROCELE

Hydrocele is an abnormal accumulation of fluid within the scrotum around the testicle and within the two layers of the tunica vaginalis.

Causes

Caused by defective or inadequate reabsorption of normally produced hydrocele fluid.

1 Secondary to local injury including hernia operation.
2 Secondary to infection.
3 Following epididymitis or orchitis; torsion.
4 As a complication of tumour of testicle.
5 In oedematous states such as congestive heart failure, cirrhosis of the liver.
6 Idiopathic.

Clinical Manifestations

1 Enlargement of the scrotum.
2 Usually painless until fluid accumulation is large enough to cause pressure.

Treatment

1 No treatment is required unless complications are present.
   a. Circulatory complications involving testicle.
   b. Painful large hydrocele which is uncomfortable and cosmetically unacceptable to the patient.
2 Surgical intervention—hydrocelectomy (excision of tunica vaginalis of testis) for removal of fluid and control of swelling.
   a. Periodic aspiration of hydrocele fluid in poor-risk patient.
   b. Open operation for eversion of hydrocele sac or removal of hydrocele sac.
3 See below, treatment and nursing management—varicocele, no. 3 for postoperative nursing support.

Complications

1 Haemorrhage into scrotal tissues.
2 Infection.

VARICOCELE

Varicocele is the dilatation, elongation and tortuosity of veins within the scrotum (varicosities usually of the distal portion of the left spermatic vein and its tributaries due to the absence of any venous valve along its route to the left renal vein.

Clinical Manifestations

1   Subfertility may occur with varicocele—may suppress spermatogenesis due to vascular and temperature changes or more likely to reflux of left adrenal corticosteroids to both testes because of intercommunication of their venous circulations.
2   A dragging sensation in the scrotum is usually the patient's chief complaint.
3   Varicocele on the right may indicate retroperitoneal tumour.

Treatment and Nursing Management

1   Patient wears a scrotal support (or suspensory) to relieve discomfort.
2   Operative intervention—ligation and excision of veins near or above internal inguinal ring through hernia or McBurney's incision.
3   Postoperative nursing support.
    a. Apply ice bag to scrotum first few hours postoperatively—relieves oedema.
    b. Apply scrotal support for comfort.

TUMOURS OF THE TESTICLE

The aetiology of testicular tumours is unknown but cryptochidism, trauma, infections and genetic endocrine factors appear to play a role in their development.

Clinical Features

1   Tumours of the testicle are usually malignant.
2   They usually develop in the 20–40 year age group.
3   Most testicular tumours metastasize early to the periaortic and pericaval lymph nodes, lungs and liver.

Clinical Manifestations

1   Painless enlargement of the testis (swelling, hardness, lump).
2   Pain in the testis (if patient has epididymitis or bleeding into tumour).
3   Gynaecomastia (enlargement of the breasts) from elaboration of chorionic gonadotrophins from testicular tumour (considered a serious prognostic sign).
4   Symptoms of metastases.
    a. Left supraclavicular or abdominal mass.
    b. Abdominal pain.
    c. Cough (lung metastases).

Diagnosis

1   Assay of urinary chorionic gonadotrophins—may be elevated—serves as a guide in evaluating extent of disease and in planning therapy.
2   Intravenous urogram to evaluate presence of enlarged lymph nodes as manifested by ureteral displacement.
3   Chest film to seek pulmonary or mediastinal metastases.
4   Lymphangiography—to assess extent of lymphatic spread of tumour.
5   Thermography—helps spot occult tumours.

Treatment and Nursing Management

Objective

To control tumour spread.

1   Orchiectomy—removal of testicle (or testes) and spermatic cord to internal inguinal ring (usually through an inguinal incision).
   a. Removal of both testes (castration) renders the patient sterile and lacking in male hormones: this is rare since tumours of the testicle are usually unilateral.
   b. Resection of iliac and lumbar lymph nodes is carried out in certain histological types.
2   Radiation therapy is used in most cases of testicular neoplasm; may be curative or palliative.
3   Chemotherapy (given in combination)—many tumours contain components of more than one cell type.
   a. Observe patient for toxic effects—nausea, vomiting, diarrhoea, leucopaenia, thrombocytopaenia, skin eruption, loss of hair.
   b. Drug(s) may have to be temporarily withheld in presence of serious toxic manifestations.
   c. See Nursing Management of Patient Receiving Chemotherapy.
4   Patient follow-up evaluation includes chest films, excretory urography and determination of urinary gonadotrophins, examination of lymph nodes—to monitor success of therapy and to detect recurrence of malignancy.
5   A patient with a history of one testis tumour is more apt to develop another than is the random patient to develop a first testis tumour.

Discharge Planning and Health Teaching

Instruct the patient as follows:

1   Carry out periodic self-examinations of the testes (see below).
2   Report for periodic physical examinations and tests as directed by the doctor.
3   Unilateral excision of a testicle will not usually lessen virility.

GUIDELINES: Self-Examination for Testicular Tumour

1   The testis is easily accessible for self-examination. Most tumours are palpable and can be detected by self-examination.
2   The hormonally-active years (15–35) are the tumour-prone years.

Procedure

Action by Patient	Explanation
1 Examine for testicular tumour periodically, preferably while showering/bathing.	
2 Use both hands to palpate (feel). Carefully examine all scrotal contents.	2 A small lump (nodule) can slip away from one hand. You can feel differences in weight between the testicles by using both hands.
3 Locate the epididymis; this is the cord-like structure at the back of the testis.	3 It is important to know what the epididymis feels like so you will not confuse it with an abnormality.
4 The spermatic cord (and vas) extends upward from the epididymis.	
5 Feel each testis between the thumb and first two fingers of each hand.	5 The testes lie freely in the scrotum, are oval shaped, $1\frac{3}{4}$ in in length, and have a spongy, uniform texture.
6 Note size, shape, abnormal tenderness.	6 An abnormality may be felt as a firm area on the front or side of the testicle.
7 Stand in front of mirror and look for changes in size/shape of scrotum.	7 Tumours or cystic masses tend to involve only one side.

EPIDIDYMITIS

Epididymitis is an infection of the epididymis which usually descends from an infected prostate or urinary tract.

Causes

1 Prostatic infection (most common cause).
2 Urinary tract infection.
3 Infection via the bloodstream with tubercle bacilli.
4 Postoperative epididymitis—complication of prostatectomy and urethral catheterization.
5 Reflux of sterile urine down the vas deferens.

Clinical Manifestations

1 Pain in the groin and scrotum.
2 Swollen, tender epididymis.
3 Oedema, redness and tenderness of scrotum.
4 Chills and fever.

Diagnosis

1 Elevated white blood count.

2 Staining of urethral discharge if preceded by urethritis (either nonspecific or gonorrhoeal); usually no discharge is present with epididymitis.

Treatment

1 Bed rest during acute phase.
2 Antibiotic therapy until all evidence of acute inflammatory reaction has subsided.
3 Scrotal support for enlarged testicle—to relieve oedema and discomfort and to take the tension off the cord. A cotton-lined athletic supporter may promote comfort.
4 Infiltration of spermatic cord with local anaesthetic agent (procaine hydrochloride)—for pain relief if patient is seen within 24 hours after onset.
5 Analgesics for pain relief.
6 Initially, intermittent cold compresses to scrotum—for pain relief.
7 Local heat or salt bath later—to hasten resolution of inflammatory process.
8 Treatment for possible abscess formation.

Discharge Planning and Health Teaching

Instruct the patient as follows:

1 Avoid straining (lifting, defaecation) and sexual excitement until infection under control.
2 It may take 4 weeks or longer for epididymis to return to normal.

ORCHITIS

Orchitis is infection or inflammation of the testis.

Clinical Features

1 Orchitis (relatively rare) is usually secondary to spread of inflammation in epididymis.
2 It may be pyogenic, viral, spirochetal, traumatic, etc., in origin.
3 Mumps is the main cause of pure orchitis that is not secondary to epididymitis.

Clinical Manifestations

1 Pain and swelling of the testicle; the scrotum becomes reddened and oedematous.
2 Fever and prostration.

Treatment and Nursing Management

1 Treat underlying disease.
2 Keep the patient at bed rest with scrotum (testis) elevated and supported. Cotton-lined athletic supporter may be used.
3 Give antibiotic therapy for specific aetiologic agent.
   Antibiotics are of no value in the treatment of mumps orchitis.
4 Apply hot and cold compresses to scrotum for symptomatic relief.

5   Traumatic orchitis with rupture of the capsule (tunica albuginea) may require surgical repair and drainage since abscess may occur.

Nursing Alert: A lump in the testis following *minor* trauma may call attention of the patient to a malignant testicular tumour.

Complications

The involved testis may become infertile due to damage to drainage system or to spermatogenic cells.

VASECTOMY

Vasectomy is the ligation and transection of a section of the vas deferens; a bilateral vasectomy is a sterilization procedure for males.

Clinical Indications

1   Performed as a sterilization procedure.
2   Performed if the patient has recurrent acute epididymitis (p. 319).

Underlying Considerations

1   A vasectomy interrupts the transportation of the sperm. This procedure has no effect on sexual potency, erection, ejaculation or hormonal production.
2   Seminal fluid is mostly manufactured in the seminal vesicles and prostate which are unaffected by vasectomy.
    a. There will be no noticeable decrease in the amount of ejaculated fluid; the sperm accounts for less than 5% of the volume. The sperm cells are reabsorbed into the body.
    b. Psychological problems have been noted in an occasional patient following this procedure.
3   A vasectomy can be done on an outpatient basis.
4   The patient should be advised that he will be sterile but that potency will not be altered following a bilateral vasectomy. Rarely is there a spontaneous reanastomosis resulting in pregnancy.
5   A vasectomy may not be reversible and should be considered permanent.
    New surgical techniques are being developed for vasectomy reversal (vasovasostomy) but more time is needed for evaluation of these techniques. Success rates are promising.
6   A legal consent form must be obtained, often from wife and patient.
7   The patient must understand sterilization.
8   Rarely is it done on the young adult without children.

Postoperative Care

1   Apply ice bags intermittently to the scrotum for several hours after surgery to reduce swelling and relieve pain.
2   Advise patient to wear suspensory for added comfort and support.

Complications

1   Pain, swelling and scrotal oedema.

2 Sperm granuloma—due to extravasation of sperm.
3 Infection.
4 Nonbacterial epididymitis.
5 Recanalization of vas deferens (very rare).
6 Bleeding and haematoma.

Health Teaching

Instruct the patient as follows:

1 The primary function of the testicle(s) is the production of hormones and of sperm. A vasectomy will not interfere with these functions but it will interrupt the descent of sperm from the testicle to the ejaculatory ducts.
2 Avoid strenuous activities for several days.
3 Sexual intercourse may be resumed as desired.
4 Contraceptives should be used until the sperm stored distal to the point of interruption of the vas is evacuated; (two negative semen specimens 1 month apart). This evacuation of sperm may take at least 12 ejaculations (often more) and at least 6 weeks. *The patient is still fertile for a variable period of time after vasectomy*. Therefore other methods of contraception must be used.
5 Absence of sperm must be demonstrated microscopically; laboratory tests confirm no sperm are present in the seminal fluid.
6 A vasectomy does not prevent venereal disease.

CONDITIONS AFFECTING THE PENIS

Ulceration of the Glans Penis

Causes

1 Cancer.
2 Syphilis.
3 Herpes progenitalis (virus existing in tissues of the glans and foreskin).
4 Chancroid.
5 Lymphogranuloma venereum.
6 Numerous benign skin lesions (e.g., psoriasis).

Clinical Manifestations

Ulceration of the penis should be suspected as being venereal in origin until proved otherwise.

Diagnosis

1 Dark field microscopic examination of smear for spirochetes.
2 Serological (blood) test for syphilis.

Treatment

Penicillin or tetracycline.

Carcinoma of the Penis

Carcinoma of the penis is a rare tumour usually involving the prepuce or glans.

Clinical Manifestations

1   Painless, warty growth; ulcer on glans or foreskin.
2   Masses in inguinal region.
3   Urine specimen frequently contaminated with red and white blood cells from tumour.
4   Bloody, foul smelling discharge (if secondary infection develops).

Preventive Measures

Circumcision in infancy since chronic inflammation of foreskin and glans penis predisposes to development of penile tumours.

Treatment

1   Local excision of lesion and irradiation therapy to small early lesions.
2   Partial or complete amputation of penis for extensive lesions; usually done with bilateral groin (node) dissections and radiation therapy.
3   Irradiation used for relief of nonresectable recurrences.

Other Conditions

Chancre

Is a venereal ulcer caused by *Treponema pallidum* (syphilis).

1   Is the primary lesion of syphilis; appears 3–4 weeks after infection.
2   Begins as a dull red, hard and insensitive papule on or near the glans penis.
3   Persists 1–5 days or longer, then heals spontaneously.
4   The treatment of syphilis is outlined in Volume 1, Chapter 6.

Balanitis

Is inflammation of the glans penis.

Phimosis

Is a condition in which the foreskin is narrowed and cannot be retracted over the glans. The treatment is circumcision.

Circumcision

Circumcision is the excision of the foreskin (prepuce) of the glans penis.

Clinical Indications

1   Usually done in infancy for hygienic purposes.

2   Phimosis (inability to retract foreskin over the glans).
3   Paraphimosis (condition in which the foreskin cannot be reduced from a retracted position).
4   Recurrent infections of glans and foreskin.
5   Personal desire of patient (or parents, if patient is a minor).

Postoperative Nursing Management

1   Watch for bleeding.
2   Change gauze dressing as directed.
3   Give analgesia as patient's condition indicates; circumcision can be quite painful in the adult male.

NOTE: *Circumcision is an important preventive measure against carcinoma of the penis.*

SEXUALLY TRANSMITTED DISEASES

See Volume 1, Chapter 6.

2. *Gynaecological Conditions*

MENSTRUATION

Menstruation is a physiological process in the female of childbearing age.

1   If conception does not occur, the ovum dies; tissue lining the endometrial cavity, which has become thickened and congested, becomes haemorrhagic.
2   Tissue lining the uterus, blood cells and breakdown-products slough off and are discharged through the cervix into the vagina.
3   This cyclic process is called menstruation and usually occurs about every 28–30 days.
4   The average flow of blood lasts about 4–5 days and totals 50–150 ml.

Menarche or onset of menstruation occurs between 11 and 15 years.

Ovulation refers to the expulsion of an ovum from the ovary—14 days before the onset of the next menstrual period.

As the endometrium is being shed, the process of repair and regrowth starts again—preparing once more for the reception of a fertilized ovum.

Disturbances of Menstruation

A relationship with feedback mechanism exists between the hormonal secretions of the ovary, adrenal, thyroid and pituitary glands. An increase or decrease in the activity of one or more glands can cause a disturbance in menstruation.

Dysmenorrhoea

Dysmenorrhoea is painful menstruation.

Occurrence

Common in umarried women and women who have not borne children.

Cause

1 Primary—due to unknown factors; thought to be intrinsic to uterus; extrinsic pathology such as polyp and fibroids may be a factor.
   May involve emotional and psychological factors.
2 Secondary—due to factors extrinsic to uterus, such as endometriosis, pelvic infection.

Symptoms

1 Pain may be due to uterine spasm caused by a narrowing of cervical canal (exaggerated uterine contractility).
2 Pain—colicky, cyclic, nagging, dull ache; usually in lower abdomen, may radiate down back of legs. May be severe enough to require bed rest for a day or two.
3 Severe dysmenorrhoea may be experienced—with chills, headache, diarrhoea, nausea, vomiting and syncope.

Aetiology

1 Endocrine.
   Some investigators believe there is a relation between release of prostaglandin from the endometrium and the symptoms of dysmenorrhoea; this has not been proven.
2 Anatomic.
   a. Some discomfort results from the passing of a cervical sound or from dilatation of the cervix; a pathological growth could produce the same symptoms.
   b. An infantile or small uterus may contribute to dysmenorrhoea but this has not been proven.
3 Constitutional.
   Chronic illnesses and general debilitation seem to be associated with a high incidence of dysmenorrhoea (anaemia, fatigue, diabetes, tuberculosis).
4 Psychogenic.
   Most studies indicate that strong underlying psychological factors cause dysmenorrhoea. Parental instruction and a healthy emotional environment for the growing young girl, in a setting where realistic family relations are cultivated, almost precludes primary dysmenorrhoea.

Treatment and Nursing Management

Since there is no single treatment for dysmenorrhoea, a three-pronged approach seems best to relieve symptoms: Combine therapies as they relate to constitutional, hormonal and psychological factors.

1 Selective, according to needs of individual and severity of problem.
   a. Proper psychological preparation of girls for menarche.

    b. Good posture; use special exercises to improve posture and correct weak musculature and imbalance.
2 Since emotional makeup may accentuate discomfort, psychotherapy or suitable drugs may be necessary.
3 Complete physical examination to rule out other physical abnormalities.
4 Instructions to patient:
    a. Usual activity is possible—should be encouraged.
    b. Mild analgesics for discomfort are permissible.
    c. Avoid use of habit-forming drugs such as narcotics and alcohol.
5 Dysmenorrhoea can usually be eliminated by oral contraceptives which block ovulation.
6 Regular exercises (as well as physical activity) are recommended.
7 If the above are unsuccessful, surgery may be necessary but this is rare.
    Presacral and ovarian neurectomy (cutting nerve fibres) may be done.
8 Psychological counselling may also benefit some individuals.

Amenorrhoea

Amenorrhoea is absence of menstrual flow.

Primary (when a girl is 16 or 17 and has not menstruated)

1 May be caused by embryonic maldevelopment.
2 Treatment is according to aetiology.

Secondary (menstruation has begun (initial menarche) but stops)

1 Causes:
    a. Normal pregnancy and lactation.
    b. Psychogenic (minor emotional upsets).
    Hypothalamic disturbances (anatomic nervous system) may also be the cause.
    Example—anorexia nervosa.
    c. Constitutional.
    Any disturbance of metabolism and nutrition. Examples—diabetes, tuberculosis, obesity.
2 Treatment: directed at cause—constitutional therapy, psychotherapy, hormone therapy, surgery.

Oligomenorrhoea

Oligomenorrhoea is markedly diminished menstrual flow—nearing amenorrhoea.

Menorrhagia

Menorrhagia is excessive bleeding during regular menstruation.

Causes

1 Endocrine disturbances.
2 Inflammatory diseases; benign or malignant pelvic tumours.
3 Emotional stress.

Treatment

1   Search for underlying cause.
2   Correct anaemia.

Metrorrhagia

Metrorrhagia is bleeding from the uterus between regular menstrual periods.
    Significant because it is usually a symptom of some disease—often cancer or benign tumours of uterus.

Polymenorrhea

Polymenorrhea is frequent and often profuse menstruation occurring at intervals of less than 3 weeks.

DIAGNOSTIC STUDIES FOR GYNAECOLOGICAL CONDITIONS

Pelvic Examination

A *pelvic examination* is an inspection of the external genitalia for signs of inflammation, swelling, bleeding, discharge or local skin and epithelial changes. A speculum is inserted to permit the examiner to visualize the vagina and cervix. (For Guidelines: Vaginal Examination by the Doctor, see p. 329).

Patient Preparation

1   Provide psychological support—patient needs reassurance, understanding and skilful consideration of her emotional as well as physical problems.
2   Instruct patient to avoid douching for 24 hours before examination; cellular deposits might wash away.
3   Encourage patient to go to bathroom before examination—micturition and bowel evacuation before the examination provide more relaxation of perineal tissues.
4   Advise patient to remove sufficient clothing to permit adequate exposure of genitalia and allow for examination of the abdomen.
5   Avoid undue exposure of the patient.

Positioning of Patient (best done on an examining table but can be achieved on a bed)

1   *Lithotomy*—knees and hips flexed; heels resting on foot rests.
    a. Drape sheet diagonally over patient so that corner may be grasped and pulled upwards to expose perineal area.
    b. When examination is done in bed, the patient may be positioned across the bed with hips extending slightly over the edge (dorsal supine position); feet are placed on examiner's knees or on two chairs placed next to the bed.
2   *Sims' position*—the patient lies on one side, usually the left, with the left arm behind her back. The right (uppermost) thigh and knee are flexed as much as possible; left leg is partially flexed.

Drape sheet over lower extremities and hips to permit easy exposure of genitalia.

3   *Knee–chest*—Patient kneels on table with feet extending over the end.
   a. Separate knees and maintain thighs at right angles to the table.
   b. Turn patient's head to one side and allow face and chest to rest on a soft pillow.
   c. Patient's arms may grasp sides of table.

Procedure for Examining the Pelvis (carried out by doctor with the nurse assisting)

1   A speculum is inserted so that the vaginal tissues and condition of cervix can be visualized (Fig. 5.14).
2   *Cytology smear* (Papanicolaou) is best made by scraping cervix directly (see Fig. 5.15).
3   *Bimanual examination*—by inserting one or two gloved fingers of the left hand in the vagina and palpating the abdomen with the right hand, it is possible to further examine the uterus and cervix.
4   *Rectal examination*—to detect abnormalities of contour, motility and placement of adjacent structures and tissues.

Nursing Support

1   Attend and support the patient by encouraging her to relax, by holding her hand, etc.
2   Focus the light and uncover examining tray with speculum, swabs, cytology necessities, etc.
3   Assist doctor by providing gloves, lubricant, etc.

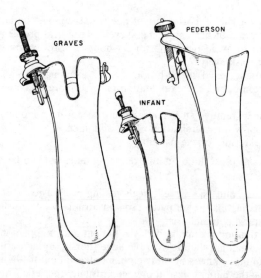

Figure 5.14. Styles and sizes of specula. (From: Green, T A (1977) Gynecology, 3rd edition, Boston, Little, Brown.)

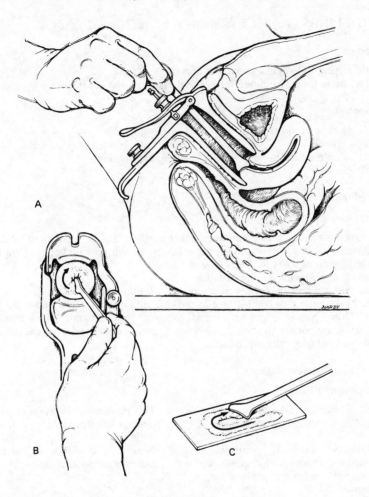

Figure 5.15. Method of using a wooden Ayre spatula to obtain cervical secretions for cytology. a. The speculum in place and the Ayre spatula in position at the cervical os. b. By rotation of the spatula, a representative sample is obtained. c. Cervical secretions are transferred from wooden spatula to glass slide in a single circular motion.

4 At conclusion of examination, wipe discharge from patient before assisting her from the table.
5 Have patient slide up on table before removing feet from stirrups.
6 Allow time for older patient to adjust to sitting position before helping her off the table.
7 Answer any questions patient may have; elaborate on doctor's instructions.
8 Assist patient with dressing if necessary.

GUIDELINES: Vaginal Examination by the Nurse/Doctor

Purposes

1 To inspect the vaginal canal and cervix.
2 To obtain tissue specimen for cervical cytology and other tests.

Equipment

Perineal drape or sheet
Vaginal specula
Water soluble lubricant
Sterile gloves

Long swab sticks
Papanicolaou smear equipment
Adequate lighting

Procedure

Preparatory Phase

1 Have woman micturate before assistant positions her on examining table.
2 Position woman on examining table (woman's slip may be kept on but other clothing from waist to knees is removed).
   a. Have buttocks at edge of table.
   b. Position feet in stirrups to assume dorsal lithotomy position.
   c. Make patient as comfortable as possible with a small pillow under her head.
   d. Drape patient to permit minimal exposure (but adequate for examiner).
3 Encourage patient to relax; tell her what you are doing and what she may feel.
4 Adjust light for maximum focus.

Nursing Action	Reason

Performance Phase

1	Be gentle and take your time; don sterile gloves; lubricate fingers.	1	This promotes relaxation of patient, making the procedure easier for both.
2	Observe external genitalia for apparent abnormalities; gently separate labia and continue visual inspection.	2	Note any evidence of irritation, infection or abnormalities.
3	To encourage relaxation in patient, gently place the tip of one or two fingers into introitus.	3	Say to patient, 'Tighten your muscles and squeeze my fingers—try hard —then relax.'
4	Identify cervix manually and depress the perineum downwards with your fingers.	4	Downward pressure is away from the more sensitive anterior structures.
5	Gently insert warm speculum horizontally, passing it over your fingers and aiming it towards the cervix.	5	If it is preferred not to initially insert gloved fingers, the speculum is introduced vertically using a downward pressure (after entering the vestibule, the speculum is slowly rotated to the horizontal position).

Nursing Action	**Reason**
6 Slowly open the speculum and lock into position. With slow manipulation, the speculum can be turned to permit visualization of the vaginal walls.	6 Walls normally are pink and moist. A pale white secretion may be noted.
7 Inspect the cervix, which should be pink in colour. Normally, the os is a dent, unless the woman has had children, in which case a slit is noted.	7 If woman is on the Pill, the cervix may be deep pink to red. A thread coming out of cervix would suggest presence of an IUD.
8 If Papanicolaou is to be done, follow procedure below.	
9 When removing speculum, hold it open until cervix is cleared; then withdraw speculum and let it close as it will.	9 By the time speculum is completely withdrawn, it will be closed.

Follow-up Phase

1 Gently wipe the perineal area with soft tissue or gauze using firm strokes from the pubic area back to beyond the rectum.	1 This will remove secretions and liquid lubricant.
2 Instruct assistant in carefully helping patient to remove feet from stirrups.	2 Both feet must be removed at the same time to reduce strain.
3 Elevate the lower third of examining table to receive legs—permits patient to assume dorsal recumbent position.	3 Keep patient covered with a sheet.
4 Assist patient in sliding towards head end of table; provide a wide-based stool for her to step on as she gets off table.	4 Do not rush patient as she is getting off the table since sudden shifting from recumbent to sitting position may cause a feeling of dizziness.
5 Assist patient in dressing (closing zippers, etc.) if necessary. Answer any queries woman may have.	

Other Diagnostic Tests

Cytology Test for Cancer (Papanicolaou)

Purpose

To screen for cervical dysplasia and/or cervical cancer. Occasionally adenocarcinoma of the endometrium will also be discovered.

Procedure (see Fig. 5.15)

1   Examination and interpretation of cytological smear as done by the pathologist.
2   Classification of cytological findings (after Papanicolaou):
    Class 1—Absence of atypical or abnormal cells.
    Class 2—Atypical cytology but no evidence of malignancy.
    Class 3—Cytology suggestive of, but not conclusive for, malignancy.
    Class 4—Cytology strongly suggestive of malignancy.
    Class 5—Cytology conclusive for malignancy.
3   If the patient has an abnormal smear of Class 2, 3 or 4, explain to her that this is not conclusive but requires additional testing such as a cone biopsy.

Cervical Biopsy and Cauterization

Purpose

To remove cervical tissue for laboratory study.

Patient Preparation

1   To be done preferably at a time when cervix is least vascular (usually a week after the end of the menstrual flow).
2   Explain the nature of the procedure to the patient.
3   Place her in lithotomy position and drape her properly.
4   Explain to her that no anaesthesia is required since the cervix does not have pain receptors.

Procedure

1   After the speculum is positioned in the vagina and the cervix properly exposed, the surgeon, under colposcopic guidance, uses biopsy forceps to take bits of cervical tissues.
2   Tissue is preserved in 10% formalin, labelled and sent to the laboratory.
3   If bleeding occurs, suturing and packing may be necessary.

Aftercare of Patient

1   A brief rest after the procedure is usually necessary before the patient leaves.
2   Discharge instructions/health teaching:
    Instruct the patient as follows:
    a. Avoid heavy lifting for 24 hours.
    b. Packing will remain in place for 12–24 hours depending on doctor's orders.
    c. There may be some bleeding; however, more than that of a normal period must be reported to the doctor.
    d. Obtain doctor's orders regarding douching and sexual relations.

Uterotubal Insufflation (Rubin's Test)

Carbon dioxide is injected under pressure through a special cannula into the cervical canal. If one or both tubes are patent, the gas will pass through the fallopian tube into the peritoneal cavity.

1   The patient is prepared as for a vaginal examination.
2   A speculum is positioned in the vagina.

3   Special cannula is passed through intrauterine canal; cervix is held tightly with a tenaculum against a rubber stopper to prevent gas leakage.
4   Tubing is connected to a machine which measures and records pressure.

Findings

1   Normal—if pressure is below 180 mmHg and gas is heard (with a stethoscope) passing through the tubes.
2   Partial obstruction—180–200 mmHg.
3   Complete obstruction—200 mmHg and above.

Culdoscopy

A *culdoscopy* is an uncommon operative, diagnostic procedure in which an incision is made into the posterior vaginal fornix so that a culdoscope can be inserted for the purpose of visualizing the uterus, tubes, broad ligaments, uterosacral ligaments, rectal wall, sigmoid and even the small intestines.

1   The patient is prepared as for any vaginal operation (see p. 336).
2   Anaesthesia may be local, general or regional.
3   The knee–chest position is best for a culdoscopy.
4   Following the examination, the scope is withdrawn and sutures placed; the patient is returned to her room.

Laparoscopy

Laparoscopy—the endoscopic visualzation of the uterine cavity by means of an endoscope through the anterior abdominal wall.

1   Earlier attempts were usually unsuccessful because uterine bleeding obscured the view.
2   Today, fibreoptic lighting and the distention of the uterine cavity with carbon-dioxide or nitrous oxide permits optimum visualization.

Indications

Primarily to complement other diagnostic procedures, chiefly staging of endometrial cancer.

1   Problem of infertility.
2   When the cause of uterine bleeding is unknown.
3   To view lesions which can be photographed and removed in some instances.
4   To diagnose and manage intrauterine adhesions.
5   For transuterine tubal sterilization.

Contraindications

1   Pelvic infection.
2   Recurrent upper genital tract infection.
3   Uterine perforation.
4   Pregnancy, because of possible disturbance of pregnancy and risk of infection.

Patient Preparation and Follow-up

1 Preparation as for general anaesthesia.
2 A small skin incision is made at the lower border of the umbilicus. A trocar and cannular is used to aid the passage of the laparoscope.
3 Following the operation, the gas is expelled by abdominal pressure before removing the cannula.
4 The small wound is closed with clips.
5 The patient may return home later the same day or next day.

Follow-up

1 Following removal of instruments, the patient is returned to bed to rest.
2 She may be discharged later the same day.

X-ray Studies–Hysterosalpingogram

A *hysterosalpingogram* is an x-ray study of the uterus and fallopian tubes following the injection of a contrast medium.

Purpose

1 To study sterility problems.
2 To determine extent of tubal patency.
3 To note the presence of pathology in the uterine cavity.

Procedure

1 Patient is placed in lithotomy position on a fluoroscopic x-ray table.
2 The bivalve speculum is introduced to expose cervix.
3 Radiopaque dye is injected into uterine cavity.
4 X-rays are taken to determine configuration of pelvic area.

GUIDELINES: Colposcopy

Colposcopy is a stereoscopic examination of the cervix using a binocular instrument with strong light illumination.

Purposes

1 To determine distribution of abnormal squamous epithelium.
2 To pinpoint areas from which biopsy tissue can be taken.

Indications

1 Following atypical vaginal or cervical cytology.
2 When suspicious cervical lesions are present.
3 Previous treatment for dysplasia or cancer of the cervix.

Advantage: Colposcopy may spare the patient a conization (D&C), which requires hospitalization. (Colposcopy can be done in the gynaecologist's surgery provided he has the instrument and possesses the skill.)

Procedure

Preparatory Phase

1 Identical to that for preparation of patient having pelvic examination (p. 327).
2 Additional explanation may be required so that the patient will know what to expect.

Action	**Reason**

Performance Phase

1 Use a long cotton applicator stick to dry cervix.
2 Swab cervix with saline using long cotton applicator.

1 This will clear away mucus and other secretions.
2 Moistening of cervical epithelium allows vascular patterns and squamous columnar junction to be visualized.

3 Examine tissue with colposcope utilizing green filter illuminator.
4 Paint cervix with 3% acetic acid.
5 Note colposcopic patterns—particularly the transformation area (where columnar epithelium is replaced by squamous epithelium).

4 This acts as a mucolytic agent and accentuates epithelial topography.
5 Acetic acid tends to draw moisture from tissues of high nuclear density—this accounts for colour changes in the cervical epithelium.

6 Biopsy (using a fine biopsy forceps) any questionable area; endocervical curettage should also be done.
7 If bleeding occurs, direct pressure or application of silver nitrate stick will usually stop it. Some clinicians prefer to apply ferric subsulphate (Monsel's solution) via applicator stick for haemostasis.

6 The cervical os has few nerve endings so the patient will experience minimal discomfort.
7 Measures to prevent or control bleeding.

8 Insert a vaginal tampon following examination.

8 To absorb discharge; may be removed after 5–6 hours.

Follow-up Phase

Similar to that following pelvic examination; see p. 327

Dilatation and Curettage (D&C)

Dilatation and curettage is a widening of the cervical canal with a dilator and the scraping of the uterine canal with a curette. The cervix is scraped first without dilatation.

Purposes

1 To secure endometrial and endocervical tissue for tissue study.

2 To control abnormal uterine bleeding.
3 To serve as a therapeutic measure for incomplete abortion.

Nursing Management

Preoperative Care

1 Inform the patient about the nature of the operation to be done (usually done by a gynaecologist).
2 Answer questions patient may have regarding D&C.
3 Ascertain whether patient has been told what to expect with regard to postoperative discomfort, drainage or incapacity following the D&C.
4 Check with doctor regarding perineal shave (some prefer no shave).
5 Prepare bladder and intestinal tract by having patient micturate and by giving a small enema, if necessary.

Postoperative Care

1 Check that perineal pad is held in place with a sanitary belt.
2 Replace each perineal pad with a sterile pad as required during the time packing is in place.
3 Report excessive bleeding.
4 Recommend bed rest for the remainder of the day, with bathroom privileges.
5 Offer mild analgesics for low back pain and pelvic discomfort.
6 Offer meals as desired.

CONDITIONS OF THE EXTERNAL GENITALIA
AND VAGINA

Contact Dermatitis of the Vulva

Nature of the Irritation

1 An inflammation of the vulvar skin is annoying because it causes itching.
2 Itching causes scratching, which presents an open lesion subject to many irritants: vaginal discharge, skin secretions, menstrual discharge, urine and faeces.
3 In addition, there is local irritation caused by close-fitting underpants, made of synthetic fibre, girdles, pantihose and slacks, and by laundry detergents.

Treatment and Health Teaching

Instruct the patient as follows:

1 Take pharmacotherapeutic agents as prescribed.
2 Carefully cleanse the perineal area with cotton wool that has been moistened in a warm bland soap solution.
3 Pat dry with a soft washcloth or dry cotton wool.
4 Dust lightly with a nonperfumed powder as an aid in keeping the area dry; cornstarch is very effective.
5 Do not use sprays, perfumed soaps, topical anaesthetic agents—they may compound the problem.

6   Replace synthetic fibre undergarments with loose cotton underclothing.
7   Avoid wearing tight garments over the cotton undergarments
8   Thoroughly wash and rinse all underclothing (use soap, not detergents).

Pruritus

Pruritus is an itching of the vulva which often accompanies chronic infections of genital tract such as trichomoniasis, gonorrhoea or yeast infection—particularly in young women.

Clinical Manifestation

1   Itching followed by scratching and a thickening of tissues.
2   Patient often appears nervous.

Treatment

1   Real cause may be difficult to discover.
2   Cleanliness must be scrupulous.
3   Glucosuria and urinary incontinence must be controlled.
4   Temporary relief is obtained from soothing lotions and ointments.

Condylomata

Condylomata are warty papillary excrescences on the external genitalia.

Cause

Irritation and infection.

Types

1   Pointed type associated with gonorrhoea.
2   Flat type considered syphilitic.

Clinical Manifestations

White discharge causing irritation.

Treatment

Directed to venereal problem.

Kraurosis Vulvae and Leucoplakia

Kraurosis Vulvae is a disease of the vulva; the skin becomes thin, dry, white and easily fissured.
   Leucoplakia is similar to kraurosis; greyish-white patchy thickening and hardening of vulvar tissues with itching and burning. Treated like kraurosis.

Clinical Manifestations

1 As disease progresses, vulva appears shrunken and leathery.
2 Marked itching.
3 May lead to cancer of the vulva.

Treatment

1 Ovarian extract, antihistaminics, vitamin A.
2 Advanced problem may require a vulvectomy (p. 339).

Vulvitis and Abscess of Greater Vestibular Gland (Bartholin's Gland)

Vulvitis is an inflammation of the vulva; the cause may be infection possibly caused by uncleanliness. Common offending organism are *Escherichia coli*, staphylococcus, streptococcus, gonococcus and *Trichomonas vaginalis*.

Clinical Manifestations

1 Burning pain which is worse with intercourse.
2 Red and oedematous tissue with profuse purulent exudate.
3 Acute throbbing pain and swelling between labia indicating vulvovaginal abscess (infection of Bartholin's glands).
4 When the acute infection subsides, the problem tends to become chronic.

Treatment and Nursing Management

1 Advise the patient to remain in bed; administer analgesics for the relief of pain.
2 Employ thermotherapy in the form of hot packs and salt baths for comfort.
3 Administer broad spectrum antibacterial agents to combat infection.
4 Prepare the patient for incision and drainage of the abscess, which will afford immediate relief.
5 Marsupialization (creation of a pouch) with or without biopsy is indicated when there are painful recurrences or obstruction at introitus.
   a. Ice packs are applied intermittently for 24 hours to reduce oedema and provide comfort.
   b. Thereafter, warm salt baths or a perineal heat lamp are comforting.

Cancer of the Vulva

Incidence

1 Most common in elderly women; cancer of the vulva represents 3–4% of all malignancies of female reproductive system.
2 Women seem reluctant to seek medical attention in early phases when ulcer is small and on the skin surface; they tend to delay until the ulcer becomes infected and painful.
3 Early radical vulvectomy with complete node dissection is curative. If the lesion is large and treatment late, cures are unlikely.

Clinical Manifestations

1 In orderly progression, symptoms are: severe vulvar pruritus, reddened, pigmented, whitish or slightly elevated lesions with ulceration.
2 Frequent site.
   a. Labia majora—mid- or anterior portion.
   b. Clitoris.
   c. Encroachment upon urethra in larger lesions.
3 Less frequent sites—fourchette and posterior labial areas.
4 As disease progresses, tissues become oedematous and lymphadenopathy is apparent.
5 Secondary infection is responsible for foul-smelling discharge.

Diagnosis

1 A biopsy is taken after procaine is injected. The entire lesion, when it is small, may be excised; but final treatment is reserved until laboratory studies are completed.
2 Superficial lymph nodes on both sides are palpated for metastasis.
3 Pelvic examination is necessary to determine the extent of the cancer (clinical stage) and to rule out other pelvic neoplastic disease.

Treatment

This depends on type and extent of malignancy:

1 Basal cell carcinoma requires superficial hemivulvectomy.
2 Carcinoma in situ (noninvasive carcinoma) is treated by simple vulvectomy.
3 Invasive carcinoma calls for a radical vulvectomy and bilateral lymph node resection—often requiring removal of the deep pelvic (retroperitoneal) nodes.

Nursing Management

Preoperative Care

1 Shave a wide area to include perineal, pubic and inguinal areas.
2 Encourage the patient to talk about her condition and to ask questions.
   a. Concerns occur regarding fear of mutilation and loss of sexual function.
   b. Possibility of becoming pregnant again may be important to the woman of childbearing age.
   c. The possibility of metastasis, and its effects, cause the cancer patient to be concerned about prognosis, suffering, relation to others in the family, etc.
3 Cleanse the vulva thoroughly 2 or 3 days prior to surgery by using salt baths twice daily.
4 Evacuate the intestinal tract before surgery to provide the advantage of no bowel movements for 2–3 days postoperatively.

Objectives of Postoperative Care

1 To maintain proper drainage and compression of tissues, connect drains to suction.

2   To promote comfort, place patient in semiprone position with legs slightly elevated with a pillow to lessen tension on sutures.
3   To minimize postoperative complications, mobilize patient on the day of surgery.
4   To prevent infection of wound and bladder, the wound may be cleaned daily with warm sterile solutions as prescribed (dilute hydrogen, peroxide, saline, antibacterial solution) and follow with warm water. Usually the raw area is left to heal by granulation.
5   Healing may be expedited by use of skin grafts in some cases.
6   To prevent straining on defecation and wound contamination, offer a low residue diet.
7   To prevent bladder infection, give meticulous care to the vagina and urethral orifice.
8   To encourage social adjustment, maintain a relationship conducive to allowing the patient to voice her concerns.
9   To promote tissue repair, salt baths may be prescribed after the 10th day.
10 To maintain continuity of care upon discharge from the hospital, a follow-up plan is devised to provide for family care, visits by the community nurse and return visits to the surgeon.

Vaginal Fistula

A *fistula* is an abnormal, tortuous opening between two internal hollow organs, or between an internal hollow organ and the exterior of the body.
   Ureterovaginal fistula is an opening between the ureter and vagina.
   Vesicovaginal fistula is an opening between the bladder and vagina.
   Rectovaginal fistula is an opening between the rectum and vagina.

Causes

Vaginal fistula may result from:

1   Obstetric injury.
2   Pelvic surgery (hysterectomy or vaginal reconstructive procedures are most common).
3   Extension of carcinoma or a complication of treatment for carcinoma.

Clinical Manifestations

1   Patient with vesicovaginal fistula will experience continuous trickling of urine into vagina.
2   Patient with rectovaginal fistula will experience faecal incontinence and flatus passed through vagina, a malodorous condition.

Diagnostic Aids in Locating Fistula Site

1   *Methylene blue test.*
      Following instillation of this dye in the bladder:

a. Methylene blue appears in vagina in vesicovaginal fistula.

b. Methylene blue does not appear in vagina in ureterovaginal fistula.

2 *Indigo carmine test*—Following a negative methylene blue test, indigo carmine is injected intravenously.

If dye appears in vagina, this indicates a ureteral fistula.

3 *Intravenous urogram*—(see p. 220) is a valuable test for determining presence of hydroureter or hydronephrosis and position or location of the fistula.

4 *Cystoscopy*—performed to determine number and location of fistulas.

Treatment and Nursing Management

Rarely, a fistula will heal without surgical intervention. The following measures may promote such healing:

1 Maintain cleanliness by encouraging frequent, soothing salt baths and deodorizing douches.

2 Use perineal pads and plastic or rubber pants if required.

3 Provide optimum skin care to prevent excoriation; bland creams or a light dusting of cornstarch may be soothing.

4 Recognize value of meeting psychosocial needs, such as feminine morale boosters (attractive hairdo, nail polish, perfume, new bed jacket, etc.); encourage visitors, diversion, recreation, activities, etc.

Preparation of Patient for Surgery

1 Fistulas recognized at time of delivery should be corrected immediately.

2 Postoperative fistulas are not treated immediately but delayed, sometimes for 2 or 3 months, to allow for treatment of inflammation.

3 Surgery is recommended if tissues are healthy.

4 Maintain adequate nutrition; increase intake of vitamins and protein content of meals.

5 Promote local cleanliness by vaginal flushing and rectal enemata.

6 Administer chemotherpeutic agents to reduce pathogenic flora in intestine.

7 If the patient is postmenopausal, oral oestrogen may be given to promote healthier, more viable tissue in the operative area.

Specific Postoperative Nursing Management

1 Rectovaginal fistula.

a. Limit bowel activity by keeping patient on clear fluids for several days; progress to a low residue, then a full diet.

b. Encourage rest because of the high degree of debilitation.

2 Vesicovaginal fistula.

a. Maintain proper drainage from indwelling catheter—otherwise, pressure may build up and be exerted against newly sutured tissues.

b. Employ gentleness in administering bladder or vaginal irrigations because of tenderness of the operative site.

c. Pay particular attention to urinary output.

Vaginal Infections

Normal Vaginal Condition

1 The vaginal secretions are acid (pH 3.5–4.5); acidity is produced by the conversion of cellular glycogen to lactic acid by Döderlein's bacilli, which normally inhibit the vagina.
2 When oestrogen production is low (before menarche and after menopause) the epithelium is inactive; the cells contain no glycogen, Döderlein's bacilli are absent and the pH is between 6 and 7.
3 *Leucorrhoea* is a whitish vaginal discharge; it is considered normal to have a slight discharge at the time of ovulation or just before menstruation.

Simple Vaginitis

Simple vaginitis is an inflammation of the vagina, with discharge; this may be due to invading organisms, irritation, poor hygiene.

Urethritis often accompanies vaginitis because of the proximity of the urethra to the vagina.

Symptoms

1 Leucorrhoeal discharge with itching, redness, burning and oedema.
2 Micturition and defecation aggravate the above symptoms.

Predisposing Factors

Trichomonas vaginalis, Candida or Monilia, *Haemophilus vaginalis*, pediculosis pubis, contact allergens, excessive perspiration, poor hygiene.

Nursing Assessment

Assessment	Reason
1 Regarding the discharge: When was it first noticed? Any other symptoms?	1 May be suggestive of other pelvic difficulty.
2 Menstrual period: Does patient have dysmenorrhoea, amenorrhoea, dysfunctional bleeding?	2 May be suggestive of other pelvic difficulty. Consider psychogenic problem.
3 Urinary tract: Does she have burning on urination?	3 Suspect cystitis or other urinary difficulties.
4 Type of itching: Is it more prevalent at night?	4 Suspect scabies.
5 Odour: Is odour offensive?	5 Indicative of poor hygiene, foreign body (lost tampon) or other infection.
6 Husband: Does he have a discharge?	6 Suspect reinfection of each other: *Trichomonas, Candida,* gonococcus.

Assessment	Reason
7 Use of deodorant spray, strong douche solution, ointment: What products does she use?	7 Suspect sensitivity, overuse of product.
8 Clothing: Is clothing too tight (girdle, pantihose?	8 Synthetics and excessive perspiration are irritating.
9 Other disease: Ask if patient has diabetes.	9 This generally is linked to vulvovaginitis.
10 Nature of discharge: Cheese-like Frothy Pus-like Thick and foul-smelling Whitish grey, scant, foul odour	Suspect: *Candida* *Trichomonas* Mixed infection Foreign body *Haemophilus vaginalis*

Objectives to Treatment

1 To stimulate the growth of Döderlein's bacilli by administering beta-lactose vaginal suppository; this dissolves with body heat and the sugar then acts.
2 To foster cleanliness by meticulous care after micturition and defecation.
3 To control infection by initiating chemotherapy: insert medication into vagina via applicator or by using a chemotherapeutic cream locally as prescribed.

Trichomonas Vaginalis

A condition produced by a protozoan which infects the vagina and which is evident as a bubbly, greenish-yellow, irritating leucorrhoea and as a red, speckled ('strawberry') cervix.

Characteristics

1 Caused by a pear-shaped mobile flagellate that thrives in an alkaline medium.
2 *Trichomonas vaginalis* is persistent and resistant.
3 Vulvar oedema and hyperaemia occur secondary to irritation of discharge.
4 Remissions may occur; the organism meanwhile remains inaccessible to treatment in the urinary tract.
5 The male partner may carry the organism in his urogenital tract and reinfect his mate.

Objectives of Treatment

1 To destroy infective protozoa give metronidazole (Flagyl) for 10 days (by mouth).
   If above cannot be tolerated or is contraindicated, insert vaginal suppositories containing trichomonocidal compounds (Tricofuron, Devegan).
2 To counteract alkaline preferred environment of infecting organisms, administer acidic vaginal douches.
3 To prevent reinfection, treat male concurrently with Flagyl (metronidazole).

Monilial Vaginitis

A fungal infection caused by *Candida albicans*.

Incidence

Five factors have been found to be significantly associated with the incidence of *Candida albicans*.

1 Drug addiction.
2 Obesity.
3 Pregnancy.
4 Antibiotic therapy.
5 Diabetes mellitus.

Characteristics

1 *Candida albicans* is a normal inhabitant of the intestinal tract and therefore a frequent contaminant of the vagina.
2 Since this fungus thrives in an environment rich in carbohydrates, it is seen commonly in patients with poorly controlled diabetes.
3 This infection is observed in patients who have been on antibiotic or steroid therapy for a while (reduces natural protective organisms in vagina).

Manifestations

1 Vaginal discharge is thick and irritating; white, patchy, cheese-like particles adhere to vaginal walls.
2 Itching is common.
3 Appearance of vulva and vagina varies from normal to that of an acute inflammation.

Objectives of Treatment

1 To eradicate the fungus, apply miconazole nitrate (Monistat) cream, one application daily at bedtime for 14 days, or
   a. Nystatin vaginal tablets twice daily, to be inserted high in the vagina, for 15 days.
   b. Treatment should be continued without interruption even during menstruation.
2 To reduce local irritation and itching apply nystatin or neomycin sulphate cream to the affected areas twice daily.
3 To treat the symptomatic or uncircumcised partner by applying econazole nitrate (Ecostan) cream to the penis twice a day for a week.
4 To discourage the wearing of clothing that tends to promote moisture and heat in the perineal area since *Candida albicans* thrives best in the presence of moisture and heat.

Atrophic (Postmenopausal) Vaginitis

This is a common postmenopausal occurrence. Because of atrophy of vaginal mucosa, the woman is prone to postmenopausal dyspareunia (painful intercourse due to a tight vagina).

1 Signs and symptoms—vesicovaginal itching, burning and pain.

2   Treatment.
   a. Since this is a manifestation of general body oestrogenic depletion, the patient should be treated with oral, water soluble, natural, conjugated oestrogen (Premarin).
   b. The condition reverses itself under treatment, which must be maintained.
   c. If infection is also present, this is treated.
   d. Oestrogenic or cortisone vaginal cream may be prescribed.

Nursing Alert: In the postmenopausal woman, if vaginal bleeding occurs, encourage patient to see her doctor immediately, because cancer may be suspected.

GUIDELINES: Vaginal Irrigation (Douche)

This procedure is only rarely performed.

Purpose

1   To cleanse or disinfect the vagina and adjacent tissues.
2   To soothe inflamed tissue.
3   Local preparation prior to vaginal surgery.

Equipment

Sterile reservoir for irrigating fluid—can or bag
Sterile irrigating fluid as ordered (1000–4000 ml) at 40.5°–43.3°C (105°–110°F)
Tubing, connecting tubes, and clamp (sterile)
Irrigating vaginal nozzle (sterile)
Bedpan or douch pan
Plastic sheet with cloth protection
Sterile cotton balls, cleaning solution
Sterile disposable gloves

Procedure (Fig. 5.16)

Nursing Action	Reason
Preparatory Phase	
1 Have patient micturate before beginning irrigation.	1 A full bladder would prevent adequate distension of vagina by solution.
2 Place patient in dorsal recumbent position.	2 To permit gravity to assist in allowing fluid to reach distal areas of vagina.
3 Drape patient.	3 To prevent chilling and undue exposure.
4 Arrange irrigating receptacle at a level just above patient's hips (not more than 2/3 m, i.e., 2 ft, above hips) so that fluid flows easily but gently.	4 The higher the fluid source, the greater the pressure.

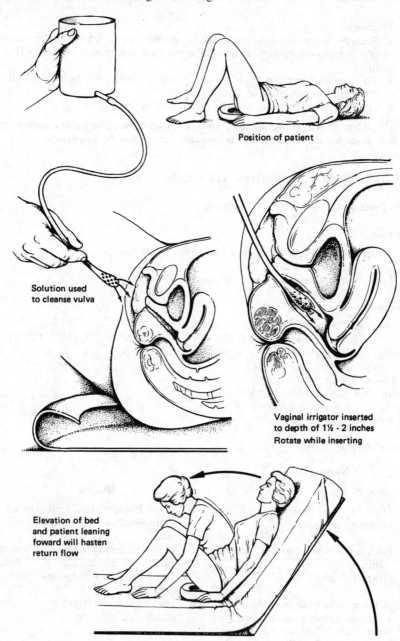

Position of patient

Solution used to cleanse vulva

Vaginal irrigator inserted to depth of 1½ - 2 inches
Rotate while inserting

Elevation of bed and patient leaning foward will hasten return flow

Figure 5.16. Vaginal irrigation.

Nursing Action	Reason

Performance Phase

1. Cleanse vulva by separating labia and allowing solution to flow over area; if insufficient, use cotton balls saturated in soap solution; cleanse from front towards anal area.
2. Allow some solution to flow through tubing and out over nozzle to lubricate it.
3. Insert nozzle gently into vagina in a downwards and backwards direction.

4. Rotate nozzle gently in the vagina during inflow.
5. Clamp tubing when solution is almost all used; remove nozzle and permit patient to sit on bedpan for return flow.

1. Materials found around vaginal meatus may be introduced into vagina and cervix. This is to be avoided.

2. Moisture provides lubrication and less resistance when one surface is moved against another.
3. When the patient is in a dorsal recumbent position, the natural anatomical position of the vagina is in the downwards–backwards direction.
4. All surfaces are irrigated when nozzle is rotated.
5. Gravity will assist in allowing return flow to drain from vaginal tract.

Follow-up Phase

1. Wipe patient dry using cotton balls in a front-to-back direction.
2. Remove bedpan from patient and apply sterile perineal pad.
3. Cleanse equipment with soap and water; dry before storing in well-ventilated area.

1. Drying the area prevents skin excoriation and promotes comfort.

3. This will prolong life of equipment.

GUIDELINES: Vulval Swabbing

Purpose

To cleanse the vulval and perineal area after urination or a bowel movement in order to minimize infection.

Equipment

Sterile jug with irrigating fluid (300–500 ml) 40.5°–43.3°C (105°–110°F)
Sterile gloves, sterile sponge forceps and gauze swabs
Bedpan
Plastic or rubber sheet with cloth protection
Paper bag for disposal of gauze swabs

Procedure (Fig. 5.17)

Preparatory Phase

1   Place patient in dorsal recumbent position with legs flexed and separated.
2   Place protecting sheet under patient.

Nursing Action	Reason
Performance Phase	
1 Pour warmed irrigating solution gently over vulva from a sterile jug.	1 Materials will be flushed from perineal area into bedpan.
2 Cleanse vulval area with gauze swabs held in a sponge holder; use a top–down direction and discard each sponge in a plastic or paper bag after one use, or use sterile gloves.	2 Friction facilitates cleansing process and the removal of soil.
3 Dry perineal area using dry gauze swabs in same fashion as for cleansing.	3 Cleansing from front to back assists in preventing intestinal organisms from entering vaginal area.
Follow-up Phase	
1 Apply sterile perineal pad and hold in place with a T-binder or netalast.	1 To maintain cleanliness and provide comfort for patient.

PROBLEMS RESULTING FROM RELAXED PELVIC MUSCLES

Cystocele

Cystocele is a downward displacement (protrusion) of the bladder into the vagina.

Aetiology

1   Associated with obstetrical trauma to fascia, muscle and ligaments during childbirth (results in poor support).
2   Often becomes apparent years later when genital atrophy associated with ageing occurs.

Clinical Manifestations

1   Fatigue and pelvic pressure.
2   Urinary symptoms—urgency, frequency, incontinence.
3   At times a marked protrusion of anterior wall outside the vulva.
4   Interference with coitus (intercourse).
5   Residual urine and urinary infection.

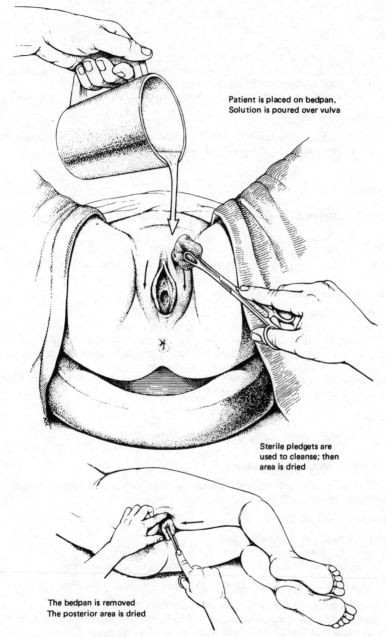

Patient is placed on bedpan.
Solution is poured over vulva

Sterile pledgets are
used to cleanse; then
area is dried

The bedpan is removed
The posterior area is dried

Figure 5.17. Vulval swabbing.

Treatment

Medical

1   Generally, nonsurgical treatment with vaginal pessaries is rarely used.
2   Pelvic floor exercises are useful and may prove beneficial in some women.
    a. Conscious contraction of the pelvic floor or levator ani muscles.
    b. This can be done many times during the day, as one sits, stands or lies in bed.

Surgical Colporrhaphy

An anterior colporrhapy, usually in conjunction with a vaginal hysterectomy and posterior colporrhaphy, is the standard surgical therapy.

Rectocele

Rectocele is displacement (protrusion) of the rectum into the vagina.

Aetiology

Similar to cystocele; however, posterior vaginal wall is weakened in a rectocele.

Clinical Manifestations

1   Disturbance of bowel function: constipation.
2   A 'bearing down' feeling—as though the 'pelvic organs were going to fall out'.
3   Difficulty in faecal evacuation; some patients state that 'they must put their fingers in the vagina to push the mass up' so that defecation can take place.
4   Symptoms disappear in the recumbent position.
5   Incontinence of gas and faeces (in patients with a complete tear between rectum and vagina).

Treatment

Posterior colporrhaphy—repair of posterior vaginal wall.

Objectives of Nursing Management

To Encourage Women who have Problems Resulting from Relaxed Pelvic Muscles to See a Gynaecologist

Patient may tend to:

1   Procrastinate and feel embarrassed.
2   Expect that time will take care of it.
3   Be resigned to the fact that this is a normal result of child-bearing.

To Enable the Patient to Relax During Preoperative Preparation Phase

1   Promote rest particularly in a patient who has been working hard.
2   Suggest semirecumbent position in bed to lessen oedema and congestion.
3   Recognize that this problem often occurs in older women.
4   Prepare intestinal tract by administering an aperient and enema.

To Prevent Pressure on the Suture Line Postoperatively, and to Prevent Infection

1   Encourage micturition to reduce pressure every 4–8 hours, so that no more than 150 ml will accumulate in bladder—catheterization or use of an indwelling catheter may be required.
2   Administer perineal care to the patient after each micturition and defecation.
3   Employ a heat lamp to help dry the incision line and enhance the healing process.
4   Utilize available sprays for anaesthetic and antiseptic effects.
5   Apply an ice pack locally to relieve congestion and discomfort.

To Recognize the Special Care Required by Patients Following Operations for a Complete Perineal Laceration

1   Encourage micturition (catheterization if necessary) to prevent pressure on suture line due to a full bladder.
2   Avoid the use of enemas or a rectal tube for several days to permit wound healing.
3   Provide liquid diet for several days to prevent necessity of a bowel movement.
4   Administer liquid paraffin/Milpar by about the 6th day and follow with an oil retention enema at sign of a possible bowel movement, if necessary.

Displacement of the Uterus

Considerations

1   Normally the cervix lies in the axis of the vagina with the corpus uteri inclined forward on the bladder.
2   Twenty-five percent of all women have, to some degree, the reverse position (retroversion).
    a. The corpus lies back in the posterior cul-de-sac, essentially against the rectum.
    b. This is in no sense pathological; it is normal for such women.

Retroversion

Symptoms

There are no symptoms produced by retroversion. Its association with salpingitis or endometriosis is due to complaints about the disease—not the retroversion.

Treatment

Retroversion is surgically treated when conservative operations are carried out for associated pathology—not the retroversion per se.

Prolapse and Procidentia

Uterine prolapse is a herniation of the uterus through the pelvic floor with a resultant protrusion into the vagina (prolapse) and at times even beyond the introitus (procidentia).

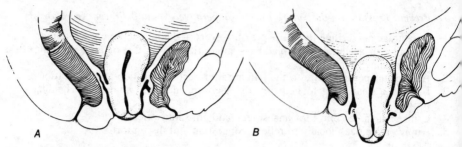

Figure 5.18. Prolapse of the uterus. a. Second degree prolapse of the uterus. Note cervix extends over perineum. b. Third degree prolapse—entire or most of the uterus protrudes. (From: Gray, L A Postgraduate Medicine, 30: 208–209.)

Prolapse

First degree—cervix, without straining or traction, is at the introitus (spread the labia and it is visible).
Second degree—the cervix extends over the perineum (Fig. 5.18a)
Third degree—the entire uterus (or most of it) protrudes (Fig. 5.18b).

Procidentia

The uterus, vaginal vault, rectum and bladder (and in some cases the posterior cul-de-sac) protrude.

Factors Aggravating the Condition

1   Obstetrical trauma.
2   Overstretching of the musculofascial supports.
3   Standing, straining, coughing, lifting a heavy object.
4   Chronic constipation.

Treatment

Surgical correction is recommended treatment.

1   Vaginal hysterectomy—combined with anterior and posterior repair.
2   Fothergill or Manchester repair—anterior and posterior colporrhaphy and amputation of the cervix.
3   For stress incontinence Marshall and Manchetti, Everard William Kelly's repair operation plus suturing the urethra and its supports and the bladder neck.

TUMOURS OF THE UTERUS

Incidence and the Importance of Patient Education

1   In the UK, malignant tumours of the uterus (cervix and endometrium) rank seventh highest among cancers in women.
2   The death rate for uterine cancer has been showing a steady decline; this is attributed to the unremitting education of women, which stresses the importance of annual checkups, including the cytology smear.

3 Nurses need to seek out the reasons why millions of women have not had cytology tests—lack of information, no transportation, inconvenient schedules of clinics, fear of results and general lack of motivation.

Cancer of the Cervix

Aetiology

1 It is most common between the ages of 35 and 55, but it can occur at any age.
2 Early cancer of the cervix is usually asymptomatic; it is almost always curable in its preinvasive stage.
3 Early sexual activity and multiple sexual partners appear to be related to the incidence of this cancer.
4 Viral and chronic infections as well as erosions of the cervix appear to be significant in the development of cancer.
5 Incidence of cancer of the cervix is higher in groups with low socioeconomic status; occurs more often in black women than in white.

Clinical Manifestations

1 There are no symptoms of early cervical carcinoma.
2 Initial symptoms of carcinoma of the cervix.
   a. Post-traumatic bleeding (coitus).
   b. Irregular vaginal bleeding or spotting—between periods (metrorrhagia) or after the menopause; at first it may be very slight, but as disease progresses, bleeding becomes more constant.
   c. Leucorrhoea—increases in amount, becomes dark and foul-smelling because of necrosis and infection of tumour mass.
3 With advanced cancer there is excruciating pain in back and legs relieved only by large doses of narcotics.
4 Later, extreme emaciation and anaemia occur; occasionally there is irregular fever due to secondary infection, peritonitis and abscesses in ulcerating mass.

Diagnosis

1 Physical and gynaecological examination plus a complete history are done initially.
2 Laboratory studies include cytology smear, routine blood examinations plus fasting blood sugar to detect diabetes, total plasma proteins for nutritional status evaluation and bleeding and clotting time.
3 Colposcopy, cone biopsy (cone and punch) are essential diagnostic aids.
4 X-rays should include chest x-ray, intravenous urogram, barium enema, proctoscopic examination and bone studies.
5 Electrocardiogram.

Treatment

1 Carcinoma in situ.
   a. Hysterectomy is usually recommended, with preservation of the ovaries.

    b. Cervical amputation, wide conization, cryosurgery are alternatives to hysterectomy but there is less assurance of complete removal of the lesion.

2 Invasive carcinoma.

    a. Treatment is individualized, depending on the state of the disease, age of patient and general physical condition.

    b. Most often invasive carcinoma is treated by radiation; radical operations are performed on some patients.

3 Health teaching and follow-up emphasis.

    Regardless of the treatment, the nurse must emphasize the necessity of follow-up visits for this patient, since they will be required for the rest of her life:

    a. To determine patient's response to treatment.

    b. To detect spread of metastasis.

    c. To maintain the best health possible.

    d. To take regular cytologic smears.

Cancer of the Corpus Uteri

Incidence

1 Carcinoma of the cervix and carcinoma of the body of the uterus occurred in the ratio of 4:1 a few years ago; at present the ratio is 2:1.

2 Endometrial cancer is most common in women past 40 (peaks at age 55).

3 Seventy-five percent of women with cancer of the corpus uteri are post-menopausal.

4 Often this malignancy occurs when the patient is also affected by obesity, hypertensive cardiovascular diseases and diabetes.

5 Forty years of statistical and laboratory experimentation have failed to show a definite relationship between oestrogen and cancer.

Clinical Manifestations

1 The first evidence is usually a serous, malodorous leucorrhoea—often this is disregarded by the patient.

2 This is followed by a bloody discharge—it may be spotty or it may be steady.

3 Pain is not a symptom until the late stages.

4 Anaemia may result if there is considerable bleeding.

Diagnosis

1 Determine source of bleeding; even if it is coming from the cervical canal, it could be caused by other than carcinoma.

    (If tampon is inserted in the vagina overnight, the place where blood is noted on the dressing may offer a clue to bleeding source, i.e., near the string could suggest bladder source, but near the tip of the tampon would suggest cervix as source).

2 Endometrial biopsy: Positive indicates cancer, whereas negative does not necessarily exclude carcinoma.

3 Fractional curettage is the most effective and accurate diagnostic aid.

Treatment

1   Hysterectomy (p. 357)—depending on stage of lesion.
2   Radiation therapy (p. 356)—depending on stage of lesion.

Myoma of the Uterus

Myomas are benign tumours of the uterus; (they are also called fibromyomas, 'fibroids', and leiomyomas).

Incidence and Characteristics

1   Such tumours occur in about 20% of women past age 30.
2   Myomas rearely develop after menopause; tumours which develop earlier may regress slightly after menopause—but the significant ones do not disappear.
3   Incidence is higher in black women than in white.
4   These tumours tend to be of dense musculofibrous structure; they are encapsulated and tend to form small or large nodules.

Clinical Manifestations

1   Small myomas do not cause symptoms.
2   After myomas (or myomata) grow, the first indication of the presence of a tumour is a palpable mass.
3   Excessive or prolonged menstruation is usually the chief symptom (with little or no change in the menstrual interval); intermenstrual or postmenopausal bleeding may also occur.
4   Pain comes with degeneration of the growth and from pressure on adjacent organs. As myomas grow there may be a sensation of weight—a heavy feeling.
5   Secondary symptoms may be a feeling of lassitude, general weakness, anaemia and lower abdominal discomfort.

Diagnostic Measures

1   These are done primarily to rule out cancer: cytology, dilatation and curettage, cervical biopsy.
2   Diagnosis is made by abdominal and bimanual palpation.

Treatment

1   If patient is of childbearing age and desires children, treatment is conservative.
    a. If small tumour—myomectomy.
    b. If large tumour—hysterectomy.
    c. Ovaries are preserved.
    d. If tumour is large with excessive bleeding—hysteromyomectomy (tumour and uterus removed).
2   For medical and nursing management, see p. 358.

Nursing Care of the Patient Receiving Radiation Therapy of the Uterus

Radiation Therapy

1   Radium, caesium-137, or radioactive cobalt is introduced into the endocervical canal and vagina for a prescribed time; radium (or caesium) is placed in tubes designed to filter out most alpha and beta rays while allowing gamma rays to penetrate into the tumour.
2   Such therapy may be supplemented by external radiation (supervoltage x-ray, telecobalt, or linear accelerator sources) directed over the pelvis in an effort to eliminate cancer spread via lymphatic system; energy may be delivered via anterior or posterior portals over lower abdomen or back, or by means of rotational therapy permitting more uniform exposure of pelvis.
3   Therapy is individualized according to stage of disease and patient's response to and tolerance of radiation.
4   A popular method of treatment involves using radiation therapy externally, then shifting to radium application, and then returning to radiation therapy. Total treatment time is 5–6 weeks.

Patient Preparation for Radium (Caesium) Implantation

1   Doctor explains to the patient the reason why such therapy is advocated; nurse can amplify or answer any questions patient may later raise.
2   Prepare the patient for various preliminary tests (may be done on an outpatient basis)—blood studies, biopsies (endometrial and cervical), chest x-ray, electrocardiogram, cystoscopy.
3   Be available for questions and conversation with the patient regarding any phase of the preliminary studies or treatment.
4   Following admission to the hospital, prepare the patient for surgery and, in addition, prepare the intestinal tract by enemata.
5   Caesium-137 has tended recently to supplant radium because it is less expensive.

Radium Application

1   The dose of caesium is carefully estimated—damage to the rectum and to a lesser extent to the bladder is easily done.
2   The caesium is put into containers in the prescribed dose and inserted into the cervical canal and the vaginal fornices. Spacers are inert and used to keep the container in position. The patient returns with a vaginal pack and an indwelling catheter.

Nursing Management

Nursing Alert: It is imperative to keep the radiation applicators in the uterine canal and to prevent change of position. The patient is nursed in bed until the caesium is removed. Adjust all nursing measures to meet this objective.

While Radium is in Place

1   Check threads from applicators which should be strapped to the patient's thigh. Usually the nurse in charge signs a receipt for the amount of caesium and is given

a lead box to receive the caesium after removal or if accidentally displaced. The threads should be checked 4 hourly.

2   Inspect catheter frequently to ensure straight drainage—a distended bladder may cause severe radiation burns. Observe vulval pad. Carry out vulval toilet and catheter care twice daily.

3   Observe for symptoms of radiation sickness, nausea, vomiting, elevated temperature. Give antiemetics as necessary.

4   Encourage patient to eat by offering small attractive meals to offset poor appetite. Maintain a high fluid intake.

5   Maintain patient on low residue diet to prevent bowel movements which might dislodge apparatus.

6   Administer prophylactic antibiotics, e.g., nitrofurantoin, as prescribed.

7   Provide back care but spend a minimum amount of time at the bedside.

8   Relieve patient of anxiety and fear by utilizing wisely the contact time with the patient. Engage in profitable conversation about her medical and nursing problems.

Radium Removal

1   Can be uncomfortable. Give analgesia, e.g., pethidine, as prescribed.

2   The radiologist will notify when it is time to remove the radium or caesium.

3   Have sterile gloves, long forceps and the lead box ready.

4   Check with the notes the number of tubes applied so that this number is accounted for on removal.

5   Observe radium precautions in handling and returning radium (caesium) to the radiotherapy department.

6   Swab vulval area and remove catheter, then the vaginal pack and finally the threads using the forceps.

7   Check the threads, rinse caesium quickly in Savlon and return to the lead box.

8   After a rest, the patient may get up and move about.

9   Check urinary output is satisfactory. A slight discharge is to be expected after removal of vaginal pack.

10   Full blood count is taken.

11   Tell the patient the importance of monthly follow-up visits to her doctor for the first 6 months, to assess the effects of radiation on the tumour.
    a. Cytological smears are taken; if positive, treatment was not successful. This may mean surgery is required.
    b. If cytology smear is negative and tissue looks satisfactory, follow-up visits after 6 months may be further apart (on a twice yearly basis).

Nursing Alert: Recognize that 5–8% of women who are followed for the treatment of a particular cancer may develop other primary cancers. Therefore, such follow-up visits are essential even though the woman is symptomless.

HYSTERECTOMY

Hysterectomy is the surgical removal of the uterus.

Types of Abdominal Hysterectomy

1   *Subtotal hysterectomy*—corpus of uterus is removed but cervical stump remains.

2 *Total hysterectomy*—entire uterus is removed, including cervix; tubes and ovaries remain.
3 *Total hysterectomy with bilateral salpingo-oophorectomy*—entire uterus, tubes and ovaries are removed.

Psychosocial Considerations

1 Patient may have deep-seated fears that cancer or venereal disease may be discovered.
2 There may be a conflict between recommended medical treatment and her personal religious beliefs.
3 Concerns may be raised regarding the possibility that all phases of her reproductive process may be disturbed.
4 She may be disappointed particularly if she never had children.
5 The patient may feel that she will no longer be able to fulfil her role and needs as a woman.
6 Depression and heightened emotional sensitivity to people and situations may have to be assessed.
7 The complexity of problems which are a mixture of physical, emotional and social factors needs to be considered by the nurse as she assists this patient.
8 Questions arise about how a hysterectomy will affect her participation in sexual relations.
9 The relationship of this woman to her mate and family should be determined.

Specific Preoperative Nursing Management

1 Record base line observations.
2 Blood is taken for grouping and crossmatching and haemoglobin estimation. If anaemia is severe, this may be corrected by blood transfusion in the preoperative stage.
3 An intravenous urogram is performed and blood urea taken if cancer of the cervix is present, in order to exclude renal tract involvement.
4 Administer an aperient or give suppositories.
5 Carry out abdominal and pubic shave followed by bath.

Postoperative Objectives of Nursing Management

See Postoperative Nursing Management (surgical section). In addition, observe the following specific objectives.

To Reduce the Possibility of Bladder Problems

Problems which occur due to the proximity of the bladder to the surgical site.

1 Monitor and record intake and output; administer parenteral fluids as prescribed.
2 Insert an indwelling catheter, if prescribed, because oedema or nerve trauma may cause temporary bladder atony.
3 Remove catheter with doctor's permission after 5 days.
4 Catheterize patient if no catheter is in place and the patient has not micturated after 48 hours, or is uncomfortable.

5 Observe urine output and determine whether there is pooling of residual urine; catheterize patient with a self-retaining catheter after each micturition and note amount. If over 400 ml leave catheter in situ for further 48 hours.

To Relieve the Discomfort of Abdominal Distension

1 A nasogastric tube may be inserted while the patient is in the operating room.
2 Fluids and food may be restricted until peristalsis has resumed.
3 The abdomen is auscultated for bowel sounds to determine onset of peristalsis.
  a. Insert a rectal tube to relieve abdominal flatus.
  b. Permit the patient to sit on edge of bed with feet supported and to get out of bed and walk.
  c. Serve additional fluids and soft diet as peristalsis returns.

To Prevent Respiratory and Cardiovascular Disorders

1 Assist patient in turning every 2 hours and encourage her to take deep breaths.
2 Observe blood loss on pad and report heavy loss.
3 Examine legs for positive Homan's sign (tenderness, pain in calf upon dorsiflexion of foot).
4 Observe legs for the presence of varicosities; promote circulation with special leg exercises.
5 Apply antiembolic stockings as a precautionary measure to promote peripheral circulation, if necessary.

To Counteract Effects Resulting From Removal of a Large Tumour or Unusual Blood Loss

1 Administer high protein diet with iron supplement to combat anaemia.
2 Recommend a girdle or apply an abdominal binder following removal of a large tumour to provide support for relaxed abdominal muscles.

Discharge Planning/Health Teaching

1 A total hysterectomy produces a surgical menopause.
2 Explain to patient the importance of hormonal replacement (prescribed) if she has had a total hysterectomy with oophorectomy/salpingectomy.
3 Advise her against sitting too long at one time, as in driving long distances, because of the possibility of pooling of blood in the pelvis and of thromboembolism.
4 Suggest that patient delay driving a car until the 3rd week postoperative, since even pressing the brake pedal may initiate slight discomfort in the lower abdomen.
5 Tell her to expect a 'tired feeling' for the first few days at home and, therefore, not to plan too many activities for the first week.
6 Have her plan an adjustment schedule in keeping with the expectation that she will be able to perform most of her usual household activities in a month; in 2 months she will feel her 'normal' self.
7 Stress that she should assume employment outside the home only when her doctor indicates; this will depend on the type of work, need for it, etc.

8   Tell her not to feel discouraged if at times during convalescence she experiences depression, feels like crying and seems unusually nervous. This is common, but will not last.

9   Remind her to ask her doctor regarding resumption of various preferred physical activities; note that some of the most strenuous tasks are hanging clothes on a line and using the vacuum cleaner. These tasks should be delayed for several weeks. The patient should not lift heavy objects for a month to 6 week, at least.

10 Determine what the doctor has told the patient regarding resumption of intercourse; reinforce this and explain that too-enthusiastic genital sex may injure the incision site and produce bleeding. In other words, she is to 'go easy' at first. Suggest coital position variation.

11 Emphasize the importance of follow-up physical and gynaecological examinations not only for peace of mind but also to detect any beginning pathology.

ENDOMETRIOSIS

Endometriosis is a disease characterized by displaced groups of cells (resembling the cells that line the uterus) growing aberrantly in the pelvic cavity outside of the uterus.

Incidence

1   Frequency of occurrence is about 25–30% in white women.
2   It is rarely encountered in women of the black race.

Characteristics

1   Pelvic endometriosis attacks many areas. Order of frequency is—the ovary, ureterosacral ligaments, the pouch of Douglas, ureterovesical peritoneum, cervix, umbilicus, laparotomy scars, hernial sacs and appendix.
2   Misplaced endometrium responds to ovarian hormonal stimulation and even depends on this for survival.
    a. When uterus goes through the process of menstruation, this misplaced tissue also bleeds; because there is no outlet for accumulated blood, pain and adhesions result.
    b. At surgery, concealed bleeding is in evidence because lesions are brown or blue-black.
    c. Ovarian cysts in which such bleeding has occurred are referred to as 'chocolate cysts', but all such cysts are not indicative of endometriosis.

Aetiology

1   Embryonic tissue remnants may cover pelvic peritoneum and ovaries and may differentiate as a result of hormonal stimulation.
2   Such tissue may be spread via lymphatic or venous channels.
3   Endometrial tissue, during surgery, may accidentally be transferred by way of instruments (uncommon).

Clinical Manifestations

1 Abnormal uterine bleeding, lower abdominal and pelvic pain, rectal pain and dyspareunia (painful intercourse).
2 Symptoms are more acute during menstruation and subside after menstruation.
3 When a cyst ruptures, symptoms mimic acute appendicitis or ruptured ectopic pregnancy—an acute abdomen is apparent.

Diagnosis

1 Manual rectal and pelvic examinations reveal fixed, tender nodular structures, ovarian abnormalities and uterus fixed by restraining adhesions.
2 X-ray studies, such as barium enema, may demonstrate constrictions suggestive of endometriosis.
3 Laparoscopy is an effective diagnostic aid because tissue can be visualized.

Treatment and Nursing Management

1 It is necessary for the patient to be included in treatment plans so that she knows why a particular method of treatment has been selected and how her role is a vital one in the success of the team effort.
2 Encourage the patient to express her concerns; often false ideas emerge—such as 'perhaps I have endometriosis because I used tampons'.
3 Hormonal therapy is initiated to interrupt ovulation—relieves dysmenorrhoea and temporarily postpones surgery.
4 Surgery when indicated is directed toward resection of cysts and lysis of adhesions.
5 Likelihood of recurrence of endometriosis is high; conservative and minor surgery is done during childbearing years.
6 Ultimate treatment requires more radical procedures when conservative measures fail (total hysterectomy).

OVARIAN CANCER

Ovarian cancer is high risk cancer of the ovary.

Incidence

1 Of women over 40, 10 out of every 1000 are affected.
2 Of the ten affected, only one or two will survive.

Diagnosis

1 Because of the high risk nature of ovarian cancer, it is important that every effort be made to diagnose this condition earlier.
2 The nurse should recognize those conditions in a woman which collectively place her in a high-risk category. High risk individuals include women who are*
   a. Infertile.

* Barber, H R K et al (1974) Ovarian cancer, CA—A Cancer Journal for Clinicians, 24: 339.

   b. Anovulatory.
   c. Nulliparous.
   d. Habitual aborters.
3 If only *one* of the above conditions is present, along with *three* of the following symptoms, the patient should be labelled as 'High Risk'.
   a. Increasing premenstrual tension.
   b. Irregular menses.
   c. Menorrhagia with breast tenderness.
   d. An early menopause.
4 Semiannual gynaecological examination and cervical cytology.
5 Investigate any ovarian enlargement by laparoscopy or laparotomy.
   This is particularly true of postmenopausal women whose ovaries should not be palpable.

Treatment

Surgical oophorectomy. Depending on extent, radiation and chemotherapy may be required.

PELVIC INFECTION

All structures in the pelvic cavity can become infected. Two types can be roughly distinguished according to the site of the infection and its spread.

Aetiology

Gonoccocal and Mixed Infection

1 Gonococcal infection originates in the urethra, cervix and/or rectum.
2 If reinfection does occur following proper treatment, the disease is self-limiting.
3 Most frequently women are reinfected, and the secondary invaders (streptococcus, staphylococcus, *Escherichia coli*, etc.) take over. Accordingly, as a rule, what started as a self-limiting salpingitis becomes a chronic process. The disease is spread by way of the uterine canal into the tube and through the fimbria (Fig. 5.19).
4 As a rule, the endometritis resulting from gonorrhoea is shortlived.
5 The largest group of infections are created by pelvic cellulitis—i.e., endometritis from a complication of pregnancy or an intrauterine device.
6 Here all the cervical and vaginal pathogens are offenders. They spread by way of the lymphatics and blood vessels.
7 Cellulitis tends to be unilateral whereas gonorrhoea is a bilateral process.
8 Tuberculous endometritis is a cause of infertility.

Clinical Manifestations

1 Abdominal pain, nausea and vomiting, temperature elevation, malaise.
2 Leucocytosis.
3 Malodorous, purulent vaginal discharge.

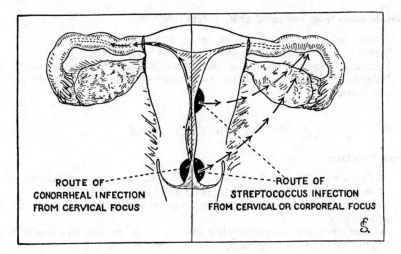

ROUTE OF
GONORRHEAL INFECTION
FROM CERVICAL FOCUS

ROUTE OF
STREPTOCOCCUS INFECTION
FROM CERVICAL OR CORPOREAL FOCUS

Figure 5.19. Two chief routes of pelvic infection. (From: Novak Textbook of Gynecology, Williams and Wilkins.)

Treatment and Nursing Management

Objectives

To control the spread of infection within the patient.
To prevent the spread of infection to others, including the nurse.

1 Place patient in a semirecumbent position to facilitate drainage.
2 Avoid the use of tampons and do not catheterize this patient in order to minimize spread of infection.
3 Support patient nutritionally with attractive, well-balanced meals.
4 Vaginal douches are occasionally prescribed to remove infected material before commencing treatment.
5 Administer appropriate antibiotics and chemotherapeutic agents as prescribed.
6 Control spread of infection by the following safeguards:
   a. Handle perineal pads with extreme precautions:
      (1) Use an instrument or gloves.
      (2) Deposit pad in paper bag for proper disposal.
   b. Wash hands carefully before and after patient contacts.
   c. Disinfect utensils, bedpans, toilet seats and linen.
      Adopt procedure appropriate for specific organism.
   d. Instruct patient in procedure to protect herself from reinfection and to prevent spread to others.
7 Record vital signs, patient responses (physical and mental) to therapy and nature and amount of vaginal discharge.
8 Reconize the depressing nature of the disease and that the patient needs support and understanding, particularly when she has discomfort and vague symptoms.

Complications from Untreated or Recurrent Infection

1   Chronic pelvic discomfort; disease becomes rampant.
2   Sterility occurs because of closing of fallopian tubes with scar tissue.
3   Ectopic pregnancy is possible if fertilized egg is unable to pass stricture.
4   Inflammatory masses may develop, eventually requiring removal of uterus, tubes and ovaries.

FERTILITY CONTROL

Basic Principles

1   The nurse should be familiar with the application, advantages and disadvantages of the various methods of contraception available.
2   The most effective method is the one a woman selects for herself and will use consistently.
3   Women are entitled to contraceptive advice as part of good medical care without the burden of moral judgement.

Contraceptive Methods

NOTE: Failure rate (pregnancy) is determined by the experience of 100 women for 1 year and is expressed as . . . pregnancies per 100 woman years.

Coitus Interruptus

This is the withdrawal of the penis from the vagina when ejaculation is imminent.

1   Indications—effective when mechanical devices are unavailable.
2   Contraindications.
    a. When male is not able to exert self-control.
    b. Ineffective when premature ejaculation occurs—this is true of almost 50% of males.
3   Undesirable effects.
    a. Failure rate is between 35–40%.
    b. Psychological ill effects for both male and female.
    c. Subsequent prostatitis has been substantiated.

Condom

Application of a rubber sheath worn over the penis by the male during coitus.

1   Procedure for use and precautions.
    a. Place condom over erect penis.
    b. Leave a dead space at the tip of the condom (from which air has been expelled) to allow room for ejaculate.
    c. Lubricate (spermicidal) exterior of condom—as an added precaution.
    d. Avoid leaving condom in vagina during withdrawal; this is facilitated by grasping ring around top of condom at time of withdrawal.
2   Advantages.
    a. Inexpensive and easy to use.

b. Protects against pregnancy and offers some protection against venereal disease.

c. May lessen premature ejaculation.

3 Disadvantages.

    a. May dull sensation somewhat for male and female.

    b. Requires an erect penis for application.

    c. Condom may tear or rupture and thus be ineffective.

    d. May cause a contact dermatitis.

4 Failure rate (pregnancy).

    Varies from 15 to 35 (various authorities) undesired pregnancies per 100 woman years.

NOTE: If condom ruptures the female should see her gynaecologist immediately to obtain 'morning after pill' (high oestrogen) for pregnancy interception.

Diaphragm

A rubber dome-shaped device with a flexible wire rim which is inserted in the vagina to fit snugly behind pubic bone and over the cervix into the posterior fornix. It is used to prevent sperm from reaching the cervical os. Spermicidal jelly is often used on both sides of the diaphragm.

1 Indications—preferred by women who:

    a. Object to a device in utero.

    b. Object to hormonal or chemical contraceptives.

    c. Do not object to insertion of the diaphragm immediately prior to intercourse.

2 Procedure for insertion and follow-up.

    a. Bimanual pelvic examination and cytology smear are preliminary to measurement for a diaphragm.

    b. Measure depth of vagina; select largest diaphragm that can be retained comfortably; if too small, the device will be displaced during intercourse.

    c. Teach the patient how to insert diaphragm behind lower edge of pubic bone; use spermicidal jelly or cream for additional contraceptive action.

    d. Instruct her to retain diaphragm for 6–8 hours after intercourse.

    e. Remind patient of annual gynaecological examination.

    f. Inform patient that a larger diaphragm may be necessary after a pregnancy.

3 Failure rate (pregnancy).

    15 undesired pregnancies per 100 woman years of using diaphragm.

Vaginal Foam

This is a spermicidal cushioning foam that is available as cream, jel, aerosol or tablet; all except the tablet are effective immediately—tablets require 5–10 min to dissolve.

1 Advantages:

    a. Requires little instruction; a favourite method with lower socioeconomic groups.

    b. May be used to advantage with coitus interruptus.

2 Disadvantage:

    Higher failure rate than other contraceptive methods.

3 Failure rate (pregnancy):
Somewhere between 35 and 45 per 100 woman years.

Intrauterine Device (IUD)

A device made of metal or plastic that fits inside the uterus; it may be in the shape of a spiral, loop, shield or ring.

Nursing Alert: It is now apparent that the IUD is more dangerous than ever antici-pated. Endometritis, ovarian abscesses, ruptured uteri and their consequences have left a trail of pelvic surgery and permanent crippling that cannot be ignored.

1 Indications:
a. When hormonal medications appear to be contraindicated.
b. When motivation and other resources are lacking, as a last resort.
2 Contraindications:
a. Inflammation or infection of cervix, uterus or uterine tubes.
b. Objections on the part of the woman to a foreign device in her uterus.
c. Severe dysmenorrhoea.
3 Procedure for insertion and follow-up:
a. A pelvic examination and a cytology smear.
b. Calibre of interior of the uterus determined by means of sounding.
c. Insertion of IUD with the aid of a plastic inserter at time of menstruation (cervix is dilated and doctor knows patient is not pregnant).
d. Patient instruction as to the nature of the device and detection of nylon thread to determine its placement.
e. Must be checked by a doctor in a month and at yearly intervals.
4 Undesirable effects:
a. Excessive staining or bleeding; irregular bleeding between periods.
b. Excessive cramps which persist.
c. Expulsion of device spontaneously. (This accounts for 20–30% of a combina-tion of expulsion and patient request for removal.)
d. Copper devices have two disadvantages
(1) Copper is a potentially toxic metal.
(2) The device must be removed and reinserted every 2 years.

Nursing Alert: If the patient is pregnant when an IUD is inserted, she may suffer septic abortion and possibly fatal septicaemic shock; hence the wisdom of having the device inserted during menstruation.

5 IUD combined with steroid (Progestasert).
This is an intrauterine device that includes hormonal action. When inserted in the uterus, the T-shaped device delivers a small daily dose of natural proges-terone for 12 months. Hormone acts locally in uterus to prevent pregnancy but not ovulation.
a. Advantage:
Progesterone does not enter patient circulation to cause systemic effects simi-lar to those occurring with oral contraceptives.
b. Disadvantages:
Similar to IUD listed above.

Oral Fertility Control—the 'Pill'

1 Basis of operation of oral contraceptives:
    Oral synthetic preparations of oestrogens and progesterone are used. It is believed that in the presence of sufficient amounts of these synthetic compounds, the hypothalamus fails to secrete the usual LH releasing factor and its stimulating product LH which normally occurs 12–14 days after the onset of the monthly menstrual cycle and is essential to ovulation.

2 Indications:
    a. For those desirous of a highly effective contraceptive with no special preparation immediately before intercourse.
    b. For women who will conscientiously adhere to a daily plan of pill-taking.

3 Contraindications:
    a. A complete physical examination is required prior to taking the 'pill' and 12-month checkups thereafter.
    b. Contraindications are debatable and often not substantiated by hard, reliable data.

4 Methods:
    a. Combined steroid therapy.
    A pill with an oestrogen and progestogen usually taken 20 days during each month beginning on the 5th day after the onset of menstruation.
    b. Microprogestational therapy.
    Low dosage of progestational drug given continuously:
        Androgens—19-carbon compounds.
        Progesterone—21-carbon compounds.
        Oestrogens—Mestranol and ethrynyl oestradiol.

5 Disadvantages:
    a. Because oral contraceptives are potent drugs there may be side-effects: increased incidence of thromboembolic disease, essential hypertension, disturbance of carbohydrate metabolism—diabetes, speeding of the process of arteriosclerosis in those with a predisposition.
    b. They require close supervision by a doctor.
    c. Interference with laboratory diagnostic procedures: sedimentation rate, thyroid test for protein-bound iodine or thyroxine, cervical smears and biopsy.

6 Side-effects—occur in approximately 1–3% of women on low-dose pill.

7 Failure rate (pregnancy)
    Combined—less than 1 pregnancy per 100 woman years.

Sterilization Procedures

Indications

1 The patient's desire:
    a. Socioeconomic reasons.
    b. Therapeutic or eugenic reasons to prevent a pregnancy that might endanger the mother's life.

2 Legal considerations:
    a. Laws much less rigid than those governing therapeutic abortion.
    b. Written consent required from a legally responsible and informed person.

3 Incidence and indications:
   a. Increasing numbers are performed annually in the UK.
   b. Done for multiparity, two or more previous caesarean sections, hypertensive cardiovascular disease.
   c. Done for other reasons: vaginal plastic procedures, for inheritable life-threatening diseases.

Tubal Sterilization

1 Types:
   a. Tubal ligation with or without resection.
   b. Tubal ligation with or without crushing.
   c. Tubal transection and burying of stumps.
   d. Cornual resection.
   e. Cornual occlusion utilizing cautery.
2 Approaches:
   a. Abdominal.
   b. After a caesarean section.
   c. Vaginally.
3 Evaluation:
   a. There are advantages and disadvantages to each of the above—the individual situation must be considered.
   b. Reversible methods of tubal occlusion or semipermanent sterilization using metal clips or chemical injections are still experimental.
4 Laparoscopy:
   a. A procedure in which coagulation and transection of the isthmic tubal segments is done through a laparoscope (an electrical current is passed for 3–5 s to cut and coagulate tube).
   b. The procedure is considered rapid, safe and effective.
   c. The patient is discharged from the hospital about 3 hours postoperatively with minimal discomfort; procedure can be done on an outpatient basis.
   d. Effectiveness:
      (1) Hysterosalpingography done 12 weeks postoperatively confirms tubal occlusion in 98% of patients.
      (2) No adverse effects occur in sex relations, menstrual function or outward bodily appearance.
   e. Hazards:
      (1) Pulmonary embolism, haemorrhage, infection.
      (2) Tubal pregnancy.
      (3) Some women are disturbed emotionally by procedure; however, 90% of patients who request this have no subsequent regret.

Vasectomy (See p. 321)

Source of information: local family planning clinics and own general practitioner.

3. Conditions of the Breast

CONDITIONS OF THE NIPPLE

Fissures and Bleeding

Clinical Identification and Manifestations

Fissure of Nipple	*Bleeding from Nipple*

A *fissure* of the nipple is a longitudinal type of ulcer that occasionally develops in the breast of a nursing mother.

a. Nipple appears sore and irritated.
b. Bleeding from nipple.

Bloody discharge—usually on edge of areola.

Causes

1 Lack of preparation of nipples in prenatal period.

2 Condition aggravated by sucking infant.

1 Most commonly due to wart-like papilloma in one of larger collecting ducts at edge of areola.

2 Occasionally a malignancy is responsible (Fig. 5.20, cytology examination).

Health Teaching

1 Keep nipple clean by washing and drying after each nursing period.
2 In prenatal period, wash, dry and lubricate nipples in preparation for nursing.

Treatment and Nursing Management

1 Wash nipples with sterile saline solution.

1 Surgery for palpable mass.
   a. Duct is identified.
   b. Papilloma is excised (or a wedge of breast from area producing the bleeding is excised if no gross papilloma is identified) through a small periareolar incision—send for laboratory analysis.
   c. Sterile dressings applied.

2 Use artificial nipple for nursing.

2 If no palpable mass, mammography and xerography.

3 If above does not initiate healing process, stop nursing and use breast pump.

Paget's Disease of the Breast

Paget's disease is a cancer that originates in the major lactiferous ductal system and extends into the nipple (Fig. 5.21).

Clinical Evidence

1   Begins as a mild eczema of the nipple: scaling, crust formation, redness, weeping and erosion.
2   Spreads from nipple to areola to part of breast and then ulcerates.
3   A palpable mass may be felt.
4   Retraction of nipple may be noted—a malignant manifestation.

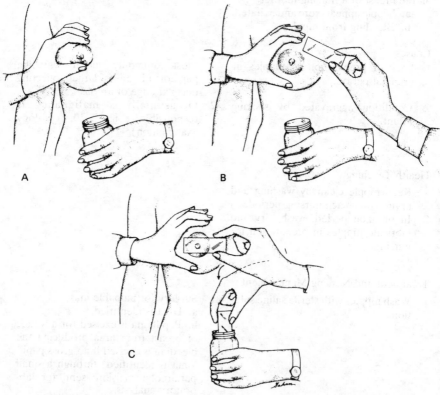

Figure 5.20. Obtaining nipple discharge specimen for cytological examination (1) Wash nipple gently with cotton swab; pat dry. (2) Gently strip duct and express fluid only until a small pea-sized drop appears on nipple. (3) Solicit assistance of patient in holding container of fixative solution near breast to receive the prepared slide. (4) Stabilize breast with fingers and thumb of one hand (a). (5) Gently place one end of slide on nipple (b) rapidly drawn slide across nipple and immediately drop into fixative solution (c). (6) This may be repeated to secure additional specimens if necessary.

Treatment and Prognosis: Nursing Implications

1   Early and total mastectomy

2 Survival Rate:*	Negative Axilla Nodes	Positive Nodes in Axilla
Without palpable mass	96–97%	80%
With palpable mass	75%	41%

* From: Howland, S (Ed) (1973) Paget's disease of the nipple, Clinical Bulletin, 3: 143

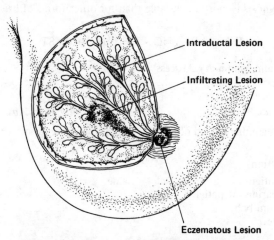

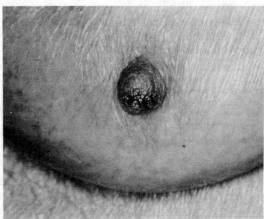

Figure 5.21. Paget's disease of the nipple originates as a cancer in the major lactiferous duct system and extends into the nipple. It is an eczematoid lesion of the nipple and is characterized by scaling and crust formation, erosion or sometimes ulceration as noted in the lower illustration. NOTE: 1. Positive results are significant. 2. Negative results may be false negatives. This test is never used alone, but in conjunction with other dianostic tests. (From: Howland, S (Ed) (1973) Paget's disease of the nipple, Clinical Bulletin, 3: 142.)

3   The nursing implication here is to emphasize the importance of *early* diagnosis.
   a. Paget's disease can usually be diagnosed at an early stage because it can be seen.
   b. Deep wedge biopsy of the nipple and underlying ducts may be done under local anaesthesia for suspicious, persistent lesions of the nipple and areola.
   c. In majority of patients with early Paget's disease in which no mass is clinically palpable and regional lymph nodes are negative, a modified radical mastectomy is done.
   d. The prognosis is more favourable than for other forms of breast cancer.

INFLAMMATION OF THE BREAST

Acute Mastitis and Mammary Abscess

Incidence

Acute Mastitis	*Mammary Abscess*
May occur at beginning or end of lactation.	Often follows acute mastitis.

Source of Infection

1 Hands of patient.	Same.
2 Personnel caring for patient.	
3 Infection from baby.	
4 Blood-borne.	

Clinical Manifestations

1 Infection attacks duct causing stagnation of milk in lobules.	1 Area is very sensitive, appears dusky red.
2 Dull pain occurs in the area affected.	2 Pus may be expressed from nipple. (See Fig. 5.20, nipple discharge for cytology.)
3 Breast feels doughy and tough.	3 Mass is palpable.
4 May also have a discharging nipple.	

Treatment and Nursing Management

1 Have patient stop breast feeding.	1 Administer antibiotics and chemotherapy as prescribed.
2 Evacuate milk by means of a breast pump.	2 Incise and drain.
3 Administer chemotherapeutic agents as prescribed.	3 Apply hot wet dressings to increase drainage and hasten resolution.
4 Give Bromocriptine to arrest secretory phase.	
5 Have patient wear firm breast support.	
6 Encourage patient to practise meticulous personal hygiene.	

FIBROCYSTIC DISEASE

Fibrocystic disease is a mammary dysplasia characterized by increased formation of fibrous tissue, hyperplasia of the epithelial cells of the ducts and breast glands and dilatation of the ducts. It is related to the cyclic stimulation of the breast by oestrogen, but represents a departure from the normal stimulation and regression pattern of this process.

Incidence

1   The most common lesion of the female breast; three to four times more prevalent than cancer.
2   Overgrowth of fibrous tissue around ducts; dilatation of the ducts to form cysts; epithelial hyperplasia in ducts on glands.
3   Occurs usually in women between 30 and 50 and is endocrine related.

Clinical Manifestations

1   Patient complains of an uncomfortable feeling in the breast.
2   Cysts or lumps are usually firm, single or multiple smooth, round masses; bilateral.
3   They are tender on palpation or pressure and slightly mobile.
4   Pain may be of the 'shooting' type and may be aggravated by congestion before a menstrual period.

Treatment and Nursing Management

1   Aspiration
    a. Patient is placed in supine position. Under aseptic precautions, skin area is cleaned with a skin antiseptic.
    b. Local anaesthesia is given.
    c. The doctor immobilizes cyst with thumb and index finger of one hand.
    d. Using a 20 ml syringe and 16 or 18 gauge needle, the cyst is penetrated and aspirated.
2   Excision.
    If cyst refills within a week or two, excisional biopsy is usually performed.
3   The nurse emphasizes the importance of frequent re-examinations.
    a. Individuals with fibrocystic disease have an increased incidence of subsequent malignancy.
    b. Self-examination is difficult in the markedly fibrotic breast.

NOTE: The palpable changes of fibrocystic disease may mask an underlying cancer.

TUMOURS OF THE BREAST

Fibroadenomata

Clinical Manifestations

1   Firm, round, movable, benign tumours of the breast.

2 Appear in breasts of girls in their late teens or early twenties.
3 No pain or tenderness.

Treatment

Removal through a small incision.

Prognosis

No malignant potential.

GUIDELINES: Examination of the Breast by the Nurse

Purpose

1 To detect abnormalities in the breasts.
2 To teach a woman how to perform breast self-examination.

Equipment

A good lamp and privacy.

Procedure

Nursing Action	Reason
Preparatory Phase and Superficial Examination	
1 Have the woman strip to her waist and sit comfortably, facing the examiner.	1 This provides an opportunity to visually observe breasts for lack of symmetry and for gross signs such as redness, irritated nipple, dimpling, orange-peel skin.
2 Wash your hands under warm water and dry them; powder if they feel 'sticky'.	2 The breast is sensitive to cold.
Examination	
1 Palpate supraclavicular area.	1 Note whether lymph nodes are enlarged, fixed, movable or difficult to locate.
2 Palpate axillary nodes; hold woman's forearm in your left palm while you check nodes with your right fingertips. Repeat on other side.	2 Same as 1 above.
3 Instruct patient to lie down with her right arm under her head. Place a small pillow under the right shoulder.	3 This will spread breast tissue evenly over chest wall.

Nursing Action	Reason
4 With the flattened surface of two or three fingers, gently palpate breast tissue beginning at the upper outer quadrant. **a.** Proceed in an orderly pattern around the breast and repeat the first quarter examined. **b.** Repeat procedure for other breast.	4 The sensitive fingers proceeding in a kneading fashion can detect thickened, lumpy or 'buckshot' tissue between the patient's skin and chest wall. Since the majority of breast lesions are in the upper outer quadrant, this segment is double checked.
5 Recognize that there is a prolongation of the axillary extension of normal breast tissue which may extend high into the axilla.	5 This is normal if symmetrical; abnormal if asymmetrical.
6 Check the areolar area for crustiness, nipple discharge, signs of infection.	6 Prepare to collect a discharge specimen for cytology if indicated (see Fig. 5.20, p. 370).
7 Record findings and report abnormalities to the doctor.	
8 Instruct the patient in performing self-examination on her own (see p. 378). Encourage her to ask questions; provide her with appropriate literature.	8 Ninety-five percent of women discover their own abnormalities.

Cancer of the Breast

Incidence

1 Breast cancer is the leading cause of cancer incidence and death in women today.
2 One of every four women having an initial breast biopsy will have a malignany.
3 Despite all efforts to date, breast cancer death rate remains high.
4 Survival rate for all breast cancer patients, treated or untreated, is roughly 50%.
5 About 95% of patients discover their condition themselves through breast self-examination:
 a. 60% will have spread to axillary lymph nodes; 5-year survival rate is 40–45%.
 b. 40% will be localized to breast; 5-year survival rate is 80–85%.

Risk Factors in Breast Cancer*

Major Risk Factors

1 Sex—99% occur in females.
2 Age—75% are clinically detectable over age 40.
3 Family history—risk very high when there is any history of breast cancer in blood relatives.
4 Parity—decreased risk three to fourfold if first birth is before 18 years of age. Decrease in risk continues, but at a declining rate, up to age 25 for first parity.
 Increased risks in unmarried women, infertile women, women with less than

* Adapted from Leis (1975) Risk factors in breast cancer, AORN Journal, 22: 723–729.

three children and women who have first child after 34. Lower incidence of breast cancer with early parity.

5   Previous cancer in one breast—risk of developing cancer in second breast after first breast is removed because of cancer is about five times greater than for women in general population.

6   Precancerous mastopathy type of fibrocystic disease.

Prominent Risk Factors

1   Prolonged total menstrual activity. Increased incidence under the following circumstances:
   a. When menarche occurs before 12 years of age.
   b. In those with 30 or more years of menstrual activity.
   c. When menopause occurs after 55.

2   Other organ cancers such as ovary, colon, endometrium.

Possible Risk Factors

1   Heavy radiation exposure.
2   Immunodeficiency.
3   Exogenous oestrogen administration.

Clinical Manifestations (Fig. 5.22)

1   Early signs are insidious.
2   A nontender lump appears in the breast, most frequently in the upper outer quadrant; it may be movable and isolated.
3   Pain usually is absent except in the late stages.
4   Retraction or dimpling of the skin over the mass may be noted.
5   On mirror examination, asymmetry may be observed—the affected breast appears more elevated than the other.
6   Nipple retraction or nipple bleeding may be apparent.
7   Later, the breast becomes more fixed to the chest wall.
8   Nodular axillary masses may appear.
9   Ulceration appears in late stages.

Diagnosis

Breast Self-examination

1   Clinical value.
   a. Experience has verified that 95% of breast cancers are found by women themselves.
   b. When women discover lumps in their breasts at a very early stage, surgery can save 70–80% of proven cases.

2   Health teaching.
   a. Encourage women to examine their breasts once a month, just after the menstrual period and, equally important, at regular monthly intervals after the cessation of menses (Fig. 5.23).
   b. The breast can be examined in the sitting or standing position noting in a mirror any contour changes and asymmetry.

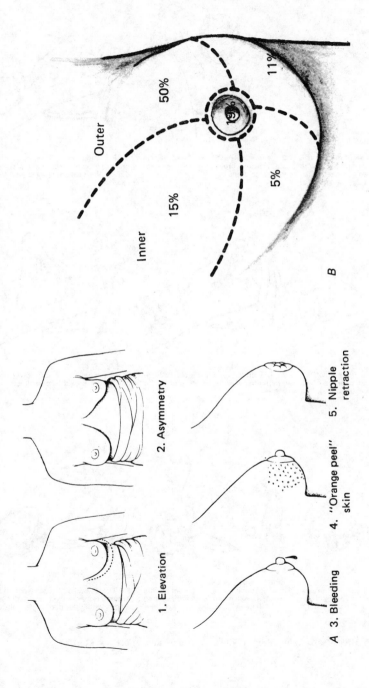

Figure 5.22. a. Signs of cancer of the breast. b. Distribution of carcinomas in different areas of breast.

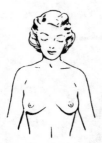

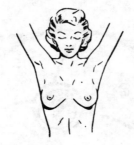

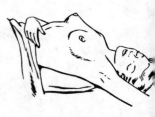

1. Careful examination of the breasts before a mirror for symmetry in size and shape, noting any puckering or dimpling of the skin or retraction of the nipple.

2. Arms raised over head, again studying the breasts in the mirror for the same signs.

3. Reclining on bed with flat pillow or folded bath towel under the shoulder on the same side as breast to be examined.

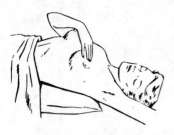

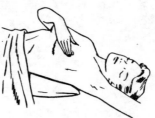

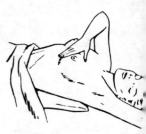

4. To examine the inner half of the breast the arm is raised over the head. Beginning at the breastbone and, in a series of steps, the inner half of the breast is palpated.

5. The area over the nipple is carefully palpated with the flat part of the fingers.

6. Examination of the lower inner half of the breast is completed.

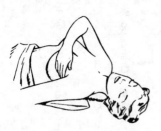

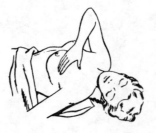

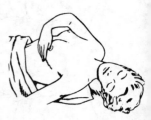

7. With arm down at side self examination of breasts continues by carefully feeling the tissues which extend to the armpit.

8. The upper outer quadrant of the breast is examined with the flat part of the fingers.

9. The lower outer quadrant of the breast is examined in successive stages with flat part of the fingers.

Figure 5.23. Breast self-examination. (Courtesy: American Cancer Society.)

c. Then the breast is examined in the supine position with the breast spread out on the chest wall; use the flattened, more sensitive surface of the fingers to gently knead breast tissue in the search for abnormalities.

d. Since most of the lesions occur in the upper outer quadrant (Fig. 5.22b), an effective pattern to follow is to start the examination in the upper outer quadrant, proceed around the breast, and repeat (at the end) the upper outer quadrant. (In this manner, five-fourths of the breast are examined.)

e. When in doubt, compare findings with opposite breast.

3   Suggestions for patients unable to or who are having difficulty doing self-examination:

a. Determine the problem:

(1) If patient complains of tenderness, gentle self-examination may be more effective and less painful than examination by someone else.

(2) For the woman who has cysts or lumps, recommend professional examination annually and instruct her in detecting changes from one month to the next.

(3) If the patient has large pendulous breasts, encourage her to lie on her back and perform self-examination slowly and in a specific pattern or order.

b. Recommend other diagnostic aids periodically—mammography, thermography, xeroradiography (below) as condition indicates.

4   Health teaching.

a. Tell women's organizations about the breast self-examination film and advise them to see it.

b. Arrange for local showings of the film.

c. Take part in the discussion of the film. Be prepared—know the signs that may mean breast cancer.

d. Help to create healthy psychological attitudes.

e. Know the resources within the community where medical help is available, the doctors' offices, nearby hospitals, cancer clinics or cancer hospitals.

Physical Examination

1   Annual physical checkup should include breast examination and palpation.

2   Twice-a-year examination recommended for women with a family history of cancer.

Mammography

X-ray of breast without injection of contrast medium; three views: (i) craniocaudal, (ii) mediolateral and (iii) axillary.

Indications: Greatest value is in detecting suspicious area before a 'lump' is felt. Hence, earlier diagnosis.

1   Breast disease evident in form of a questionable lump.

2   Family history of breast cancer.

3   Previous breast biopsy.

4   Lumpy or very large breasts which are difficult to examine.

5   Screening the opposite breast in a woman with a mass on one side.

6   Cancerophobia (fear of cancer).

NOTE: How frequently the patient can be exposed to mammography radiation is still controversial. Newer techniques are reducing the amount of radiation exposure.

Current trend is to avoid mammography as a routine screening procedure in young menstruating women.

Thermography

Infrared photography which may detect signs of abnormal circulation (of limited value).

1 By using heat sensing equipment, minute amounts of heat generated in and around areas of increased blood supply may be detected.
2 Official statement about thermography made Dec. 1975 by the American Thermographic Society:
'Thermography is a complementary diagnostic tool that may be useful in the evaluation of breast disease when combined with both physical examination under the supervision of a qualified physician and mammography by a trained radiologist.'

Xerography

A special x-ray in which a selenium-coated plate is subjected to an electrical charge; after the x-ray exposure is made, the plate is carefully developed. The xerogram portrays all tissue in bas-relief, like a 'positive' film instead of the 'negative'.

Transillumination

By using a powerful cold light in a completely darkened room, breast tissue can be illuminated and a cyst or neoplasm can easily be demonstrated. The method is not satisfactory in fibrosis because of the density of tissue.

Ultrasound Holography

A more recent low-cost noninvasive technique that is still being evaluated.

Biopsy

1 *Aspiration* (performed by doctor).
Purpose: This is a simple, rapid and accurate procedure to detect breast cancer.
a. Tumour or cyst is immobilized between two fingers to stabilize it during needle insertion (Fig. 5.24)
b. A vacuum is gently created in syringe by pulling back and forth on plunger; allow pressure to equalize before withdrawing needle.
c. The contents of the needle are spread on a glass slide; a further specimen is spread with a second glass slide held at right angles.

NOTE: Positive results are significant. Negative results are ignored; other clinical evaluations must be done.

2 *Incisional.*
A piece of tissue is obtained in the operating room and sent to the laboratory for frozen section, which is then stained and examined under the microscope.

Classification of Breast Tumours
See table 5.2.

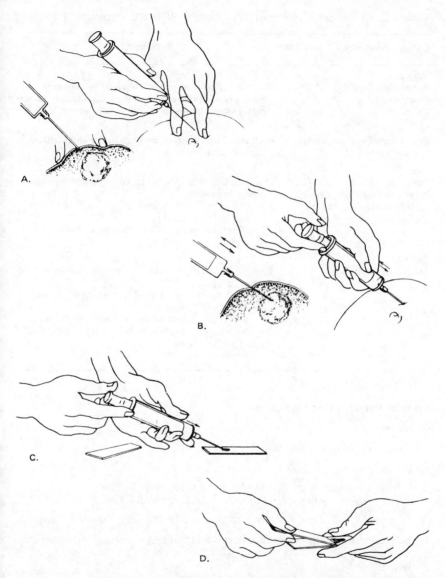

Figure 5.24. Aspiration cytology. a. Tumour is immobilzed with two fingers before the needle is inserted. b. A vacuum is created by withdrawing the plunger slowly but forcefully several times. Before removing the needle, the pressure is allowed to equalize. c. Contents of the needle are placed on a glass slide. d. The smear is spread forward gently with a glass slide inclined at an angle of 35°, with an up and down movement. (From: Zajdela, A (1975) The value of aspiration cytology in the diagnosis of breast cancer, Cancer, 35, Feb.)

Table 5.2. Classification of Breast Tumours and Preferred Method of Treatment

Clinical Anatomic Observation	Treatment
Stage I Breast mass localized; all nodes negative	Modified radical mastectomy preferred by most surgeons. Some prefer simple mastectomy plus irradiation. Others prefer simple mastectomy with irradiation
Stage II Breast mass localized; axillary nodes positive	Modified radical mastectomy preferred with or without postoperative irradiation
Stage III Breast mass locally extensive; axillary supraclavicular and internal mammary nodes positive	This is considered inoperable for cure. Variable depending on extensiveness: 1 Simple mastectomy with radiation, chemotherapy and hormone therapy 2 Radiation therapy, chemotherapy and hormone therapy
Stage IV Distant metastasis	Variable, depending on location of metastasis (bone, soft tissue, etc.) 1 Radiation therapy for primary lesion or metastasis 2 Hormonal therapy **a.** Systemic—oestrogens, androgens or steroids **b.** Ablation—oophorectomy, adrenalectomy, hypophysectomy 3 Chemotherapy

Treatment and Nursing Management

Objective

To remove or destroy whole tumour.

Prognosis

1   When malignancy is confined to breast: 5-year survival—85%.
2   When malignancy has spread to axilla: 5-year survival—45%.

Seek Optimal Physical and Psychosocial Approach in Preparing Patient for Surgery

1   Begin emotional support when patient is told that hospitalization and biopsy may be required.
2   Dispel fear by:
    a. Listening to patient's concerns and dispelling misconceptions.
    b. Emphasizing successful programme of rehabilitation and use of prosthesis.
    c. Having a patient who made a satisfactory postoperative adjustment visit present patient.
    d. Soliciting support of the husband.
    e. Providing encouragement and reassurance.

3   Minimize delay before operation.
   a. Determine physical and nutritional needs.
   b. If radical surgery is anticipated, have blood replacement available.
   c. Administer hypnotic to minimize concerns of patient.
4   Prepare skin adequately.
   When skin graft is anticipated, shave and clean donor area (usually anterior aspect of thigh).

The Selection of a Surgical Approach Aims to Remove Malignancy, Minimize Disfigurement and Prevent Spread of Cancer Cells

1   *Simple mastectomy*—removal of breast without lymph node dissection.
2   *Classical radical mastectomy*—removal of breast and underlying muscles down to chest wall; also removal of nodules and lymphatics of axilla. This is rapidly being replaced by *modified radical mastectomy*—pectoral muscles are spared. Results appear comparable—less disfiguring and better for an external or internal prosthesis, depending on preference of doctor and patient.
3   Pressure dressings usually applied to reduce serum collection, prevent haemorrhage, lessen oedema and enhance wound healing.
4   For drainage, portable suction (vacuum type) has almost completely replaced simple drain—minimizes serum collection by constant aspiration.

When Radiation Therapy is Utilized, Follow Principles of Care (p. 356)

Initiate Postoperative Surveillance to Minimize Complications and Hasten Recovery

1   Assess blood pressure and pulse status since they are valuable indices in detecting shock and haemorrhage.
2   Inspect dressings for bleeding under axilla and shoulder.
3   Upon recovery from anaesthesia, administer analgesic for relief of pain.
4   Encourage turning and deep breathing to prevent pulmonary complications.
5   Check dressings for constriction so that lung expansion is not hampered.
6   Ensure that portable suction initiated in the operating room is functioning properly. Monitor frequently to be certain that vacuum is powered and aspirated material emptied.
7   Position patient in upright position; if arm is free, elevate on a pillow; gravity aids in removal of fluid via lymphatic and venous pathways.
8   Ambulate patient early as determined by individual patient; diet as preferred and tolerated.

Discharge Planning and Health Teaching

1   Talk to and listen to patient; encourage questions and provide helpful answers.
2   Prepare the husband for his role in providing the necessary emotional support.
3   Initiate active exercise on the affected side 24 hours postoperatively for hand and elbow. Check with doctor on extent of exercise for each individual patient. Exercises will increase daily and the patient will do more of her own activities such as hair combing, teeth brushing, etc. (Table 5.3).

NOTE: Be cautious in exercising the shoulder during the first week after surgery. Excessive abduction of the arm at the shoulder can lift skin flaps from chest wall and increase serous formation.

Table 5.3. Exercises for the Rehabilitation of the Patient Following Radical Mastectomy

Exercise	Equivalent Daily Exercise
1 Stand erect Lean forward from waist Allow arms to hang Swing arms from side to side together; then in opposite direction Next, swing arms from front to back together; then in the opposite direction	Broom sweeping Vacuum cleaning Mopping floor Pulling out and pushing in drawers Weaving Playing golf
2 Stand erect facing wall with palms of hand flat against wall; arms extended Relax arms and shoulders and allow upper part of body to lean forward against hand Push away to original position; repeat	Pushing self out of bath tub Kneading bread Breast stroke swimming Sawing or cutting types of crafts
3 Stand erect facing wall with palms of hand flat against wall Climb the wall with the fingers; descend; repeat	Raising windows Washing windows Hanging clothes on line Reaching to an upper shelf
4 Stand erect and clasp hands at small of back; raise hands; lower; repeat Clasp hands back of neck; reach downwards; upwards; repeat	Fastening brassiere Buttoning blouse or dress Pulling up a dress zipper Fastening beads Washing the back
5 Toss a rope over the shower curtain rail Hold the ends of the rope (knotted) in each hand and raise arms sideways Using a see-saw motion and with arms outstretched, slide the rope up and down over the rail	Drying the back with a bath towel Raising and lowering a window blind Closing and opening window drapes
6 Flex and extend each finger in turn	Sewing, knitting, chrocheting Typing, painting, playing piano or other musical instrument

    a. Exercise should not be painful.
    b. Bilateral activity should be emphasized.
    c. Proper posture should be maintained.
    d. If the patient has had a skin graft or if the skin was approximated under tension, exercises will be limited.
4   Care of wound:
    a. Explain how the wound will gradually change.
    b. Note that the newly healed wound may have less sensation due to severed nerves.
    c. Bathe gently and blot carefully to dry.

d. Recognize signs of infection—pain, tenderness, redness, swelling; if these are present, report to doctor.
5 Use of a prosthesis—sponge rubber, air-filled or fluid-filled.
   a. Type and style are suggested on an individual basis; skilled fitters from reliable companies are most helpful (or representative from Appliance Department).
   b. Observe effect of prosthesis on incision; to prevent irritation, sheepskin padding may be used.
   c. A prosthesis should not be worn unless authorized by the doctor.

Complication–Lymphoedema of the Arm

Lymphoedema is an obstruction to the lymph flow in the arm on the operated side producing a chronic swelling of the part, particularly if it is in a dependent position. Lymphoedema is due to lymph node removal and compression of axillary vein by tumour or scar.

Prevention

1 Exercises should be done as indicated above.
2 The affected arm should be massaged 3 or 4 months postoperatively to increase circulation and lessen oedema.
3 The affected arm should be elevated frequently to prevent dependent oedema.
4 The arm and operative site should be kept scrupulously clean to prevent infection.
5 Nonconstrictive clothing should be worn to permit adequate circulation.

Treatment

1 May include a diuretic.
2 An intermittent compression unit with pressurized sleeve may be used to force fluid back into venous system.

Importance of Follow-up Visit

1 Incision healing evaluated.
2 Rehabilitative effort assessed.
3 Effectiveness of prosthesis determined.
4 Patient's psychosocial adjustment evaluated.
5 Possible recurrence detected.

Recurrent or Metastatic Breast Cancer

Modalities of Endocrine Therapy

Theory and objective: Malignant tumour cells depend on hormonal function in the host; deprivation of hormones reduces tumour's growth. Currently tumour removal at operation is tested for oestrogen receptors. If positive, the use of hormonal therapy or ablation can be carried out on a more rational basis than heretofore with an anticipated good response.

Ablative Procedures

1   Bilateral salpingo-oophorectomy.
   a. This is often the initial treatment of choice for premenopausal patients with metastatic breast cancer.
   b. Remission lasts from 3 months to several years (median—1 year).
   c. If signs of reactivation of tumour growth occur, further endocrine therapy may be done (hypophysectomy or adrenalectomy).
2   Hypophysectomy—done microsurgically (transnasal or trans-sphenoidal).
   a. This is done for postmenopausal patients with metastatic breast cancer.
   b. Remission lasts from 6 months to several years (median—$1\frac{1}{2}$ years).
   c. Upon signs of reactivation of tumour growth, cytotoxic chemotherapy is initiated.
3   Adrenalectomy.
   a. Bilateral adrenalectomy is usually combined with bilateral salpingo-oophorectomy.
   b. This is often recommended for postmenopausal patients with metastatic breast cancer.
   c. Remission lasts from 6 months to several years (median—1 year).
   d. Women who have had oophorectomy and adrenalectomy and who show signs of recurrence are given cytotoxic chemotherapy.

Hormones

1   Oestrogens
   a. Most commonly used in women who are 5 or more years postmenopausal with recurrent breast carcinoma.
   b. Ethinyl oestradiol is oestrogen used.
   c. Remissions last 3 months to several years (median—1 year).
   d. With initial exacerbation of the disease, hormone therapy is immediately terminated.
   e. Recurrence of this disease following remission is treated with hypophysectomy or adrenalectomy.

Nursing Alert: Observe for fluid retention following oestrogen therapy; this can be prevented with dietary sodium restriction and use of diuretics.

2   Progestogens (medroxyprogesterone acetate).
   a. Useful in about 30% of postmenopausal women with metastatic carcinoma.
   b. Remission is about 8 months.
   c. Failure with progestins suggests a change to other modalities of endocrine therapy.
3   Androgens (fluoxymesterone).
   a. Useful in about 20% of postmenopausal women.
   b. Remissions last about 6 months.
   c. When no longer effective, other kinds of endocrine therapy may be useful.
   d. Side-effects:
      (1) Fluid retention, which can be prevented by restricting sodium and using diuretics.
      (2) Virilization (development of secondary male characteristics).

4 Corticosteroids (prednisone, dexamethasone).
   a. Not usually used in primary management of postmenopausal women with metastatic breast cancer because of the possibility of Cushing's syndrome.
   b. Useful as:
   (1) An adjunct to radiation therapy in patients with cerebral metastasis.
   (2) An adjunct to cytotoxic chemotherapy in patients with advanced liver and pulmonary metastasis.

Cytotoxic Chemotherapy

Alkylating agents: 5-fluorouracil, methotrexate, vincristine.

1 Remission lasts about 6 months (in 20% of patients).
2 Five-drug combination can boost remission rate to about 9 months (in 65% of patients)—5-fluorouracil, methotrexate, vincristine, cyclophosphamide, prednisone.
3 Recommended for patients who have metastasis to liver or lungs and are poor surgical risks for endocrine ablative surgery.
4 Recommended for premenopausal patients who are not benefiting from oophorectomy or hypophysectomy.
5 Doxorubicin hydrochloride (Adriamycin) usually used when 5-drug chemotherapy fails.

FURTHER READING

Books

Berlyn, G M (1978) A Course in Renal Diseases, 5th edition, Blackwell
Blandy, J P (1971) Transurethral Resection, 2nd edition, Pitman
Blandy, J P (ed) (1976) Urology (2 vol), Blackwell
Blandy, J P (1977) Lecture Notes on Urology, 2nd edition, Blackwell
Blandy, J P (1978) Operative Urology, Blackwell
Boyarski, S et al (1979) Care of the Patient with Neurogenic Bladder, Little, Brown & Co
Brundage, D J (1980) Nursing Management of Renal Problems, 2nd edition, Mosby
Cameron, J S et al (1976) Nephrology for Nurses: A Modern Approach to the Kidney, 2nd edition, Heinemann
Corry, R J and Thompson, J S (1977) Renal Transplantation Case Studies, Medical Examination Publishing Co
Curtis, J R and Williams, G B (1975) Clinical Management of Chronic Renal failure, Blackwell
Davison, A M (Ed) (1978) Dialysis Review, Pitman
Davison, A M (1981) A Synopsis of Renal Diseases, Wright
De Wardener, H E (1973) The Kidney. An Outline of Normal and Abnormal Structure and Function, 4th edition, Churchill Livingstone
Gabriel, R (1977) Postgraduate Nephrology, 2nd edition, Butterworth
Gabrield, R (1981) Renal Medicine, 2nd edition, Baillière Tindall
Harvey, R J (1974) The Kidneys and the Internal Environment, Chapman & Hall
Jackle, M and Rasmussen, C (1980) Renal Problems, A Critical Care Nursing Focus, Prentice-Hall

Jameson, R M (1976) Management of the Urological Patient, Churchill Livingstone
Kunin, C M (1979) Detection, Prevention and Management of the Urinary Tract Infections, 3rd edition, Lea & Febriger
Lancaster, L E (1979) The Patient with End Stage Renal Failure, Wiley
Mandelstam, D (1977) Incontinence—A Guide to the Understanding and Management of a Very Common Complaint, Heinemann
Mitchell, J P (1980) Urology for Nurses, 3rd edition, Wright
Montgomery, E (1974) Regaining Bladder Control, Wright
Morel, A and Wise, G J (1979) Urologic Endoscopic Procedures, 2nd edition, Mosby
Newsam J E and Petrie, J J B (1981) Urology and Renal Medicine, 3rd edition, Churchill Livingstone
Oberley, E T and Oberley, T D (1979) Understanding Your New Life with Dialysis: Patient Guide for Physical and Psychological Adjustment to Maintainance Dialysis, 2nd edition, Charles C Thomas
Pitts, R F (1974) Physiology of the Kidney and Body Fluids. An Introductory Text, 3rd edition, Year Book Medical Publishers
Schlotter, L (Ed) (1973) Nursing and the Nephrology Patient: A Symposium on Current Trends and Issues, Medical Examination Publishing Co
Scott, R et al (1982) Urology Illustrated, 2nd edition, Churchill Livingstone
Stirling, M W and Scott, R (1981) Urology, 2nd edition, Heinemann
Sturdy, D E (1974) Essentials of Urology, Wright
Uldall, R (1978) Renal Nursing, 2nd edition, Blackwell
Wing, A J and Magowan, M (1976) The Renal Unit

Articles

Breckman, B (1981) Stoma care after cystectomy and ileal conduit formation: the role of the stoma care nurse, Nursing Times, 77: 1110–1114
Chan, M K et al (1981) Three years experience of continuous ambulatory peritoneal dialysis, Lancet, 1: 1409–1412
Chang, M (1981) Peritoneal dialysis. No more needles. (How patients are trained in CAPD technique), Nursing Mirror, 153: 22–25
Datta, P K (1981) The post prostatectomy patient, Nursing Times, 77: 1759–1761
Davies, J G (1981) Emergencies in the home. Urinary tract emergencies, British Medical Journal, 282: 111–113
Hadfield, J (1981) Clinical forum: Urological emergencies, Nursing Mirror, 152: VI–XIV
Perston, Y (1981) Urinary incontinence—ways to help solve a sensitive problem, Nursing Mirror, 153: 38–42
Practitioner Symposium (1981) Renal disease, Practitioner, 225: 959–1038

Gynaecological Conditions

Books

Bailey, R (1975) Obstetric and Gynaecological Nursing, 2nd edition, Baillière Tindall
Barnes, J (1980) Lecture Notes on Gynaecology, 4th edition, Blackwell
Burnett, C W F (1974) A Summary of Gynaecology, 2nd edition, Faber

Clayton, Sir S G and Newton, J R (1979) A Pocket Gynaecology, 9th edition
    Churchill Livingstone
Clayton, Sir S G et al (Eds) (1980) Gynaecology by Ten Teachers, 13th edition,
    Arnold
Farrer, H (1979) Gynaecological Care, Pitman
Fream, W C (1979) Notes on Gynaecological Nursing, Churchill Livingstone
Garrey, M M et al (1978) Gynaecology, Illustrated, 2nd edition, Churchill Living-
    stone
Green, T H (1977) Gynaecology: Essentials of Clinical Practice, 3rd edition, Little,
    Brown & Co
Hector, W (1980) Modern Gynaecology with Obstetrics for Nurses, 6th edition,
    Heinemann
Hudson, C N (1978) The Female Reproductive System, Churchill Livingstone
Jeffcoate, Sir N (1975) Principles of Gynaecology, 4th edition, Butterworth
Lanson, L (1977) From Woman to Woman: A Gynaecologist Answers Questions
    About You and Your Body, revised edition, Penguin
Law, B (1973) Family Planning in Nursing, Crosby Lockwood Staples
Llewellyn-Jones, D (1978) Everywoman. A Gynaecological Guide for Life, 2nd
    edition, Faber
Llewellyn-Jones D (1978) Fundamentals of Obstetrics and Gynaecology. Volume
    2—Gynaecology, 2nd edition, Faber
Paletta, J L and Essoka, G C (Eds) (1978) Gynaecological Nursing, Medical
    Examination Co
Quixley J M E and Cameron, I D (1980) Obstetrics and Gynaecology, 4th edition,
    Hodder and Stoughton
Roberts, H (Ed) (1981) Women, Health and Reproduction, Routledge & Kegan
    Paul
Shorthouse, M A and Brush, M G (1981) Gynaecology in Nursing Practice, Ballière
    Tindall

Articles

Barker, G (1981) Treating dysmenorrhea (report of recent conference), World
    Medicine, 16:
Burke, M and Gregory, M (1981) Infertility—Can I ever have children?, Nursing
    Mirror, 153: 49–51
Lancet (1981) Premenstrual syndrom, Lancet, 2: 1393–1394
Savage, J (1982) Gynaecology: no sex please Mrs Smith (need for counselling of
    women on sex after surgery), Nursing Mirror, 154: 28–32

INDEX

The Index covers all three volumes of *The Lippincott Manual of Medical-Surgical Nursing*. The figures printed in **bold** type before each entry or group of entries indicate the volume in which that page number or numbers will be found. The page numbers in italic indicate a figure, and page numbers followed by 't' indicate a table.

abdomen, regions and incisions **1** 71
abdominal hernia **2** 447–448
abdominal injuries
    blunt trauma **1** 164–165
    emergency treatment of **1** 163–165
    penetrating **1** 163–164
abscess
    Bartholin's gland **3** 338
    brain **3** 43–44
    greater vestibular gland **3** 338
    lung **2** 326–328
    mammary **3** 372
    pancreatic **2** 516
    perianal **2** 473–474
Acetest **2** 563
acetone, tests for **2** 563
achalasia **2** 389–390
acid–base balance **2** 364–365
acne vulgaris **1** 316–320
actinic cheilitis **2** 317
actinic trauma, to eye **3** 109
actinomycosis **1** 249–252
Addison's disease **2** 568–571
Addisonian crisis **2** 570
adenitis, acute cervical **2** 178
adrenal glands **2** 564–565
    Addison's disease **2** 568–571
    medulla, hyperfunction of **2** 565–568
        Cushing's syndrome **2** 566–568
        phaeochromocytoma **2** 565–566
        primary aldosteronism **2** 571
adrenalectomy **2** 571–572
adrenocorticosteroids **2** 576t
aged
    care in long-term accommodation and
        geriatric ward **1** 61–62
    and drug therapy **1** 59
    foot care **1** 60
    medical and nursing management of **1**
        56–57
    nutritional considerations **1** 58
    skin and eye care of **1** 65–66

ageing
    bodily changes associated with **1** 51–54
    disease aspects of **1** 55–56
    psychosocial influence on health **1** 54–55
agranulocytosis (granulocytopaenia) **2**
    205–207
air embolism, in blood transfusion **2** 195
airway management **1** 155–156
    artificial **2** 287–300
        endotracheal intubation **2** 287–300
        tracheostomy **2** 289–300
alcoholic hallucinosis **1** 199
alcoholism **1** 199–200
    acute **1** 199
    delirium tremens (alcoholic hallucinosis) **1**
        199
aldosteronism, primary **2** 571
Allen test **2** 155, 156
allergic conjunctivitis **1** 390–391t
allergic reactions **1** 379–381
    in blood transfusions **2** 193–194
    hypersensitivity **1** 380
    immunoglobulins **1** 380–381
    rhinitis **1** 385–392
allergy
    management of patient **1** 392–393
    tests for, and immunotherapy **1** 381–385
        guidelines for **1** 382–383
        intradermal tests **1** 384
allografts (homografts) **1** 376–377
amenorrhoea **1** 326
ametropia **1** 100
amoebiasis (amoebic dysentery) **1** 267–268
amphetamine overdose **1** 195–196
amputation
    lower limbs **3** 182–186
        prosthesis fitting **3** 185
    upper limb **3** 186–189
anaemia **2** 196–203
    aplastic **2** 201–203
    iron deficiency **2** 197–199
    megaloblastic **2** 199

pernicious **2** 199–201
anaesthetic
    recovery room scoring guide **1** 86–88, 89
anaphylactic shock **1** 163
    reaction to **1** 183–185
anaphylaxis **1** 384–385
aneurysm
    aortic **2** 158–160
    cerebral **3** 41–42
    thoracic and abdominal **2** 158, 159
angina pectoris **2** 40–43
angiocardiography **2** 10
angiography **2** 156
    cerebral **3** 2–3
    in pulmonary disease **2** 240
    renal **3** 222–223
angiomas **1** 340
anorectal conditions and treatments **2**
    473–481
    haemorrhoids **2** 474–476
    perianal abscess **2** 473–474
    pilonidal sinus **2** 476
anorexia **2** 398–402
anticoagulant therapy **2** 128–136, 131t
coumarin derivatives **2** 133–134
antiepileptic drugs **3** 50t
antihypertensive drugs **2** 172t
antistreptolysin titre **2** 12
aorta, diseases of **2** 157–160
    aortic aneurysm **2** 158–160
    aortitis **2** 157–158
aortic aneurysm **2** 158–160
aortic insufficiency **2** 63–64
aortic stenosis **2** 63
aortitis **2** 157–158
aortography **2** 10
aphasia **3** 38–40
aplastic anaemia **2** 201–203
appendicitis **2** 442–443
arm cast **3** 155–156
arterial blood gas evaluation **2** 245–247
arterial embolism **2** 150–151
arterial puncture, guidelines for **1** 99–100
arteriography, coronary **2** 10
    musculoskeletal **3** 142
arteriosclerosis **2** 151–153
    obliterans **2** 153–154
arthritis, rheumatoid **3** 196–205
    drugs in **3** 201–202t
    gouty **2** 584–586
    paraffin hand both for **3** 204, *205*
arthroplasty
    hip **3** 189–193
    total knee **3** 193–194

arthrosis **3** 205–207
artificial ventilation **1** 155–156, **2** 25
ascariasis (roundworm infestation) **1**
    272–273
aspiration
    bone marrow **2** 186–189
    chest (thoracentesis) **2** 248–251
    iliac crest **2** 189
    in pneumonia **2** 321–323
    tracheal **2** 247
    transtracheal **2** *243*
    sternal **2** 188
aspirin (salicylate) poisoning **1** 198
asthma
    acute severe (status asthmaticus) **1**
        389–392
    bronchial **1** 386–389
    aspirin-induced **1** 389
    drugs used in **1** 390–391t
astigmatism **1** 101
atherosclerosis **2** 151–153
atherosclerotic heart disease **2** 40–54
    angina pectoris **2** 40–43
athlete's foot (tinea pedis) **1** 322–323
atrial fibrillation **2** 105–107
atrial flutter **2** 103–105
atrioventricular (AV) block, and ECG **2**
    107–110
audiogram **3** 83, 84
audiologist **3** 81
auscultation
    chest **2** 237–239
    heart **2** 6
autografts **1** 374–376

bacillary dysentery (shigellosis) **1** 240–241
bacterial contamination, in blood
    transfusions **2** 193
bacterial diseases **1** 221–249
    botulism **1** 241–242
    endocarditis **2** 54
    gas gangrene **1** 229–231
    gonorrhoea **1** 242–245
    Gram-negative infection **1** 233–236
    meningococcal meningitis (cerebrospinal
        fever) **1** 245–246
    salmonella infections (salmonellosis) **1**
        238–239
    shigellosis (bacillary dysentery) **1** 240–241
    staphylococcal **1** 231–232
    streptococcal **1** 232–233
    tetanus (lockjaw) **1** 221
    tuberculosis **1** 247–249
    typhoid fever **1** 236–238

bacterial infections **1** 320–322
  carbuncles **1** 321
  furuncles **1** 320–321
  impetigo **1** 321–322
balanitis **3** 323
bandages and slings **1** 130–134
  types of **1** 131–134
barbiturate intoxication **1** 196–197
barium enema **2** 434–435
Bartholin's gland, abscess of **3** 338
basal cell and squamous cell carcinoma **1** 383–344
basic monitoring, postoperative **1** 85–86
bedbug infestation **1** 329
Bell's palsy **3** 26–28
  keratitis in **3** 28
biliary system, diseases of **2** 503–512
  diagnosis **2** 504–505
blackhead (comedo) extraction, guidelines for **1** 319–310
bladder
  cancer of **3** 295–297
  injuries to **3** 284–285
  neurogenic **3** 289–294
bleeding disorders **2** 223–224
  vascular purpuras **2** 223
blepharitis **3** 114
blood
  cellular components **2** 182–184, 190–191
    erythrocytes and leucocytes **2** 182
    platelets (thrombocytes) **2** 184
  disorders, problems of **2** 183t
  specimens **2** 184–189
    skin puncture and syringe methods **2** 185
  transfusion therapy **2** 189–196
    administering **2** 191
    air embolism in **2** 195
    allergic reactions in **2** 193–194
blood pressure
  determination of **2** 170
  factors affecting **2** 162–163
blood studies in cardiac investigation **2** 12
body temperature, helping to maintain **1** 40
bone, Paget's disease of **3** 210–212
bone marrow
  aspiration **2** 186–189
  specimens **2** 184–189
  transplantation **2** 203
bone scanning **3** 142
bone tumour, malignant **3** 207–208
botulism **1** 241–242
bougienage **2** 391–393
bradycardia, sinus and ECG **2** 96–98
brain scan **3** 3

brain abscess **3** 43–44
brain tumour **3** 44–47
breast
  cancer **3** 375–387
    recurrence of metastatic **3** 385
    signs of **3** 377
  examination of **3** 374–375, 378
  inflammation of **3** 372
  mammography **3** 379
  Paget's disease of **3** 369–372
  tumours **3** 373–387
    classification of **3** 382
    fibroadenomata **3** 373–374
breathing exercises **2** 255–261
  diaphragmatic **2** 256
bronchitis, chronic **2** 330–331
bronchogenic cancer **2** 342–344
bronchography **2** 240
bronchopulmonary disease **2** 234–237
  cough and sputum production in **2** 234–235
bronchoscopy **2** 241
bronchus, ruptured **1** 170
burns **1** 356–377
  evaluation chart **1** 358
  methods of treating **1** 368
  skin grafting **1** 373
  systemic changes **1** 361

caesium 137 **3** 356
cancer
  bladder **3** 295–297
  bone **3** 207–208
  brain **3** 44–47
  breast **3** 375–387
  bronchogenic **2** 342–344
  cervical **3** 352–354
  colonic **2** 466–468
  corpus uteri **3** 354–355
  gastric **2** 418–420
  lips **2** 376–377
  lung **2** 342–344
  mouth **2** 379–382
  oesophageal **2** 396–398
  pancreatic **2** 517–518
  prostate **3** 309–311
  skin **1** 342–343
  thyroid **2** 536–537
  tongue **2** 377–378
  vulva **3** 338–339
cancer treatment
  chemotherapy for **1** 279–289
    anti-cancer drugs **1** 281–287t
  general nursing considerations **1** 277–279
    benign and malignant tumours **1** 278t

warning signs 1 277–278
radiation diagnosis and therapy 1 289–292
cane use
  purpose of 1 34
  technique 1 36
carbon monoxide, poisoning, emergency management of 1 189–190
carbuncles 1 321
carcinoma
  basal and squamous cell 1 343–344
  care of patient with advanced 1 297–300
cardiac arrest, cardiopulmonary resuscitation for 2 23–28
cardiac arrhythmias 2 32–40, 117–118t
  classification of 2 34
  ECG interpretation of 2 95–120
cardiac catheterization 2 10
cardiac compression, external 2 25–27
cardiac investigations, in heart disease 2 6–9
cardiac tamponade 1 170, 2 20
cardiogenic shock 2 49–50
cardiopulmonary resuscitation, drugs used in 2 28t
cardioversion, synchronized 2 118–120
casts 3 150–160
  application of 3 156–158
  arm 3 155–156
  brace 3 173, 174–175
  cutter 3 159
  pressure areas in 3 151
  removal of 3 158–160
  spica, arm and leg 3 153–155
  types of 3 152
CAT scan 3 2, 142
cataracts 3 123–130
  extracapsular and intracapsular extraction 3 124
  phacoemulsification 3 126–127
catheterization
  cardiac 2 10
  of self, intermittent 3 292–294
  of urinary bladder 3 230–238
    in male 3 234–237
  subclavian 2 426
catheters
  central venous and pulmonary artery 1 85–86, 2 16–19
  indwelling 3 237
  oropharyngeal, oxygen therapy by 2 265–267
  plastic 1 102–104
  through needle (IntraCath) 1 104–105
  triple-lumen 3 238–240
central venous catheterization 1 85–86

central venous pressure (CVP) 2 13–16
cerebral angiography 3 2–3
cerebral circulation, impairment of 3 30–31
cerebral vascular accident (CVA) (stroke) 3 31–38
  rehabilitation in 3 32–38
cerebrospinal fever (meningococcal meningitis) 1 245–246
cerebrovascular disease 3 30–31
cerumen, in ear canal 3 85–86
cervical adenitis, acute 2 178
cervical biopsy and cauterization 3 332
cervical disc 3 68, 7
cervical traction 3 69
cervix, cancer of 3 352–354
chalazion 3 114
chancre 3 323
chest
  auscultation of 2 237–239
  flail 1 169
  physiotherapy 2 252–261
  trauma 2 344–348
    haemothorax and pneumothorax 2 345–346
    rib and sternum fracture 2 346
    sucking wounds 2 346
    wet lung syndrome 2 347
chest drainage, water seal 2 354–361
chest injuries
  emergency management 1 166, 168–170
    flail chest 1 169 2 347
    haemothorax 1 169–170, 2 345–346
    ruptured bronchus and cardiac tamponade 1 170, 2 347
    tension pneumothorax 1 169, 2 345–346
chest pain
  in bronchopulmonary disease 2 236–237
  in heart disease 2 4
cholangiography 2 505
cholecystitis 2 503–504
cholecystography 2 504
choledochostomy 2 506
cholelithiasis 2 503
cholesterol
  in foods 2 153
  low, in diets 2 152
circulation time, in cardiac investigation 2 12
circulatory overloading in blood transfusions 2 192
circumcision 3 323–324
cirrhosis
  hepatic 2 493–498
clavicle fracture of 3 166
Clinitest 2 562

clotting defects **2** 225–228
  coagulation, acquired defects **2** 226–228
  disseminated intravascular coagulation
    (DIC) **2** 225–226
  haemophilia **2** 226
coagulation
  acquired defects in **2** 226–228
  disseminated intravascular (DIC) **2**
    225–226
coitus interruptus **3** 364
cold injuries **1** 182–183
colitis, ulcerative **2** 448–453
colon, cancer of **2** 466–468
colonoscopy **2** *437*, 438–440
colostomy **2** 468–473
  irrigating **2** 472
  stoma in **2** 468
colporrhaphy **3** 350
colposcopy **3** 324–325
coma
  diabetic **2** 550–552
  hepatic **2** 490–493
comedo (blackhead) extraction, guidelines
  for **1** 319–310
communicable diseases **1** 209–220, 222–229t
  classification of **1** 216–220
    isolation **1** 216, 220
    precautions **1** 217–218
  control and management of **1** 209–216
  notifiable **1** 210
  nursing care **1** 212–215
computerized axial tomography (CAT) in
  neurology **3** 2
  in musculoskeletal conditions **3** 142
  in urology **3** 223
condom **3** 364
condylomata **3** 337
conjunctival irrigation **3** 107–108
conjunctivitis
  allergic **1** 390–391t
  drugs used in treatment of **3** 114–115
contusions **3** 145
constipation, postoperative **1** 136
  and diarrhoea **2** 402–404
contact lenses, removing **3** 111–114
convulsions, management of **3** 22–23
cor pulmonale **2** 336–338
cordotomy **3** 75–76
corneal abrasion **3** 110
corneal transplantation **3** 119–121
corneal ulcer **3** 116
coronary arteriography **2** 10
corpus uteri, cancer of **3** 354–355
cough **2** 352

and sputum production in
  brochopulmonary disease **2** 234–237
coumarin derivatives, in anticoagulant
  therapy **2** 133–134
counterpulsation (mechanical cardiac
  assistance) **2** 51–54
countershock, in ventricular fibrillation **2** 29
CPAP, in oxygen therapy **2** 280–281,
  302–303
cranial nerve involvement **2** 26–30
  Bell's palsy **3** 26–28
cranial nerve tests **3** 7t
craniectomy **3** 23
cranioplasty **3** 23
craniotomy **3** 23
C-reactive protein (CRP) **2** 12
crush injuries **1** 164–167
crutch walking
  crutch gait **1** 32–34, *35–37*
  preparation for **1** 30
  stance **1** *33*
culdoscopy **3** 333
Cushing's syndrome **2** 566–568
cyanosis, in heart disease **2** 5–6
cystitis **3** 272–274
cystocele **3** 348–350
cystometrogram **3** 221
cystostomy, suprapubic drainage **3** 240–242,
  299
cystoscopic examination, in urology **3** 223
cystourethrogram **3** 221
cytology
  aspiration **3** *381*
  exfoliative **2** 386
  'Pap' smear **3** 328, 331–332
  urine specimen for **3** 231
cytotoxic chemotherapy, in metastatic breast
  cancer **3** 387

decubitus ulcers (*see* pressure sores)
defibrillation **2** 29, 30
deformity, in orthopaedic conditions **3** 141
delirium tremens (alcoholic hallucinosis) **1**
  199
defaecation, helping the patients with **1** 24–25
dermabrasion **1** 355–356
dermatitis
  contact **1** 331–332, **2** 371
    patch testing in **1** 332
  of the vulva **3** 336–337
  exfoliative (generalized erthroderma) **1**
    337–338
dermatology, nursing responsibilities in **1**
  308–310

dermatosis 1 314–315
  seborrhoeic 1 315–316
Dextrostix 2 564
diabetes insipidus 2 580–581
diabetes mellitus 2 541–564
  complications of 2 550–554
    infection 2 552–553
    ketoacidosis and coma 2 550–552
    long-term 2 553–554
  dietary treatment in 2 545
  health teaching in 2 555–564
    insulin self-injections in 2 558–562
    urine testing for glucose and ketone 2
      562–564
  insulin therapy in 2 546–550
  surgery 2 554–555
  types of 2 542
diabetic retinopathy 2 553–554
dialysis, peritoneal 3 251–258
diaphragm, vaginal in birth control 3 365
diarrhoea, and constipation 2 402–404
Diastix 2 563
diet
  low cholestrol 2 152, 153
  reduced calcium and phosphorous in
    urolithiasis 3 285t
  sodium-restricted, in congestive heart
    failure 2 74–75t
  varying in residue 2 451t
digitalis therapy, in congestive heart failure 2
  64–70
dilatation and curettage (D and C) 3 335–336
disability
  causes and psychological implications of 1
    11
  emotional reactions of patient to 1 11–12
  prevention of 1 13
disaster conditions, emergency nursing in 1
  204–206
  triage in 1 204
disc, prolapsed intravertebral (slipped) 3
  67–70
discography 3 5
disseminated intravascular coagulation
  (DIC) 2 225–226
diuretics, in congestive heart failure 2 70–72
diverticulitis 2 458–461
diverticulosis 2 458–461
Doppler ultrasound 2 124
dorsal fracture of the spine 3 175–176
dressing
  changing a surgical 1 117–120
  for skin conditions 1 313–314
  laparotomy 1 *116*

occlusive (pressure) for burns 1 369–370
open wet, in skin disorders 1 310
drug abuse, emergency management of 1
  192–198
  amphetamines 1 195–196
  acute reaction to 1 193
  anti-cancer 1 281–287t
  barbiturate intoxication 1 196–197
  hallucinogens 1 195
  narcotic 1 193
    heroin withdrawal syndrome 1 194–195
  non-barbiturate sedatives 1 197–198
  salicylate (aspirin) 1 198
drugs
  antiepileptic 3 50t
  antihypertensive 2 172t
  for parenteral treatment of hypertension 2
    173t
  in asthma, rhinitis and conjunctivitis
    treatment 1 390–391t
  in cardiopulmonary resuscitation 2 28t
  in glaucoma 3 132
  in hyperthyroidism 2 528–529
  in Parkinson's disease 3 53
  in rheumatoid arthritis 3 201–202t
  nebulized, in oxygen therapy 2 262
duodenal drainage 2 428–432
dying patient
  psychosocial support of 1 301–305
  psychotherapeutic agents in 1 304
dysentery
  amoebic 1 267–268
  bacillary (shigellosis) 1 240–241
dysmenorrhoea 3 325
dyspnoea
  in bronchopulmonary disease 2 236
  in heart disease 2 3–4

ear care specialists 3 81
ear disorders
  examinations and diagnostic procedures 3
    82–83
  external, problems of 3 85–87
ear hygiene 3 83–85
ear irritation 3 *88*
eardrum, perforation of 3 91–94
ecchymoses 2 223
ECG
  and cardiac arrhythmias 2 95–120
    atrial fibrillation 2 105–107
    atrial flutter 2 103–105
    atrioventricular (AV) block 2 107–110
    paroxysmal atrial tachycardia (PAT) 2
      101–103

premature atrial contractions (PACs) **2** 99–100
premature ventricular contractions (PVC) **2** 110–112
sinus arrhythmia **2** 98–99
sinus bradycardia **2** 96–98
sinus tachycardia **2** 95–96
ventricular fibrillation **2** 114–118
ventricular tachycardia **2** 112–114
echocardiography **2** 9
echoencephalography **3** 4
ECP (external counterpulsation pressure) **2** 51, *52*
eczema **1** 333–334
EEG (electroencephalography) **3** 6
electrocardiography, essentials of **2** 87–120 (*see also* ECG)
electrolyte, and fluid imbalance **3** 244–246
embolism
air, in blood transfusions **2** 195
arterial **2** 150–151
cerebral **3** 31
pulmonary **2** 338–340
emergency nursing
airway management of artificial ventilation **1** 155–156
obtaining history **1** 154
psychological management **1** 155
EMG (electromyography) **2** 6, 142
emmetropia **3** 100
emphysema, pulmonary **2** 331–337
empyema **2** 325–326
encephalitis, viral (arthropod-borne) **1** 259–260
endocardial disease **2** 54–56
endocarditis **2** 54–56
endolymphatic hydrops (Ménière's disease) **3** 96–98
endometriosis **3** 360–361
endoscopic retrograde pancreatico-cholecystography (ERCP) **2** 508–512
endoscopy procedures **2** 241–242
bronchoscopy **2** 241
fibre optic **2** 411–412
oesophageal **2** 385–386
endotracheal and tracheostomy tubes in oxygen therapy **2** 274–275, 287–300
epididymitis **3** 319–320
epilepsy **3** 47–52
status epilepticus **3** 51–52
epileptic seizures, international classification of **3** 48–50
erythnaemia (polycythaemia vera) **2** 203–205

erthrocyte sedimentation rate (ESR) **2** 12
erthrocytes (red blood cells) **2** 182
exercises, movement **1** 14–18, 20–23, 28–29
principles of body alignment **1** 26–27
therapeutic **1** 27–28
exfoliative cytology **2** 386
exophthalmos, in hyperthyroidism **2** 530–531
eye
actinic trauma to **3** 103
conditions requiring surgery **3** 117–135
cataracts **3** 123–130
detached retina **3** 121–123
glaucoma **3** 130–135
keratoplasty **3** 119–121
examination and diagnostic procedures for **3** 101–106
inflammatory conditions of **3** 114–116
superficial lid infections **3** 114–115
sympathetic ophthalmia **3** 115–116
uveitis **3** 115
eye care, of elderly **1** 65–66
eye care specialists **3** 99–100
eye injuries
emergency treatment of **1** 179–181
removing contact lenses **3** 111–114
removing a particle from **3** 110
types of **3** 109–112
eyedrops, administering **3** *105*, 106–107
eyelid, superficial infections of **3** 114–115

faecal impaction **2** 478–480
femoral phlebitis **1** 143
femur, fractures of **3** 171
fertility control **3** 364–369
contraceptive methods **3** 364–367
sterilization procedures **3** 367–368
fever, tepid sponge for **2** 16–18
fibroadenomata **3** 373–374
fibrocystic disease **3** 373
fibroids **3** 355
fibula, fractures of **3** 172
fissure in ano **2** 473–474
fistula
in ano **2** 473–474
vaginal **3** 340–341
flail chest **1** 169
flossing technique **2** *370*
fluid and electrolyte imbalance **3** 244–246
fluoroscopy, in cardiac investigations **2** 10
foot care, in vascular disorders **2** 138–139
fractures
cast-brace in **3** *173*, 174–175
clavicle **3** 166
complications of **3** 149–150

emergency management of 1 176–177
hip 3 177–180
lower limb 3 171–174
  femur 3 171
  tibia, fibula and knee 3 172
lumbar and dorsal spine 3 175–176
mandibular 2 374–375
maxillofacial 2 373–375
pelvis 3 176–177
spinal 3 63–67, 3 175–176
treatment of open 3 148
types of 3 146–147
upper limb 3 166–171
  elbow 3 169–170
  hand 3 171
  humerus 3 168–169
  radius, ulna and wrist 3 170–171
supracondylar 3 169
fungal infections 1 268–269, 1 322–324
mycoses and histoplasmosis 1 268–269
tinea capitis 1 323–324
tinea corporis (circinata) 1 324
tinea pedis (athlete's foot) 1 322–323
furuncles 1 320–321

gallbladder
  cholecystitis 2 503–504
  diseases of 2 503–512
  surgery 2 506
gangrene, gas 1 229–231
gas exchange, physiology of 2 361–362
gas gangrene 1 229–231
gastrectomy, partial and subtotal 2 418, 419
gastric cancer 2 418–420
gastric lavage 1 187–189
gastric resection 2 420–422
gastroduodenal conditions, diagnostic studies
  2 404–412
  treatment for 2 412–432
    peptic ulcer 2 412–417
gastrointestinal disturbances 2 398–404
  anorexia, nausea and vomiting 2 398–402
  fibroscopy 2 411–412
gastrointestinal symptoms, and urological
  disease 3 219
gastrojejunostomy and vagotomy 2 418
gastrostomy 2 423–428
  feedings 2 423–424
  total parenteral nutrition (TPN)
    (hyperalimentation) 2 425–428
gelatin compression boot 2 145, 146
genitalia
  conditions of external 3 336–348
  contact dermatitis of the vulva 3 336–337

genitourinary tracts, disorders of 3 217–219
gingivitis 2 372
glaucoma 3 130–135
  acute 3 131–133
  chronic 3 133–135
glomerulonephritis, acute 3 278–279
glucocorticoids, effects of 2 572–573
glucose
  blood testing for 2 564
  urine testing for 2 562–564
gonioscopy 3 103
gonococcal infection 3 362
gonorrhoea 1 242–245
  urethritis from 3 305–306
gout 2 583–586
gouty arthritis 2 584–586
Gram-negative infections 1 233–236
granulocyte infusions 2 190
granulocytic leukaemia, chronic 2 213–214
granulocytopaenia (agranulocytosis) 2
  205–207
granulomatous colitis 2 455t
gynaecological conditions, diagnostic studies
  for 3 327–336
  dilatation and curettage (DIC) 3 335–336
  pelvic examination 3 327–330
  vaginal examination 3 329–330

haematoma, in wound complication 1
  148–149
in eye 3 109
haemodialysis 3 258–263
  dietary management in 3 260–261
  medical problems in 3 261
  psychosocial problems in 3 262
haemolytic reactions, in blood transfusions 2
  194
haemophilia 2 226
haemoptysis
  in bronchopulmonary disease 2 235
  in heart disease 2 5
haemorrhage
  and cerebrovascular disease 3 30
  emergency management of 2 157–158
  following radical neck dissection and
    mouth surgery 2 384–385
  postoperative 2 142–143
  pressure points for control of 2 159
  subarachnoid 3 40–41
  with wound complications 2 148–149
haemorrhoids 2 474–476
haemothorax 1 169–170, 2 345–346
hallucinogen overdose 1 195

hand
  fractures of **3** 71
  psoriasis of **1** *335*
Hashimoto's thyroiditis **2** 535–536
head injuries **1** 170–171, **3** 11–14
hearing, physiological principles of **3** 92
heart auscultation **2** 6
heart disease
  atherosclerotic **2** 40–54
  cyanosis in **2** 5–6
  diagnosis in **2** 6–19
  manifestations of **2** 3–6
  pulmonary (cor pulmonale) **2** 336–338
  rheumatic **2** 57–58
  valvular **2** 62–66
heart disorders **2** 3–86
heart failure, congestive **2** 66–75
  diet in **2** 73–75
  digitalis therapy in **2** 69–70
  dieuretics in **2** 70–72
heart physiology, and the EGG **2** 87–94
  wave significance **2** 90–94
heart surgery **2** 78–87
  complications following **2** 84–86
  health teaching after **2** 86–87
heartburn (pyrosis) in peptic ulcer **2** 414
heat stroke **1** 181–182
helminthic infestations **1** 269–275
  ascariasis (roundworm infestation) **1** 272–273
  hookworm disease **1** 271–272
  Oxyuris vermicularis (threadworm) **1** 273–275
  trichonosis **1** 269–270
heparin therapy, monitoring of **1** 78
  as a cause of bleeding **2** 227–228
  sodium **2** 131
  subcutaneous injection of **2** 135–136
hepatic cirrhosis **2** 493–498
hepatic coma **2** 490–493
hepatitis **2** 487–490
  type A **2** 488
  type B **2** 489–490
hernia, abdominal **2** 447–448
herniated (slipped) disc **3** 67–70
heroin withdrawal syndrome **1** 194–195
herpes simplex **2** 317–372
herpes zoster **1** 329–331
hiccups (singultus), controlling **1** *147*, 148
hip
  arthroplasty (total hip replacement) **3** 189–193
  fracture of **3** 177–180
  spica cast **3** 153–155

histoplasmosis, and mycoses **1** 268–269
hoarseness, in bronchopulmonary disease **2** 235–236
Hollander test, for gastric analysis **2** 409–410
homografts (allografts) **1** 376–377
hookworm disease **1** 271–272
hordoleum (stye) 114
hormones
  in metastatic breast cancer **3** 386–387
humerus, fracture of **3** 168–169
hydrocele **3** 316
hydronephrosis **3** 280–281
hyperalimentation **2** 425–428
hypercalcaemia, after heart surgery **2** 83
hypercapnia **2** 364
  in blood transfusions **2** 195
hyperkalaemia, after heart surgery **2** 83
  in blood transfusions **2** 195
hypermetropia **3** 100
hyperparathyroidism **2** 537–539
hyperpituitarism **2** 579–580
hypersensitivity
  in allergic rhinitis **1** 385–392
  in allergic reactions **1** 380
  respiratory **1** 385
hypertension **2** 162–177
  classification of **2** 163–164
  evaluation and treatment of **2** 167–170
  factors affecting blood pressure **2** 162–163
  phases of **2** 165–167
hypertensive crisis **2** 170–173
hyperthyroidism **2** 526–531
  exophthalmos in **2** 530–531
  pharmacotherapy in **2** 528–529
hypocalcaemia, after heart surgery **2** 83
hypoglycaemia, in diabetes **2** 547–549
hypoglycaemic agents, oral **2** 549–550t
hypoglycaemic analysis (Hollander test) **2** 409–410
hypokalaemia, after heart surgery **2** 82
hyponatraemia, after heart surgery **2** 83
hypoparathyroidism **2** 540–541
hypophysectomy **2** 582
hyposensitivity **1** 381–385
hypothermia **1** 182–183
hypothyroidism **2** 524–526
hypovolaemia, after heart surgery **2** 84
hypoxaemia causes of **2** 364
hysterectomy **3** 357–360
hysterosalpingogram **3** 334
hysteroscopy **3** 333–334

idiopathic thrombocytopaenia purpura **2** 223–224
ileostomy **2** 453, **2** 455–458
iliac crest aspiration **2** 189
immunity **1** 215
immunization, and vaccination procedures 214t
immunoglobulins, in allergic reactions **1** 380–381
immunotherapy
  in cancer **1** 290–297
  and allergy tests **1** 381–385
impetigo **1** 321–322
incompatibility, in blood transfusion **2** 194
indwelling catheter **3** 237
infection
  process of **1** 208–209
infectious mononucleosis **1** 258–259
influenza **1** 255–257
infusion therapy
  'butterfly' set in **1** 105–106
  fluid flow in **1** 96
insect stings, emergency management of **1** 190–191
insulin
  complications of **2** 549–550
  hypoglycaemia in **2** 547–549
  self-injection **2** 558–559
  therapy, in diabetes **2** 546–550
intestinal conditions and treatment **2** 432–473
  surgery **2** 441–442
    abdominal hernia **2** 447–448
    appendicitis **2** 442–443
    Crohn's disease **2** 453–455
    Meckel's diverticulum **2** 443–444
    peritonitis **2** 444–445
    ulcerative colitis **2** 448–453
intestinal obstruction, postoperative **1** 146–147, **2** 462–466
intra-aortic balloon pump **2** 51, *53*
IntraCath **1** 104–105
intracranial aneurysm **2** 41–42
intracranial pressure, increased **3** 16–18
intractranial surgery **3** 23–26
intraocular lens **3** 128
intrauterine device (IUD) **3** 366
intravenous therapy **1** 88
  bolus **1** 107–108
  complications of **1** 108–114
    circulatory and drug overloads **1** 115
    infection **1** 108
    mechanical failure **1** 110
    nerve damage in **1** 114

pyogenic reaction and infiltration **1** 111–112
thrombophlebitis and air embolism **1** 113
IPPB (intermittent positive pressure breathing) **2** 281–284
IPPT (intermittent positive pressure ventilation) **2** 301–302
iridectomy **3** 133
iridencleisis **3** 133
iron deficiency anaemia **2** 197–199
irrigation system, continuous **3** 238–242
ischaemia **2** 121
ischaemic attacks, transient (TIA) **2** 30–31

jaundice **2** 483–487
  cholestatic **2** 486–487
  haemolytic **2** 483
  hepatocellular **2** 483–484
joint dislocation **3** 143–144

keratoplasty **3** 119–121
keloids **1** 341
keratitis **3** 116
  in Bell's palsy **3** 28
ketoacidosis **2** 550–552
Ketodiastix **2** 563
ketones, urine testing for **2** 562–564
Ketostix **2** 563
kidney
  injuries to **3** 287–289
  needle biopsy of **3** 223–225
  transplantation **3** 263–267
  tuberculosis of **3** 276–277
  tumour of **3** 286–287
knee arthroplasty **3** 193–194
knee surgery **3** 172–173
kraurosis vulvae **3** 337–338
Kveim test, in sarcoidosis **2** 341

laminectomy **3** 71–72
laparoscopy (hysteroscopy) **3** 333–334
laparotomy dressings **1** *116*
Landry-Guillain-Barre syndrome **3** 62
leg cast **3** 155
leucocytes (white blood cells) **2** 182
leucoplakia **2** 337–338
  buccalis (smoker's patch) **2** 375–376
leukaemia **2** 207–214
  acute **2** 208
    chemotherapy in **2** 209
  chronic granulocytic **2** 213–214
  chronic lymphocytic **2** 212–213
Levin tube, in nasogastric intubation **2** 404–410

levodopa therapy, in Parkinson's disease 3 53
lips
  cancer of 2 376–377
  lesions 2 371
liver, disorders of 2 480–498
  biopsy 2 481–483
  diagnosis 2 481–483, 484–485t
  hepatic cirrhosis 2 493–498
  hepatic coma 2 490–493
  hepatitis 2 487–490
  jaundice 2 480–481, 483–487
lumbar disc 3 69–70, 71
lumbar fracture of spine, 3 175–176
lumbar puncture 3 7–10
lung
  abscess 2 326–328
  biopsy procedures 2 244–245
  cancer of 2 342–344
  chronic obstructive disease (COLD) 2 329–330
lupus erythematosus, systemic (SLE) 1 347–349
lymph node biopsy 2 177
lymphangiography 2 177
lymphangitis 2 177
lymphatic system 2 177–179
lymphocytic leukaemia, chronic 2 212–213
lymphoedema 2 178, 384
lymphoma 2 210
  malignant 2 214–222
    Hodgkin's disease 2 215–218
    lymphocytic 2 218

malaria 2 264–267
mammary abscess 3 372
mammography 3 379
mandibular fractures 2 374–375
Maslow's hierarchy of needs 1 47
mastectomy, radical 3 385t
mastitis, acute 3 372
mastoiditis 3 90–91
mastoidectomy 3 90
maxillofacial fractures 2 373–375
maxillofacial surgery 1 354–355
Meckel's diverticulum 2 443–444
megaloblastic anaemia 2 199
melanoma, malignant 1 345–346
menarche 3 324
Ménière's disease (endolymphatic hydrops) 3 96–98
meningococcal meningitis (cerebrospinal fever) 1 245–246
menorrhagia 3 326
menstruation, disturbances of 3 324–327

amenorrhoea 3 326
dysmenorrhoea 3 325
menorrhagia 3 326
metrorrhagia 3 327
oligomenorrhoea 3 326
polymenorrhoea 3 327
metastatic breast, recurrence of 3 385
metrorrhagia 3 327
micturition
  changes in 3 218–219
  helping the patient with 1 24–25
mitral insufficiency 2 65
mitral stenosis (regurgitation) 2 64
moles 1 341
monilial vaginitis 3 343–344
mononucleosis, infectious 1 258–259
mouth
  tongue, cancer 2 377–378
  conditions of 2 369–370
  lesions 2 371–372
    premalignant 2 375–376
  lip cancer 2 376–377
  lips, lesions of 2 371
  salivary glands 2 373
  tongue cancer 2 377–378
multiple injuries, emergency management of 1 173–176
multiple sclerosis 3 55–58
muscle spasm, in low back pain 3 194
musculoskeletal arteriography 3 142
musculoskeletal disorders, diagnosis of 3 142
musculoskeletal trauma 3 143–150
  contusions, sprains and joint dislocation 3 143–144
  fractures 3 144–150
    complications of 3 149–150
    treatment of open 3 148
    types of 3 146–147
myasthenia gravis 3 58–62
  crises in 3 60–61
  thymectomy in 3 60
mycoses, and histoplasmosis 1 268–269
mycosis fungoides 2 219–220
myelography 3 5
myeloma, multiple 2 220–222
myocardial infarction 2 43–49 45
  and ECG 2 94–95
  incidence of in UK 2 43
myocardial ischaemia 2 41–42
myocarditis 2 59–60
myoma, of uterus 3 355
myopia 3 100
myringoplasty 3 93
myringotomy 3 89

naevi pigmented (moles) **1** 341
nasal cannula, oxygen therapy by **2** 264–265
nasogastric intubation **2** 404–410
nasointestinal intubation **2** 433–434
nausea **2** 398–402
  in peptic ulcer **2** 414
  in pregnancy **2** 401
nebulizer
  slipstream **2** 284–285
  ultrasonic **2** 285–287
neck, dissection of, radical **2** 382–385
nephroptosis **3** 281–282
nephrostomy **3** 299
nephrotic syndrome **3** 279–280
nephrotomogram **3** 222
neurogenic bladder **3** 289–294
  flaccid **3** 290
  spastic **3** 289
neurological conditions, diagnosis of **3** 2–11
neuromodulation **3** 76
neuropathy, in diabetes **2** 554
nipple
  conditions of **3** 369–372
  fissures and bleeding **3** 369
  Paget's disease of **3** 369–372
non-barbiturate sedative overdose **1** 197–198
nursing history
  family and medical **1** 3
  general principles of **1** 2
  identifying problems **1** 6–8
  information needed **1** 2
  information recording **1** 5
  personal and social **1** 2–3

oedema
  acute pulmonary **2** 76–78
  in heart disease **2** 3
oesophageal dilatation **2** 391–393
oesophageal diverticulum **2** 394–395
oesophageal varices and perforation **2** 395–396
oesophagus, conditions of **2** 385–398
  achalasia **2** 389–390
  cancer of **2** 396–398
  diffuse spasm **2** 390–391
  oesophagitis **2** 387–389
  trauma **2** 387
oligomenorrhoea **3** 326
oophorectomy **3** 362
ophthalmia, sympathetic **3** 115–116
ophthalmic optician **3** 100
ophthalmologist **3** 99
ophthalmoscopic examination **3** 103

optician **3** 100
orchidectomy, in prostate cancer **3** 310
orchitis **3** 320–321
oropharyngeal catheter, oxygen therapy by **2** 265–267
orthopaedic conditions, problems in
  deformity **3** 141
  pain **3** 140
  psychosocial problems **3** 141
orthopaedic surgery **3** 180–182
oscillometry **2** 123
osteitis deformans (Paget's disease of the bone) **3** 210–212
osteoarthritis **3** 205–207
osteoporosis **3** 209–210
otitis **3** 85
otitis media
  acute **3** 87–89
  chronic and mastoiditis **3** 90–91
  serous (glue ear) **3** 89–90
otolaryngologist **3** 81
otosclerosis **3** 94–96
ovarian cancer **3** 361–362
ovulation **3** 324
oxygen therapy **2** 261–281
  by aerosol mask **2** 269–271
  by Ambu-bag and bag-airway systems **2** 278–279
  by endotracheal and tracheostomy tubes **2** 274–275
  by nasal cannula **2** 264–265
  by non-rebreathing mask **2** 273–274
  by oropharyngeal catheter **2** 265–267
  by partial rebreathing mask **2** 271–272
  by tent **2** 276–278
  by tracheostomy collar **2** 275–276
  by venturi mask **2** 267–269
  delivery systems **2** 263
  nebulized drugs **2** 262t
  with CPAP **2** 280–281
Oxyuris vermicularis (threadworm) **1** 273–275

pacemaker
  artificial **2** 109–110
  complications of **2** 38
  implantation **2** 37–39
  malfunctioning **2** *110*
  permanent **2** *39*
  temporary **2** *35*
  types of **2** 37
Paget's disease, of bone **3** 210–212
  of the breast **3** 369–372

pain
  chest, in bronchopulmonary disease 2 236–237
  chest, in heart disease 2 4
  in genitourinary disorders 3 217–219
  in orthopaedic conditions 3 140
  in peptic ulcer 2 414
  intractable 3 74–78
  low back 3 194–196
  postoperative 1 136
palpitation, in heart disease 2 4
pancreas, pseudocysts of 2 516–518
pancreatic abscesses 2 516
pancreatic cancer 2 517–518
pancreatitis
  acute 2 512–514
  chronic 2 515–516
'Pap' (Papanicolaou) smear 3 328, 331–332
paraffin hand bath, for rheumatoid arthritis 3 204, 205
paracentesis, abdominal 2 496–498
paraplegia 3 72–74
parasitic infection 1 267–268
  amoebiasis (amoebic dysentery) 1 267–268
parasite skin diseases 1 324–331
  pediculosis capitis, corporis, pubis 1 324–326
Parkinson's disease 3 52–55
  levodopa in 3 53
  physiotherapy in 3 55
parotitis 2 373
partial pressure, concept of 2 361–363
paroxysmal atrial tachycardia (PAT) and ECG 2 101–103
patch testing, in contact dermatitis 1 332
patient
  preparation for transfer of 1 29, 31
pediculosis capitis 1 324–326
pediculosis corporis 1 326–327
pediculosis pubis 1 327
pelvic examination 3 327–330
  lithotomy and Sims' position 3 327
pelvic infection 3 362–364
pelvic muscles, problems resulting from 3 348–352
  cystocele 3 348–350
  rectocele 3 350–351
  uterus displacement 3 351–352
pelvis, fractures of 3 176–177
pemphigus 1 338–340
penis, conditions affecting 3 322–324
  balanitis 3 323
  carcinoma of 3 323
  chancre 3 323
  circumcision 3 323–324
  phimosis 3 323
  ulceration of glans penis 3 322–323
peptic ulcer 2 412–417
percussion, technique for 2 254–255
perianal abscess 2 473–474
periarteritis nodosa (polyarteritis) 1 349–350
pericardiocentesis (pericardial aspiration) 2 19–23
pericarditis 2 60–62
perineal swabbing 3 347–348, 349
peritoneal dialysis 3 251–258
peritonitis 2 444–445
petechiae 2 223
phacoemulsification 2 126–127
phaeochromocytoma 2 565–566
phimosis 3 323
phlebitis, femoral 1 143, 2 140–145
phlebography 2 123, 144–145, 2 147–148
phlebothrombosis 2 139, 140–145
phonocardiogram 2 9
physiotherapy, chest 2 252–261
'Pill', in birth control 3 366–367
pilonidal sinus 2 476
pituitary, disorders of 2 579–582
  diabetes insipidus 2 580–581
  hyperpituitarism 2 579–580
  hypophysectomy 2 582
  hypopituitarism (Simmond's disease) 2 580
  tumours 2 581–582
planigraphy 2 10
plastic reconstructive surgery 1 351–355
  causes of graft failure 1 353
  cosmetic 1 353t
  maxillofacial surgery 1 354–355
plesiotherapy, in cancer 1 293–294
pleural effusion 2 324–325
pleural fluid, and pleural biopsy 2 244
pleurisy 2 323–324
pneumatic dilatation 2 393–394
pneumoencephalogram 2 3
pneumonia 2 314–323, 2 314–317t
  aspiration 2 321–323
pneumothorax 2 345–346
poisoning, emergency management of 1 185–192
  food 1 191–192
  gastric lavage 1 187–189
  inhaled 1 189–190
    carbon monoxide 1 189–190
  injected 1 190–191
    insects 1 190–191
    snake bite 1 191
  salicylate (aspirin) 1 198

skin contamination 1 190
swallowed 1 185-189
    corrosive and non-corrosive 1 186
polyarteritis (periarteritis nodosa) 1 349-350
polycythaemia vera (erythnaemia) 2 203-205
polymenorrhoea 3 327
polyneuritis, acute infectious 3 62
polypectomy 2 441
postphlebitic syndrome 2 142-145
postural drainage 2 252-253
premature atrial contractions (PACs) and
    ECG 2 99-100
premature ventricular contractions (PUCs) 2
    110-112
presbyopia 3 101
pressure gradient therapy 2 128
pressure, partial, concept of 2 361-362
pressure sores (decubitus ulcers), prevention
    and treatment 1 41-44
    causes of 1 42
    preventive measures 1 42
    risk assessment scoring system 1 43
procidentia and prolapse, of uterus 3 352,353
prostate, conditions of 3 306-316
    benign prostatic hyperplasia (hypertrophy)
        3 306-307
    prostatitis 3 307-309
    cancer of 3 309-311
    surgery 3 311-316
prostatectomy 3 311-316
prostatitis 3 307-309
prosthesis, in lower limb amputation 3 185
protozoan diseases 1 265-267
    malaria 1 264-267
pruritus 3 337
pseudocysts, of the pancreas 2 516-518
psoriasis 1 335-337
    of the hands 1 335
psychiatric emergency 1 201-202
    behavioural manifestations 1 201
psychological distrubances, postoperative 1
    150-151
psychosocial problems, in orthopaedic
    conditions 3 141
psychotherapeutic agents, for dying patient 1
    304
pulmonary artery catheterization 1 85-86
    by Swan-Ganz catheter 2 16-19
    complications, postoperative 1 144-145
    embolism, postoperative 1 145
pulmonary embolism 2 338-340
pulmonary emphysema 2 331-337
pulmonary function studies 2 245
pulmonary heart disease 2 336-338

pulmonary oedema, acute 2 76-78
purine metabolism, disorders of 2 583-586
    diet in 2 585t
    gout 2 583-586
purpuras, vascular 2 223-224
pyelography
    infusion drip 2 220
    retrograde 3 221
pyelonephritis 3 274-276
pyrogenic reactions, in blood transfusions 2
    192-193
pyrosis (heartburn), in peptic ulcer 2 414

Q fever 1 263-264
quadriplegia 3 72
Queckenstedt test 3 10

rabies 1 260-263
    post-exposure treatment of 1 259-260
    prophylaxis 1 261
radiation diagnosis and therapy for cancer 1
    289-292, 3 356-359
    relative penetration of alpha, beta, and
        gamma 1 294
radiculography 3 5
radiography
    gastrointestinal tract 2 410-411
    in bronchopulmonary disease 2 239-240
    in urological disease 3 219-223
    of the colon 2 434-435
    upper gastrointestinal 2 385
    radioiodine, in thyroid function tests 2
        523-524
    radioisotope therapy, for cancer 1 293-296
    lung and ventilation scan 2 240
    teletherapy and plesiotherapy 1 293-294
radiological investigations, in heart disease 2
    9-12
    in neurological conditions 2 2-6
radius, fracture of 3 170
Raynaud's disease 2 160-161
Raynaud's phenomenon 2 160
rebreathing mask, partial, in oxygen therapy 2
    271-273
rectal problems 2 476-478
rectocele 3 350-351
red blood cells 2 182
Reed-Sternberg cell 2 215
regurgitation (mitral stenosis) 2 64
rehabilitation
    helping to avoid dangers in the
        environment 1 45
    helping to maintain body temperature 1 40

helping to protect the integument 1 40–41
helping with clothing 1 39
helping with communication 1 45–46
helping with defaecation 1 24–25
helping with eating and drinking 1 19
helping with micturition 1 24–25
helping with mobility 1 26–34
helping with practising religion 1 46–47
helping with recreational activities 1 49
helping with rest and sleep 1 36–38
helping with work 1 47
nursing functions 1 10–11
team 1 10
renal angiography 3 222–223
renal failure
acute 3 246–249
chronic 3 249–263
renal function tests 3 226
renal surgery 3 267–271
renogram 3 222
renoscan 3 222
respiration
helping the patient with 1 12–19
respiratory conditions
diagnostic procedures for 2 237–248
respiratory failure, and insufficiency 2
257–261
respiratory system
control of 2 233
functions and anatomical components of 2
232–233
resuscitation
mouth-to-mouth and mouth-to-nose 1 156
cardiopulmonary, drugs used in 2 28
retina, detached 3 121–123
retinopathy, diabetic 2 553–554
retroversion, of uterus 3 351
rheumatic heart disease 2 57–58
streptococcal infection in 2 57
rheumatic fever 2 57
rheumatoid arthritis 3 196–205
drugs in 3 201–202t
paraffin hand bath for 3 204, 205
rhinitis, allergic 1 385–392
drugs used in 1 390–391t
rhizotomy 3 75
rickettsial infections 1 263–264
Q fever 1 263–264
ringworm 1 322–324
Rinne test 3 82
roundworm infestation (ascariasis) 1
272–273
Rubin's test 3 332–333
Rule of Nine chart 1 357

salicylate (aspirin) poisoning 1 198
salivary calculus (sialolithiasis) 2 373
salivary glands, conditions of 2 373
salmonella infections (salmonellosis) 1
238–239
sarcoidosis 2 340–341
Schilling test 2 200
Schiøtz tomometry 3 104, 105
scleroderma (progressive systemic sclerosis) 1
350–351
sclerosis, multiple 3 55–58
seborrhoeic dermatoses 1 315–316
Sengstaken-Blakemore tube, to control
oesphageal bleeding 2 500, 501
serum enzyme tests 2 12
sexual assault, emergency management of 1
202–204
sexual potency, after prostate surgery 3
314–316
shigellosis 1 240–241
shock
anaphylactic 1 163
burn 1 363
cardiogenic 2 49–50
emergency management of 1 158–161
postoperative 1 139–142
sialolithiasis 2 373
sigmoidoscopy 2 435–438
Simmond's disease 2 580
sinus arrhythmia, and ECG 2 98–99
sinus bradycardia and ECG 2 96–98
sinus tachycardia and ECG 2 95–96
skin
acne vulgaris 1 316–320
bacterial infections 1 320–322
carbuncles 1 321
furuncles 1 320–321
impetigo 1 321–322
cancer of 1 343–344
malignant melonama 1 345–346
types of 1 343–344
contact dermatitis 1 331–333
contamination, emergency management of
1 190
dermatosis 1 314–315
seborrhoeic 1 315–316
fungal infections 1 322–324
tinea capitis, corporis, pedis 1
322–324
grafting of burn site 1 373–377
allografts and autografts 1 374–377
removal of eschar 1 373–374
herpes zoster 1 329–331
lesions 1 309–310

non-infectious inflammatory dermatoses 1 333–340
eczema 1 333–334
exfoliative dermatitis (generalized erythroderm) 1 337–340
pemphigus 1 338–340
psoriasis 1 335–337
nursing responsibilities in dermatology 1 308–310
parasitic diseases 1 324–329
bedbug infestation 1 329
pediculosis capitis, corporis, pubis 1 324–327
preparation of for surgery 1 78
prick testing 1 383–384
surgery 1 351–356
dermabrasion 1 355–356
plastic reconstructive 1 351–355
systemic diseases 1 347–351
lupus erthematosus 1 347–349
periarteritis nodosa (polyarteritis) 1 349–350
scleroderma (progressive systemic sclerosis) 1 350–351
ulcers and tumours of 1 340–346
moles (pigmented naevi) and keloids 1 341
verrucae and angiomas 1 340
treatments 1 311–314
baths 1 311
open wet dressings 1 310
topical medications 1 313–314t
sleepnessness, and restlessness, postoperative 1 135
snake bite, emergency management of 1 191
sodium-restricted diet, in congestive heart failure 2 74–75t
specula, styles and sizes of 3 328
spica cast 3 153–155
spinal cord injury 1 171–173
spine, fractures and dislocations 3 63–67, 175–176
spirochetal infections 1 253–255
syphilis (lues) 1 253–255 3 323
splenectomy 2 228–229
sprains 3 143
sputum
and cough production in bronchopulmonary disease 2 234–237
examination of 2 242–243
stapedectomy 3 95–96
staphylococcal disease 1 231–232
stasis ulcers 2 144
status asthmaticus 1 389–392

stenosis
aortic 2 63
mitral 2 64
tricuspid 2 65
sterilization, in birth control 3 369
tubal 3 369
vasectomy 3 369
sternal aspiration 2 188
steroid therapy
in adrenal disorders 2 572–579
classification of 2 572
glucocorticoids in 2 572–573
side-effects of 2 574–575
stoma, in colostomy 2 468
stone formation, kidney 3 282
stool specimen 2 432–433
streptococcal disease 1 232–233
beta-haemolytic 1 232
poststreptococcal 1 232–233
streptococcal infections, in rheumatic heart disease 2 57
stroke 3 31–38
rehabilitation in 3 32–38
stye 3 114
subarachnoid haemorrhage 3 40–41
surgery
initial assessment of patient in 1 71–74
effect of specific conditions on 1 72–74
types of 1 70
supracondylar fracture 3 169
suture, removal 1 119, 128–130
for simple wound closure 1 126–128
Swan-Ganz catheter, measuring pulmonary artery pressure by 2 16–19
insertion of 2 17, 18
sympathectomy 3 76
syncope and fainting, in heart disease 2 5
syphilis (lues) 1 253–255, 3 323

tachycardia
paroxysmal atrial (PAT) 2 101–103
sinus, and ECG 2 95–96
ventricular 2 112–115
telangiectasia 2 223
teletherapy in 1 293–294
testicle, tumours of 3 317–319
self-examination for 3 318–319
tetanus (lockjaw) 1 221–229
prophylaxis, in emergency wound care 1 161–162
thalamotomy 3 76
thermography 3 381
thermotherapy 2 126–128
thirst, postoperative 1 136

thoracentesis 2 248–251
thoracic surgery 2 348–361
  water seal chest drainage 2 354–361
    bottle systems 2 356–358
threadworm (*Oxyuris vermicularis*) 1
  273–275
thromboangiitis obliterans (Buerger's
  disease) 2 154–157
thrombocytes (platelets) 2 184
thrombophlebitis postoperative 1 143, 2
  140–145
thrombosis, cerebral venous 3 31
  prophylaxis to prevent 1 77–78
thymectomy, in myasthenia gravis 3 60
thyroid
  cancer of 2 536–537
  crisis 2 531–533
  function tests of 2 522–524
thyroidectomy, subtotal 2 529–530, 533–534
thyroiditis
  chronic (Hashimoto's) 2 535–536
  subacute 2 535
tic douloureux 3 28–30
tibia, fracture of 3 172
tinea capitis 1 323–324
tinea corporis (circinata) 1 324
tinea pedis (athlete's foot) 1 322–323
toenails, trimming in elderly 1 64–65
tongue, cancer of 2 377–378
  anterior 2 377
  posterior 2 378
tonometry 3 103–105
  Schiøtz 3 104, *105*
  tourniquet, application of rotating 2 31–32,
  33
TPN (total parenteral nutrition) 2 425–428
trabeculectomy 3 133
tracheostomy 2 289–300
  performing 2 293–294
  removal 2 300
  tubes 2 291, 294–297
transfusion therapy 2 189–196
transillumination 2 380
transplantation, kidney 2 263–267
traction 3 160–166
  Buck's extension 3 163–166
  principles of 3 162–163
  Thomas's leg splint in 3 *172*
Trendelenburg test, in varicose veins 2
  146–147
triage (sorting of casualties) 1 204
trichonosis 1 269–270
tricuspid inefficiency 2 66
tricuspid stenosis 2 65

trigeminal neuralgia (tic douloureux) 3 28–30
triple-lumen catheter 3 238–240
tuberculosis 1 247–249
  drug therapy in 1 250–251t
  of the kidney 3 276–277
  transmission 1 247
tumour
  of kidney 3 286–287
  of testicle 3 317–319
  of uterus 3 352–357
  pituitary 2 581–582
tuning fork, in hearing assessment 3 82
tympanoplasty 3 92–94
  types of 3 93t
typhoid fever 1 236–238

ulcer
  corneal 3 116
  peptic 2 412–417
  stasis 2 144
ulcerative colitis 2 448–453
ulna, fractures of 3 170
ultrasonic scan 3 222
ultrasound examination, in gall bladder
  disease 2 505–506
ultrasound holography 3 381
unconscious patient, case of 3 18–22
ureteroileostomy 3 297, 298, 299
ureterosigmoidostomy 3 297, 298, 300
ureterostomy 3 297, 299, 300
urethra, injuries to 3 294–295
  problems affecting 3 303–306
urethral stricture 3 303–304
urethritis 3 304–306, 342
urinary difficulties, postoperative 1 145–146
urinary diversion 3 297–303
urinary tract infections 3 271–277
  cystitis 3 272–274
  pyelonephritis 3 274–276
urine retention 3 242–244, *245*
urine testing 3 226–230
  for glucose and ketones 2 562–564
  midstream specimen of 3 229–230
urography, excretory 3 220
urolithiasis 3 282–286
  stone formation in 3 282, 286
urological disease 3 219–230
  diagnostic investigations 3 219–230
  surgery 3 267–271
uterotubal insufflation (Rubin's test) 3
  332–333
uterus
  displacement of 3 351–352
    retroversion 3 351

prolapse and procidentia **3** 352, *353*
tumours **3** 352–357
  cancer of cervix **3** 352–354
  cancer of corpus uteri **3** 354–355
  myoma **3** 355
  radiation therapy **3** 356–357
uveitis **3** 115

vaccination and immunization procedures **1** 214t
vagina, conditions of **3** 336–348
vaginal examination **3** 329–330
vaginal fistula **3** 340–341
vaginal foam, in birth control **3** 365
vaginal injections **3** 342–348
vaginal irrigation (douche) **3** 345–347
vaginalis, Trichomonas **3** 343
vaginitis **3** 342–346
  atrophic (postmenopausal) **3** 344–345
  monilial **3** 343–344
  simple **3** 342–343
vagotomy **2** *418, 419*
  and pyloroplasty **2** *419*
valvular heart disease **2** 62–66
  aortic stenosis **2** 63
varicocele **3** 317
varicose veins **2** 146–150
  Trendelenburg test in **2** 146–147
vascular disorders **2** 120–178
  foot care in **2** 138–139
  general management of **2** 125–139
  ischaemia **2** 121
  pathophysiological manifestations of **2** 121–124
  peripheral disease (PVD) **2** 120
  peripheral problems **2** 137–138
  thrombus and embolus formation **2** 120
vascular purpuras **2** 223
vasectomy, bilateral **2** 311, 321–322, 369
vectorcardiography **2** 9
veins
  superficial **1** 92
  varicose **2** 146–150
venepuncture, criteria for **1** 91
  'butterfly' set in **1** 105–106
  guidelines to **1** 97–99
  methods **1** 92
  venous insufficiency (postphlebitic syndrome) **2** 142–145
  venous thrombosis, prophylaxis to prevent **1** 77–78
ventilation
  artificial **2** 287–300
  mechanical **2** 300–312

techniques **2** 301–309
ventilator types **2** 300–301
weaning modalities **2** 309–311
weaning step **2** 311–312
  Briggs adapter (T-tube) **2** 310
  IMV **2** 309
ventilatory function tests **2** 246t
ventricular fibrillation, procedure for **2** 29–31, 114–118
ventricular tachycardia **2** 112–115
ventriculogram **3** 4
venturi mask, oxygen therapy by **2** 267–269
verrucae **1** 340
vestibular gland, greater, abscess of **3** 338
viral encephalitis, arthropod-borne **1** 259–260
viral infections **1** 255–263
  arthropod-borne viral encephalitis **1** 259–260
  infectious mononucleosis **1** 258–259
  influenza **1** 255–257
  rabies **1** 260–263
vision
  colour test for **3** 102
  normal and refractive errors **3** 100, 103
  visual fields test **3** 102
  vitamin K deficiency **2** 226–227
  vomiting **2** 398–402
  in peptic ulcer **2** 414
  in pregnancy **2** 401
  postoperative **1** 134
vulva
  cancer of **3** 338–339
  contact dermatitis of **3** 336–337
vulvitis **3** 338

water seal chest drainage **2** 354–361
Weber test **3** 82
white blood cells (leucocytes) **2** 182
wound care
  complications, postoperative **1** 148–150
  dressing of draining **1** 120–121
  emergency **1** 161–162
  factors affecting healing **1** 115
  infection **1** 125–126
  irrigation **1** 124
  portable suction **1** 121–125
  purpose of dressings **1** 115–117
  tetanus prophylaxis **1** 161
wrist, fracture **3** 170–171

xerography **3** 380

Zimmer Mesher **1** 375